PARTIAL DENTURES

*Dedicated to the memory of
John Osborne*

OSBORNE & LAMMIE'S PARTIAL DENTURES

REVISED BY

GEORGE ALEXANDER LAMMIE
PhD, DDS, BSc, FDS, HDD, FACD

*General Dental Practitioner,
Formerly Senior Lecturer in Dental Prosthetics,
University of Liverpool, and Consultant Dental
Surgeon, United Liverpool Hospitals; and Lecturer
in Dental Prosthetics, University of Birmingham.
Visiting Associate Professor Northwestern
University Dental School, Chicago.*

AND

W.R.E. LAIRD
DDS, HDD, FDSRCPS (Glas)

*Professor of Dental Prosthetics,
University of Birmingham
and Consultant in Restorative Dentistry,
Central Birmingham Health Authority.
External Examiner to the Universities of
Liverpool and Wales, Royal College of
Physicians and Surgeons of Glasgow and
Royal College of Surgeons of England.
Formerly Senior Lecturer in Prosthetic
Dentistry, Victoria University of Manchester.*

FIFTH EDITION

BLACKWELL SCIENTIFIC PUBLICATIONS
OXFORD LONDON EDINBURGH
BOSTON PALO ALTO MELBOURNE

© 1968, 1974, 1986 by
Blackwell Scientific Publications
Editorial offices:
Osney Mead, Oxford, OX2 0EL
8 John Street, London, WC1N 2ES
23 Ainslie Place, Edinburgh, EH3 6AJ
52 Beacon Street, Boston
  Massachusetts 02108, USA
667 Lytton Avenue, Palo Alto
  California 94301, USA
107 Barry Street, Carlton
  Victoria 3053, Australia

All rights reserved. No part of this
publication may be reproduced, stored
in a retrieval system, or transmitted,
in any form or by any means,
electronic, mechanical, photocopying,
recording or otherwise
without the prior permission of
the copyright owner

First published 1954
Second edition 1959
Reprinted 1962
Third edition 1968
Fourth edition 1974
Reprinted 1978
Reprinted 1981
Fifth edition 1986

Photoset by Enset (Photosetting),
Midsomer Norton, Bath, Avon
and printed and bound
in Great Britain by
Butler & Tanner Ltd
Frome and London

DISTRIBUTORS

USA
  Year Book Medical Publishers
  35 East Wacker Drive
  Chicago, Illinois 60601

Canada
  The C.V. Mosby Company
  5240 Finch Avenue East,
  Scarborough, Ontario

Australia
  Blackwell Scientific Publications
  (Australia) Pty Ltd
  107 Barry Street
  Carlton, Victoria 3053

British Library
Cataloguing in Publication Data

Osborne, John, *1911–1984*
  Osborne & Lammie's partial dentures.—
  5th ed.
  1. Partial dentures
  I. Title   II. Lammie, George Alexander
  III. Laird, W.R.E.   IV. Osborne, John,
  1911–1984. Partial dentures
  617.6′92   RK664

ISBN 0-632-01698-5

CONTENTS

Preface, vii

1 A Historical Overview of Partial Denture Prosthetics, 1
2 Partial Denture Classification, 13
3 Aims in Partial Denture Construction and a Consideration of Alternatives, 20
4 Physiology and Pathology of Occlusion, 41
5 The Reaction of the Dental Apparatus to Loading, 73
6 A Perspective on Periodontal Disease, 98
7 Treatment Planning and Mouth Preparation, 129
8 Cast Surveying, 173
9 Materials Used in Partial Denture Construction, 189
10 The Component Parts of a Partial Denture, 198
11 The Bilateral Free-end Saddle (Kennedy Class I), 289
12 The Unilateral Free-end Saddle (Kennedy Class II), 324
13 The Bounded Saddle (Kennedy Class III), 330
14 The Anterior Bounded Saddle (Kennedy Class IV), 347
15 Impression Taking, 361
16 Registration of Jaw Relations, 380
17 The Trial Denture, 397
18 Aesthetics, 405
19 Denture Insertion, 418
20 Rebasing, 432
21 Periodontal Prostheses and Mouth Protectors, 441
22 Instructions to Patients, 446
23 Clinical and Laboratory Sequences in Partial Denture Construction, 455

Index, 463

PREFACE TO FIFTH EDITION

The predominant feeling in writing the preface to the fifth edition of this textbook must be one of sadness. John Osborne, its senior author, died in November 1984. His services to dentistry have been eulogized by others and their unanimous verdict does not overstate the stature of the man.

But my personal concern is not to record a catalogue of John's achievements but humbly to state for all to read that I have lost a good friend and colleague. He never treated me with anything but great kindness and, what is more, I never knew him to be mean in his behaviour towards any colleague regardless of his position in the 'pecking order'. I suppose it was the consistency and predictability of his warm goodwill that endeared him universally throughout the profession. Gatherings of dental prosthetists the world over will be the poorer for his absence.

The silver lining lies in the happy outcome that Per Saugman, Chairman of Blackwell Scientific Publications, and I were able to persuade Professor W.R.E. Laird, John's successor to the Chair of Dental Prosthetics in the University of Birmingham, to share in the extensive revision of this book. For me this has been a specially fortunate event since this may well be the last edition in which I make a substantial contribution. I would look forward to handing over a more senior role to one who has my confidence and admiration.

In this event perhaps the readership will forgive me for presenting a few contrary viewpoints. I do not expect universal applause and would feel more genuinely rewarded if the balanced presentation of controversial issues was followed by debate in our dental schools and our professional meetings. This is always an essential ingredient of good education. The other point is that indoctrination and its assured outcome is retrogression, not progress. In particular, the aetiology of periodontal disease is an issue which has attracted polar viewpoints; it is entirely possible that a synthesis of these apparently insular hypotheses will provide the productive clinical model. Certainly a resolution of the problem of periodontal disease would result in advances in partial denture prosthetics and dental medicine as a whole. I am specially indebted to Professor N.M. Naylor of Guy's Hospital for criticism in this area; he always conferred with characteristic courtesy but never acquiescence.

A special word of thanks is likewise due to Professor D.C.A. Picton of University College London, world authority on the reaction of the teeth and their supporting structures to loading. Professor Picton made available all his published and unpublished work with a generosity that I have seldom seen in the scientific dental community. Viewpoints advanced are largely those he pioneered and grateful thanks are accorded.

Lastly a personal and special recognition of the generous help always accorded to me by Mr Per Saugman, Chairman of Blackwell Scientific Publications Ltd. It is fitting to record here that when the late Sir Basil Blackwell sought in the early fifties to expand the role of his publishing house he had only one book under contract—this one. That Blackwell's is now one of the largest medical publishers in the country with international repute is largely the work of Per Saugman; his prodigious capacity for work, professional excellence and personal concern have always been greatly appreciated.

G.A. LAMMIE

1
A HISTORICAL OVERVIEW OF PARTIAL DENTURE PROSTHETICS

Professor John Osborne qualified as a dental surgeon in 1934. When he died in 1984 he had influenced change in his profession and speciality for fifty years. He had also, as senior author of this textbook, overseen its development over thirty years. The present writers felt that as a tribute to John Osborne, some history of partial denture prosthetics covering the period he practised would be interesting to the reader. However the additional and considerable reason for presenting this review is the conviction that a science which loses an appreciation of its own history is liable to lose its direction.

In terms of history these fifty years were momentous times; probably more change has been concentrated into these decades—socially, politically, economically and culturally—than in any similar period in history. Individual success in this period has required above all else an adaptability and an ability to cope with change. This is no less true professionally and there has been a constant challenge to embrace technical change in dentistry.

However, it is only when one sits down to record the changes in partial denture prosthetics that one becomes truly appreciative of the magnitude of these changes. It may be the anticipation of the reader that this essay will be a catalogue of steady advance, but in common with most histories of progress, development has come in phases of rapid change followed by longer periods of consolidation. Most change comes as a result of new ideas and a period of change must necessarily have as its precursor not only the birth of a new idea but its acceptance by the professional body.

It is proposed to consider the development of partial denture prosthetics under three headings:
(i)   Organization.
(ii) Materials and techniques.
(iii) Conceptual basis and research.

(i) Organization

In the thirties virtually all of the dentures supplied were made in general dental practice by private contract. The aims of the service were restricted by the current state of knowledge and by the hard facts of economics. The patient sought treatment much as he does today to improve appearance or facilitate mastication. The dentist acted entirely to serve these ends; most certainly no thought was given to the preservation of the dentition. However a bigger factor in limiting the provision of partial dentures was economic. This country and the Western world entered the thirties in a state of economic depression and although by the end of the decade the quality of life had greatly improved, comparatively these were still hard times. In the poverty of the thirties many peoples' concern was with continuing existence rather than the niceties of appearance. When one is starving one's dreams are of bounteous food, not of one's image. Such was the influence of personal economics that dentures nearly always meant complete dentures; the decision to extract all the natural teeth was not so much a clinical decision as a request by the patient whose health had become noticeably limited. Also very many people had all their teeth removed without being able to afford the luxury of subsequently having complete dentures. In these many cases, people adapted the physical nature of their diet or adapted physiologically to chew in the edentulous state. It was not uncommon to find a middle aged person with well developed alveolar ridges covered with a thick mucosa who could masticate a varied diet surprisingly well. Partial dentures were made mainly for the not so large and more affluent middle classes, and the demand was accordingly relatively low.

The Second World War affected the life of this country in many ways. All members of the armed services received dental examination and dental care. In the services the prevalent attitude was that some teeth had to be preserved to serve as abutments for splints in the event of jaw injury. This was a restricted approach and in most cases did not result in the provision of partial dentures following the extraction of grossly diseased teeth. Appearance was accorded no place in the decision to construct partial dentures; the ability to masticate the hard rations of an army in action was the criterion of assessment and this was based on regulation covering the number of occluding teeth remaining. This, however, was a considerable advance on the position during the Boer War when the fitness of soldiers was severely hampered by their inability to chew their food; the military solution was to send out mincers for their food rather than dentists!

Several combatant classes were recognized where the highest attainable standard of dental fitness was considered necessary for effectiveness in military duty. The largest of these special classes was air crew. Flying at 20,000 feet with little in the way of oxygen supply, demanded that the pulpal condition had to be perfect, to avoid the distraction of pain in an anoxic state. Clear speech was considered essential and the construction of partial dentures was encouraged to that end. Standards of dental technology were high; at the end of the war partial lower dentures with wrought stainless steel lingual bars and clasping were constructed routinely.

War service left a large number of demobilized personnel who had been introduced to the considerable benefits of dentistry as a means to general health and well being. Also the appearance of the nation had smartened up and people had been encouraged to look tidy and well kept. The demands for the construction of partial dentures and for the restoration and even enhancement of appearance became a large factor in the need for a partial denture service.

It is fair to say that the serving members of the armed forces in war time had paved the way for the enthusiasic reception accorded to the Beveridge Report which heralded the introduction of the National Health Service. It has always been fashionable to criticize the National Health Service and to emphasize its shortcomings, but there can be no doubt that it has provided the citizen with a high standard of health care. The hard economic fact, however, is ever present; there is no end to luxury in medical care and it is a very difficult matter to resolve where the division between necessary treatment and luxury should be drawn. Partial denture prosthetics is not exempt from this imposition. The National Health Service just cannot afford to provide some of the very expensive courses of treatment embracing sophisticated, fixed and removable restorative dentistry that might be considered in the best interests of the patient. Yet such a service should rightly be available to those whose preference is to pay for it on the basis of private contract and its provision on a limited scale is also an important research endeavour. But when thirty-seven years of the operation of the National Health Service is reviewed in special relation to partial denture prosthetics there can be no doubt that the line demarcating division between necessary treatment and luxury has moved continually in favour of substantially improved standards of treatment. One evidence of this is that the requirement of the general dental practitioner to seek prior approval for more complex and expensive forms of treatment has been considerably relaxed over the years. But there is the additional conviction that we do best what we do regularly. The certain outcome of this is that our routine standards increase in large measure as we come to undertake a class of work on a routine basis. This is especially true in the construction of the cast metal partial denture, bearing in mind that the laboratory procedure as well as the surgery endeavour has been the object of technical refinement and productivity.

(ii) Materials and Techniques

When we think of advances in dentistry our first thoughts are of great progress. But further analysis leads us to conclude that the substantial advances have been in fields of materials and techniques; it cannot be stressed too strongly nor too often that in spite of the expenditure of vast amounts of money, the two diseases with which dentistry is concerned, remain diseases of unknown aetiology. These facts are specially well illustrated in partial denture prosthetics.

In the thirties it was not possible to take an accurate impression of the mouth with consistency. The only impression materials routinely available were compound and plaster of Paris, and both had severe limitations, especially when the reproduction of tooth and tissue undercuts was concerned. The procedure with plaster of Paris was to fracture the impression immediately after its primary set and before the development of significant strength. The drawbacks were that reclaiming all the fractured pieces was difficult and that re-assembling the fractured impression was not always an accurate matter. All too often the surface detail of the impression was impaired by the reflex exudate of mucus from the discrete glands of the cheeks and palate and the copious flow of saliva from the main salivary glands; the detail of the fractured surfaces was also impaired. Further surface loss was incurred in 'soaping the impression' to create a separating layer before casting and damage to the surface of the cast could readily be incurred when separating the impression from the cast. Because of these drawbacks most operators preferred to use impression compound when taking impressions of the partially edentulous mouth. It is certain that where the convenience of the patient and operator was concerned the preference was fully justified and it is equally certain that in the great majority of cases a less accurate impression was obtained. Compound remains today, a thermoplastic material which shows varying degrees of elastic recoil when deformed in removal from undercut surfaces; moreover the concerned physical property is variable with the material used and the temperature at which it is withdrawn. On removal from an undercut surface, compound drags and is distorted in varying degree so that it is impossible to obtain an accurate impression of the dentulous mouth. But the aim of these few clinicians who were able to use the material well was not to obtain an accurate impression but one which compensated for the undercut surfaces while still procuring an accurate reproduction of those surfaces not involved in the undercut. A cast of the mouth was obtained therefore which was not accurate in all detail but which had incorporated in it the compensated modification such as would nowadays result after surveying and eliminating all redundant undercuts. Since clasps were always made by bending wrought gold wire or plate these were finally fitted with reference to the natural teeth at the insertion stage. Judging the temperature or the time of removing the impression, selecting and maintaining a path of withdrawal and controlling the force used in this, all played their important roles. All were the subject of clinical judgement and it is not surprising that masters of the technique were few indeed, and more commonly grossly distorted impressions were used in the fabrication of partial dentures. It is true that in the United States of America reversible hydrocolloids had been introduced, and these elastic materials gave highly accurate impressions comparable with those obtained routinely today. But these materials were expensive and channels of commerce were not widely open; thus for practical purposes those materials never became available in the United Kingdom.

A huge advance in partial denture prosthetics was made when the alginate impression materials became widely available at the end of World War II. Reasonably accurate impression materials became available for the first time, and the alginates which we currently use employ the reaction of the same chemicals as were originally compounded. Modifications of filler content has resulted in improvement in dimensional stability, surface texture and working viscosity, and as well as providing a material capable of giving an accurate reproduction, the flow of the newly mixed impression material is such as not to displace the soft tissue reflection at the level of its junction with the alveolar ridge. A reasonably accurate representation of the resting position of the mucosal reflection is therefore reproduced in impression taking and this permits the accurate development of saddle flanges and peripheries.

In addition to the alginates, synthetic rubber impression materials have since been developed. Silicone and thiokol rubber bases were used with appropriate catalysts, but the superiority of the thiokol base has now been recognized. Not only does this impression material give an unequalled reproduction of surface detail, it also gives an impression which is dimensionally more stable in storage.

The advance in impression materials used in partial denture fabrication has been remarkable. But having said this the story is still incomplete, for the routine availability of accurate models paved the way for two extremely important technical developments. The first was cast surveying. The aims of cast surveying remain the same as they were at the time of introduction of the technique to dentistry, namely the localization, measurement and elimination of tooth and tissue undercuts, especially the former. This permitted the accurate design of clasps related to the physical properties of the chosen metal alloy.

The second was the technical development of the one piece cast metal denture incorporating all clasping and stress breaking. There was a great advance in terms of productivity. Today, accurate one piece cast metal dentures can be routinely produced with some confidence and in terms of cost of materials and weight there is now a preference for the cobalt chromium range of alloys over the previously favoured gold alloys. However, as far as clasping and stress breaking components are concerned the physical properties of gold remain superior. If a weak spot in the technique were to be highlighted, the dependability of the so-called reproduction impression materials used to obtain a duplicate model in refractory material would be questioned. These are aqueous gels from which loss of water is, at least theoretically, liable to take place.

Consideration of these two developments would be incomplete without generously according appreciation to the dental manufacturing houses, especially those in America, for the enterprise shown in their original production. Surveying was introduced by the J.M. Ney Company, who not only produced the original instrument but also published excellent literature on its use in partial denture design and construction. Much conceptual refinement has gone on since, but the basic tenets of model surveying remain those published by Ney. Cobalt chromium alloys, too, were first developed as a commercial enterprise in America. The pioneering work in this field of metallurgy was carried out by Elwood Haines who developed the stellite group of alloys in the first decade of the present century, and it is believed that the first dental casting of cobalt chromium alloys was done by Krupps prior to 1929. In that year Erdle and Prange of the Austenal Laboratories in New York introduced their Vitallium alloy and casting technique under patent, and dentures were made of this material. These examples illustrate the great indebtedness of the profession to the free enterprise of the manufacturing companies. As dentists we are all too prone to accept credit and many believe that the introduction of new materials and techniques should be accredited to the dental materials departments of our universities; these departments have been much more concerned with the physical testing of already developed materials and the enunciation of appropriate physical standards.

The other major development was the introduction of acrylic resin as a denture base material. In the thirties, other than rarely used gold and stainless steel plate, vulcanite was the only denture base material in routine use. It was produced by compounding natural rubber and sulphur and vulcanizing in pressurized steam. Many of its physical qualities were admirable and in terms of durability, vulcanite dentures provided many years of service. The great disadvantage of the material was its unaesthetic quality; but it was not this failing that prompted the need for the development of another denture base material, it was the precarious supply position of natural rubber from Malaya in World War II that gave stimulus to the search. The first man to use methyl methacrylate by the dough technique in the fabrication of dentures was the late Harold M. Vernon of the Vernon–Benschoff Company. Here too it is specially fitting to accord to John Osborne our indebtedness for his research into the use of acrylic resin in the forties. With its several shortcomings acrylic resin has remained the material of choice, virtually unchallenged; it has done this because of its high aesthetic potential and its very simple laboratory technique. Other materials with more favourable flexural fatigue property have been advocated but confined to use in special cases where strength is specially required; these have necessitated the use of a more costly injection moulding technique.

As well as being used as a denture base material, acrylic resin is now used in the production of artificial teeth used on so many of the dentures made today. However, it must immediately be conceded that acrylic resin teeth have several deficiencies and that porcelain teeth which were exclusively used at the beginning of the fifty year period under review still remain serious contenders for preference especially in special situations.

This review illustrates that in the field of dental materials and techniques great advances have been made in the last half century.

(iii) Conceptual Basis and Research

A consideration of this most important aspect must be based on personal opinion much more heavily than was the case when considering organization and materials and techniques. These depended on acknowledged and confirmable fact in substantial measure. Certainly when considering the conceptual basis there is a record of original papers written at different stages. But the earlier writers were few in number, strongly individualistic and concerned with their own special interests. Above all no allegiance to a paradigm was required; in fact none existed. There is therefore justification for placing more reliance on observation of attitudes and concerns over the period than on publications. Some may dispute the accuracy of these observations and more especially the judgements which stem from them, but no apology is made for expressing these ideas, which the reader is even encouraged to dispute.

In the period before the Second World War there was no biological concern in the construction of partial dentures. Those who had special interest in the field were primarily concerned with what was then called dental mechanics, and with simply producing dentures which fitted first the cast and then the mouth. The acknowledged leaders in the field were rather ingenious men who loved tinkering around 'the workshop'. It was the laboratory rather than the surgery which was the scene of creative endeavour. Some of these men were gifted craftsmen and artists and were capable of producing 'jewellery' of very high quality. Many of their approaches have not stood the test of time but by and large they gave an appreciated service to their patients. Swaging gold and stainless steel denture bases is an art long since suspended. Soldering wrought gold wire and hand crafted gold plate clasps was a routine procedure. The use of tube teeth at the back of the mouth and Steel's facings at the front are examples of work most modern dentists will not even have heard of; then they were commonplace. The basic partial denture service lay in the construction of partial dentures made in vulcanite with porcelain teeth; these were always tissue borne dentures but the use especially of wrought wire clasps fashioned from half round or round gold wire was commonplace; above all a denture had to fit and be well retained. In fact it is probable that more clasping was used on these dentures than is commonly used on similar dentures today. No design analysis was made, no undercuts were measured, clasps were distributed with largesse upon abutment teeth. Many of these dentures gave exceptional service, probably because the partially edentulous state had been arrived at more through extraction following caries than periodontal disease. It is salutory to be reminded that the large majority of dentures produced in this country today are identical with those produced fifty years ago except that they are fabricated in different materials.

It is not surprising that one of the great interests of those early prosthetists was in the reproduction of jaw movements in the laboratory. Most dentures then, as now, were made on a simple hinge articulator; this articulator simply held the casts of opposing jaws in fixed relation in the tooth position. It was simply a reliable mechanical device for repeatedly replacing the casts into occlusion after periods of working on the individual casts as in 'setting up'. But it came to be appreciated that in function the teeth occluded in positions other than 'centric occlusion' and the demand arose to develop instruments capable of reproducing essential movements of the mandible when the teeth were held in occlusion.

For several decades the prime concern of dental prosthetics was the reproduction of jaw movements on articulators; some of the instruments produced were manufactured to very precise engineering standards. But in essence all of these instruments sought to reproduce protrusive and lateral mandibular movements. Although the prime stimulus to development derived from complete denture prosthetics where the stability of the lower denture in particular derived from absence of impedance in forward and sideways mandibular movements in function, the same instruments were routinely used in partial denture construction. The principle harnessed in using these 'anatomical' articulators was that the direction of jaw movement was rigidly controlled by the form of the glenoid fossa as the condyle of the mandible moved across it. In some articulators, known as average value instruments, it was assumed that for practical purposes it was sufficient that the condyles were directed forwards on the path of the glenoid fossa and this was generally inclined at an angle of 45 degrees to the horizontal. It was further assumed that the path of movement was a straight line. Instruments of this class were capable of reproducing lateral as well as protrusive movements, simply by accepting the assumption that on the 'working' side the condyle was fixed in its most retruded condylar position but was permitted to make a rotation about a vertical axis. On the contralateral or balancing side the condyle made a downward and inward compensatory movement directed again by the pitch of the inferior surface of the glenoid fossa. Such instruments were commonly used in the teaching hospitals of this country. To those who sought more sophistication, however, the adjustable anatomical articulator aimed to reproduce the actual pitch of the glenoid fossa on the instrument. The condylar paths on the instrument were adjustable and the angles were set with reference to a protrusive wax record, which defined the position of the condylar heads when the jaw was fully protruded again assuming a straight line path of movement for the condylar head. But another component of lateral jaw excursion was also incorporated in many of the more complex articulators. The discovery of a bodily lateral translation of the mandible in the execution of a lateral mandibular slide was made by a distinguished London dentist, Sir Norman Bennett, and this complicating component was reproduced on an adjustable basis by taking two lateral wax records of the mandibular positions at the extremity of right and left lateral slides. The design of the conventional fully adjustable articulators incorporated all of those movement potentials set to the individual anatomical form of the articulating temporo-mandibular joint surfaces. The most famous fully adjustable articulator ever produced, the Hanan Model H, was almost universally used in the dental schools of North America; probably it still is. The Dentatus articulator produced much later in Sweden was engineered on a similar design based on the same principle. Other designs and refinements were incorporated in many well known articulators, but none gained the universal popularity of the original Hanan Model H. It must be appreciated in retrospect that claims were made for all these instruments that were not devoid of commercial interest; the development of articulators was more the province of ingenious engineers than dentists. One exception to this general comment was the McCollum Gnathoscope, which was developed by two Californian dentists, McCollum and Stewart. Let it be said that they were both superb engineers but their biological appreciation was hardly commensurate with their precision craftsmanship.

The great concern of dental prosthetists with articulators in the first half of the present century was restricting; it was not surprising that the man whose delight was tinkering in the laboratory was not greatly concerned with the fact that the patient was made of changing, adaptable living tissue rather than rigid metallic components. But the fact should be acknowledged that we still use articulators today as a convenience in developing the first stages of the occlusal patterns of our partial dentures. However nobody today would consider that the final reference for the adjustment of occlusion both of the natural and artificial teeth should be done other than in the mouth. The preoccupation with articulators took no cognizance of the biological nature of the tissue components of the temporomandibular joint. This joint is encompassed by a capsular ligament which permits some distraction of the surfaces of the joints in functional movements of the mandible. The bony surfaces of the joints have a covering of somewhat compressible cartilaginous tissue and an articular cartilage occupies the joint space. In fact the tooth form, muscular habit and physical nature of a food bolus have more influence on the path of functional jaw movement than the joint form; a substantial amount of adaptability is present in the functioning of the joint. Moreover the masticatory movements have only a short range of interocclusal contact and this may not accord with the extreme average indications derived from the boundary mandibular positions recorded on articulators. A fundamental misconception is incorporated into the occlusal concept behind the use of all articulators; the mandibular position in which the healthy teeth interdigitate maximally does not coincide with the most retruded position of the mandible. In practice it is abundantly clear that concepts of ideal occlusal form derived from articulator concepts in full denture work do not pertain in the healthy mouth. Ideas of spreading the occlusal load should be based on the elimination of individual hypercontacts and the restriction of sharing the load within a particular segment. Still to this day, full coverage bridge work is undertaken to shape the occlusal surfaces to a form dictated by those articulators designed so many years ago.

It was, in retrospect, inevitable that there should be a conceptual revolution away from the mechanistic concepts of dental prosthetics concerned first with denture production and then with articulator theory. The biological revolution came in the fifties at a time when several young dentists had completed a biological training after the war and at a time when enthusiastic teachers of anatomy and physiology in the dental schools sought to apply their fundamental biological knowledge. It is probable that the centre of this revolutionary thinking was in Chicago; Northwestern University was then the Mecca of dentistry. The basic concept postulated a balance between the teeth, the neuromuscular system and the temporomandibular joint. The idea was first developed to account for the temporomandibular syndrome but it became clear almost immediately that it had reference to periodontology, orthodontics and partial denture prosthetics. Briefly, muscular behaviour was found to be modified by the form of the occlusal surfaces and the relationship of joint structures. The role of the brain in linking the sensory input with the motor discharge, has now been carefully studied and although much remains to be elucidated, it is abundantly clear that variables act on receptors, central mechanisms and motor discharge. The concept rationalized adjustment of the occlusion as a means of treating temporomandibular syndrome. Change occurs in all of the three components of the stomatognathic system with ageing, and oral health requires that change in each should be in harmony. It was not coincidental that the physiological technique of electromyography became available at this time and its use was widely applied during this period of development. Those working with the technique at the time envisaged the extension of its use from research to clinical practice, but this event did not materialize.

At this time too the significance of basic positions of the mandible became apparent. In the vertical plane the rest position and the tooth position were defined whereas in the horizontal plane the ligamentous position, the muscular position and the tooth position were differentiated. In particular the relationship of these positions to anatomical and physiological criteria made an analysis of the functional movements of the mandible possible and meaningful. Masticatory movements, swallowing movements and empty movements were described in detail and their significance to oral physiology and pathology became apparent. The concept of occlusal analysis was a logical outcome from these percepts and the effects of overloading the tissues were examined.

All this represents a huge step forward and a shift of emphasis from the mechanical to the biological. Hopes for the sixties and seventies ran high but consolidation rather than continued progress was to follow. It became apparent, however, that there was a positive limitation to the clinical advance that was to be achieved. In particular, hopes that these concepts might prove the forerunner to elucidation of the nature of periodontal disease were quite ill-founded. It seemed that there was at least one missing biological component the discovery of which would herald a comprehensive understanding of a unified aetiological dogma. What was lacking was ideas, especially those relating to biology. On reflection, the hiatus that succeeded the period of intensive biological progress might have been forecast. The biological revolution had been the product of a few men; but an idea is the product of one person's mind, and that person must be one of a rare breed, one capable of really creative thought. They must at the same time have large clinical experience and wide biological education. It was not all going to happen immediately.

During the sixties and seventies research work in partial denture prosthetics proceeded. It was by nature 'ordinary' science rather than 'revolutionary' science. It was characterized by a sophistication and refinement of method. What better example could illustrate this point than Watt's development of stereostethoscopy of the stomatognathic system. Cruder methods of palpation had always been used to glean information on tooth jiggling but refinement was accomplished by Watt's method. Another more universal example of progress in partial denture prosthetics was the sophisticated analysis of load distribution referable to the design of partial dentures. Such issues as tissue and tooth loading, stress breaking, direct and indirect retention, direct and indirect loading were all analysed in some detail and certainly the outcome has been better partial denture design. But a word of warning is necessary; complacency must be avoided because in all this work assumptions and approximations are made about the physical properties of the tissues involved especially the bone, mucosa and periodontal membrane. These tend to be regarded as homogenized, finite entities of static value, a system amenable to vectorial analysis. In fact the opposite is true, living tissues being in a constant state of change, their form and structure are always variable over short and long periods of time. Above all it is quite misleading, indeed wrong, to assume that a mouth treated for periodontal disease is not subject to later change. Berry's recent work showing how the occlusal form changes after a very short period of rest emphasizes the dynamic state of the oral condition.

It remains a conviction that the division of dentistry into a substantial number of specialities largely based on technique may have facilitated the organization of teaching but it has certainly had a significant part to play in retarding advance in our understanding of the aetiology of dental disease. Nowhere is this more apparent than placing a departmental barrier between the study and treatment of periodontal disease and the provision of a partial denture service. Major progress in the field of partial denture prosthetics can now only follow an elucidation of the cause of periodontal disease. We must accept a role for inflammation in the aetiology of periodontal disease, but the exclusive viewpoint of 'environmental determination' must be abandoned for one which embraces a dual role for age changes and inflammation, accepting too the ever present complication of traumatism. The aetiology is a much more complex matter than has been envisaged in the past two decades; the realization of this is hopeful even though the relative importance of the three contributory parameters can only be tentative.

However, the writers are happy to be able to conclude this brief review on a highly optimistic note because of recent advances in the field of dental implants. This is not a new area of endeavour; reports on the method go back to the fifties. The stimulus for the new clinical approach was doubtless the introduction of the cast cobalt chromium partial denture and the assurance gained from orthopaedic surgery of the biocompatibility of the alloy. At the time of introduction there was a confidence founded on ignorance, so that in retrospect it is not surprising that the life of some of the appliances was short. What was satisfactory, however, was the acceptability to the patient and that patients who had reasonably extensive success sought a similar new appliance rather than resorting to the older conventional removable partial denture. Many of these early appliances were largely subperiosteal and as bone changes took place movement of the implant was permitted and the chances of a 'periodontal' infection greatly increased. But now the position has changed hugely. Biological research has revealed the principles involved in biocompatibility and endosteal placement of the implant with osseo-integration has led to a rigid immovable implant. Above all the appreciation that bone form is a response to vascularity provides conceptual hope for this endosteal method and the confident hope that partial denture prosthetics will use the method increasingly.

Even this introduction to the development of the speciality will focus attention on the great need for encouraging biological endeavour in a field which is undoubtedly complex. Men of quality must be encouraged to be courageous and consider the final words of Sir Karl Popper:

'The advance of science is not due to the fact that more and more perceptual experiences accumulate in the course of time. Nor is it due to the fact that we are making ever better use of our senses. Out of uninterpreted experiences science cannot be distilled, no matter how industriously we gather and sort them. Bold ideas, unjustified anticipations, and speculative thought are our only means for interpreting nature; our only organon, our only instrument, for grasping her. And we must hazard them to win our prize. Those among us who are unwilling to expose their ideas to the hazard of refutation do not take part in the scientific game.'

References

BERRY D.C. and SINGH B.P. (1983) Daily variations in occlusal contacts. *J. pros. Dent.* **50**, 386.

BERRY D.C. and SINGH B.P. (1984) Effect of electromyographic biofeedback therapy on occlusal contacts. *J. pros. Dent.* **51**, 397.

WATT D.M. (1981) *Gnathosonic diagnosis and occlusal dynamics.* Praeger, Eastbourne.

2

PARTIAL DENTURE CLASSIFICATION

In this book partial dentures are defined as restorations capable of being removed from the mouth by the patient.

Before considering systems of partial denture classification it is necessary to define the term *saddle*. The saddles are those parts of a partial denture which replace lost alveolar tissue and carry artificial teeth; they may be either free-end or bounded. In the former (Fig. 2.1) an abutment tooth is present at only one end

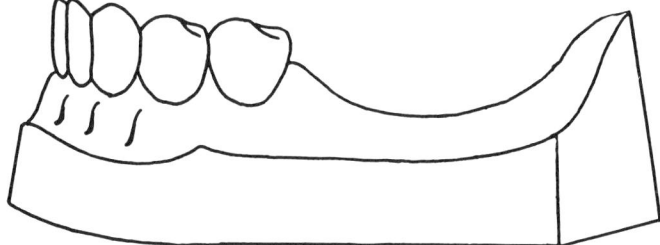

Fig. 2.1. A free-end saddle having an abutment tooth at one end only.

of the saddle, and in the latter (Fig. 2.2) abutment teeth are present at both ends. In the first case a considerable part of the masticatory pressure is resisted by the alveolar bone supporting the saddle; in the second, the abutment teeth may support the saddle almost completely. This differentiation is of great importance when treatment by partial dentures is considered, and more than one system of partial denture classification is based upon the presence, position, and number of free-end and bounded saddles.

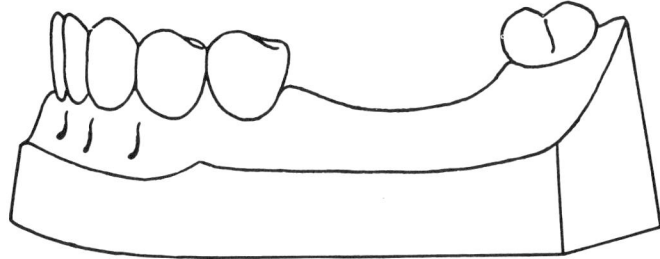

Fig. 2.2. A bounded saddle having abutment teeth at both ends.

An examination of the literature reveals that several criteria have formed the basis of partial denture classification. Classification in itself facilitates case history recording and the exchange of views between practitioners, always provided there is general acceptance of the particular system. Given this agreement some order may be created from the vast combinations of standing teeth and saddle areas that are possible as a result of the random extraction of teeth over a number of years. In addition, a classification should give some clues to the treatment and design problems of the particular patient. A design that functions successfully for a denture of a given classification can, in many instances, be used with only slight modification for another denture of the same class.

Throughout the past seventy years many systems of partial denture classification have been suggested. The ones that have received the most attention are those of Cummer (1920), Beckett (1940), Kennedy (1942), Godfrey (1951), Skinner (1959), and Applegate (1965).

At the present time Kennedy's system is the most widely used, together with the amendments to it suggested by Applegate. Beckett's system finds decreasing favour in Australia, and is not used elsewhere.

The Kennedy classification

Preference is given to the Kennedy classification since it is the most universally used and quoted. Kennedy describes four classes of upper or lower jaw conditions, and each of the first three of these may show one or more modifications.

Class I. Class I is that type of case where the saddles are bilateral and lie posterior to the standing teeth. Alternatively, this Class can be described as requiring treatment by a denture having two free-end saddles (Fig. 2.3). This is the type of partial denture that is required most frequently, and its highest incidence is in the mandible. In this Class a modification is produced if another bounded saddle is required; such a case with two free-end and one bounded saddle would be described as a Class I, modification 1 (Fig. 2.4). If two bounded saddles are

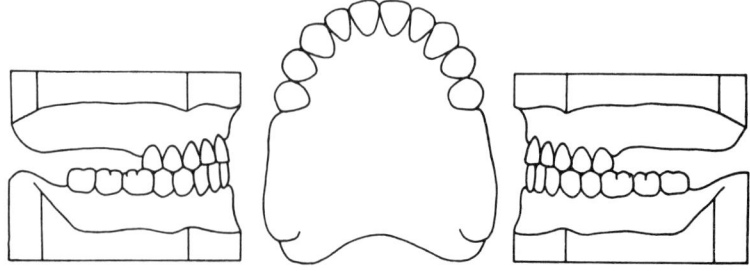

Fig. 2.3. A Class I (Kennedy) case requiring two free-end saddles.

Partial Denture Classification   15

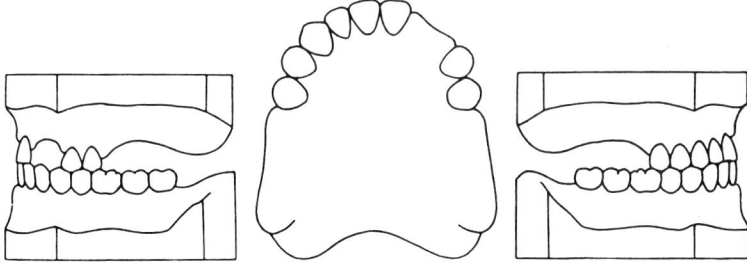

Fig. 2.4. A Class I modification 1 (Kennedy) case requiring two free-end saddles and one bounded saddle.

present in addition to the two free-end saddles the case would be a Class I, modification 2 (Fig. 2.5), and so on for increasing numbers of bounded saddles.

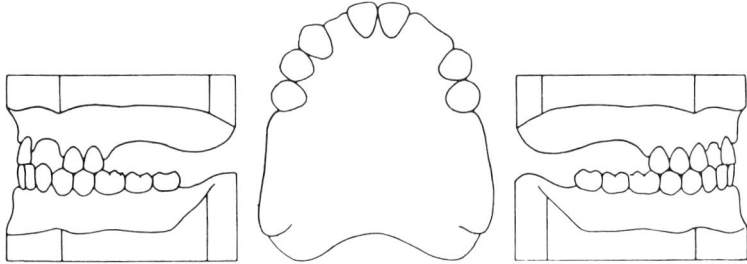

Fig. 2.5. A Class I modification 2 (Kennedy) case requiring two free-end saddles and two bounded saddles.

Class II. Class II is that type of case where the saddle is unilateral, and lies posterior to the standing teeth; in this condition the missing teeth are confined to one side of the mouth (Fig. 2.6). A partial denture in this Class would consequently have a unilateral free-end saddle. If, in addition to this single free-end

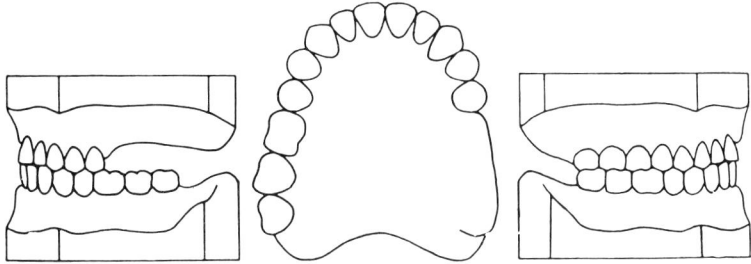

Fig. 2.6. A Class II (Kennedy) case requiring one free-end saddle.

saddle, a single bounded saddle is present, then we have a Class II, modification 1, case (Fig. 2.7), and so on (Fig. 2.8).

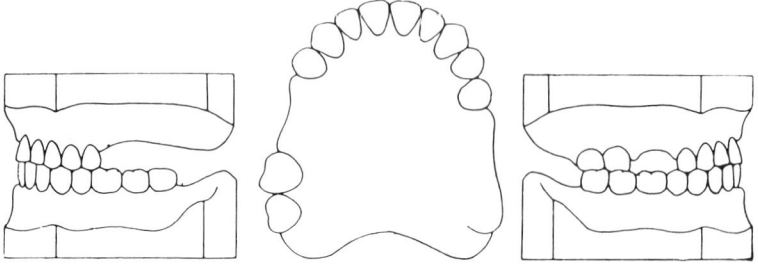

Fig. 2.7. A Class II modification 1 (Kennedy) case requiring one free-end saddle and one bounded saddle.

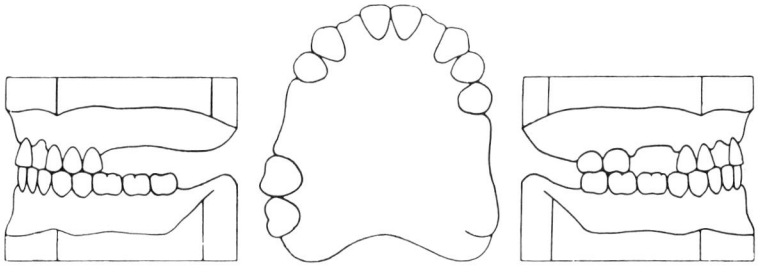

Fig. 2.8. A Class II modification 3 (Kennedy) case requiring one free-end saddle and three bounded saddles.

Class III. Class III is that type of case where teeth are missing on one side of the mouth, the saddle having support anteriorly and posteriorly (Fig. 2.9). A denture of this Class, therefore, has one bounded saddle on one side of the mouth. Here again modifications can be, and usually are, present (Fig. 2.10).

Applegate considers the Kennedy classification to have many excellent features, but points out that, since considerable variations of treatment plan may

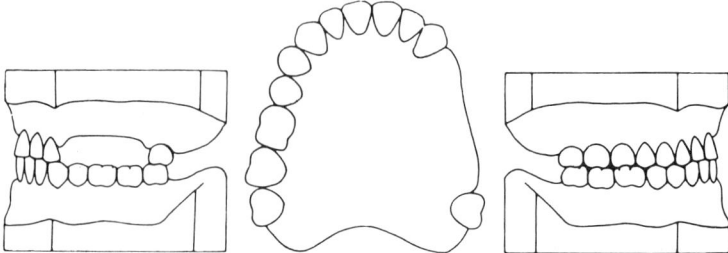

Fig. 2.9. A Class III (Kennedy) case requiring one bounded saddle.

Partial Denture Classification

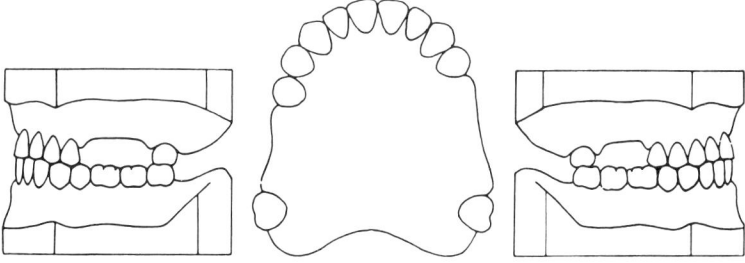

Fig. 2.10. A Class III modification 1 (Kennedy) case requiring two bounded saddles.

be required with Class III cases, it is desirable to have two additional groups within this class. These are intended to designate different structural and anatomical situations which will require dissimilar designs. Further consideration is given to these groups in Chapter 13.

Class IV. Class IV is that type in which a single saddle lies entirely anterior to the attachments (Fig. 2.11). This Class has no modifications.

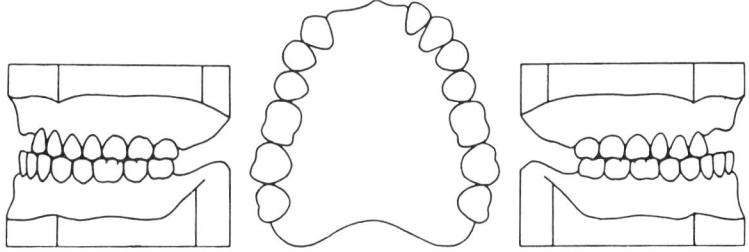

Fig. 2.11. A Class IV (Kennedy) case requiring a single saddle lying anterior to the abutments.

A classification depending on distribution of load

A simple classification depends on the tissues which bear the masticatory load in function. Vertical and horizontal components of the force placed on the occlusal surface of a partial denture are, in the end, resisted by standing teeth and their supporting structures, or by the bony tissues of the edentulous ridge or hard palate, which are covered by a mucosa. In the first instance the partial denture is referred to as *tooth borne*, in the second as *mucosa borne*. An often quoted classification which refers to the denture as a whole is:

Class I   mucosa borne,
Class II   tooth borne,
Class III combination of mucosa and tooth borne.

The Beckett classification

Beckett's classification is based on the load distribution of the individual component saddles of the partial denture. His classification has the great merit of providing a guide to design. Utilization of his classification, however, implies acceptance of his theories on design. Beckett claims that any individual saddle of a denture should be either entirely tooth supported or entirely mucosa supported; any attempt to share the load between the two is considered unsound since 'it is impossible to transmit varying occlusal stresses in determined proportions to tissues whose supporting value can only be estimated approximately instead of measured with accuracy'. Further, he rightly contends that even if a finite distribution of load could be obtained, in time, the ratio in which the forces were distributed between tooth and tissue would be altered by reactions in these living tissues.

In Beckett's classification the individual saddles of any partial denture are divided into three groups:

Class 1 saddles are those that are entirely tooth supported (Fig. 2.12). As a result of clinical and X-ray examination it is assessed that the teeth at either extremity of the saddle can fully support the additional load.

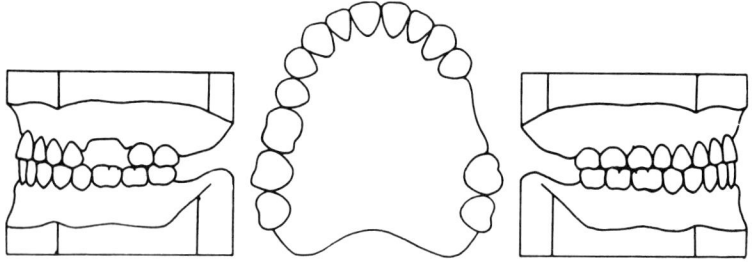

Fig. 2.12. A Class 1 (Beckett) saddle which would be entirely tooth borne.

Class 2 saddles are those that are entirely mucosa supported. Two types of saddle are found in this class:
1   All free-end saddles (Fig. 2.1).
2   Those bounded saddles where obviously the length of saddle and/or the condition of the abutment teeth contra-indicates a tooth-borne saddle. Beckett treats these saddles as mucosa borne by using a stress-broken design.

Class 3 saddles are those bounded saddles about which a problem exists (Fig. 2.13). Saddles are placed in this class only temporarily while it is considered if

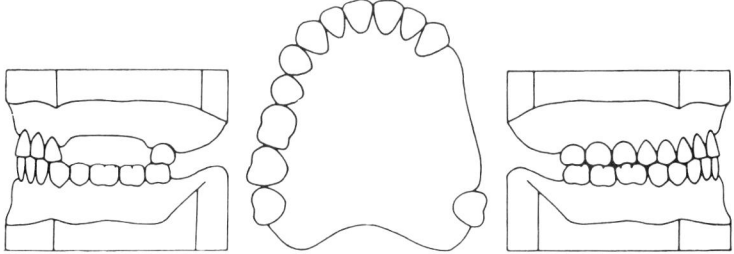

Fig. 2.13. A Class 3 (Beckett) saddle presenting a problem. This saddle would eventually be classified as Class 2 on account of its length.

they should fall into Class *1* or *2*. Such factors as the anatomy and pathology of the abutment teeth, the length and position of the saddle in the arch and the nature of the alveolar bone and covering mucosa, will eventually influence the decision as to whether such bounded saddles be tooth or mucosa supported.

The Kennedy classification has been preferred in this book since it is the most universally used system, has the merit of simplicity, and differentiates between bounded and free-end saddle cases.

References

APPLEGATE O.C. (1960) The rationale of partial denture choice. *J. pros. Dent.* **10,** 891.

APPLEGATE O.C. (1965) *Essentials of removable partial denture prosthodontics*, 3rd ed. W.B. Saunders Co., Philadelphia.

BECKETT L.S. (1940) Some fundamentals of partial denture construction. *Aust. J. Dent.* **44,** 363.

CODY L.G. (1948) Broken stress partial dentures for the general practitioner. *Fortnight. Rev. Chicago dent. Soc.* **16,** 8.

CUMMER W.E. (1920) Possible combinations of teeth present or missing in partial restorations. *Oral Health,* **10,** 421.

GODFREY R.J. (1951) Classification of removable partial dentures. *J. Amer. Coll. Dent.* **18,** 5.

KENNEDY E. (1942) Partial denture construction. *Dent. Items of Interest.* Publishing Co. New York, 3.

MILLER E.L. (1970) Systems for classifying partially dentulous arches. *J. pros. Dent.* **24,** 25.

SKINNER C.S. (1959) A classification of removable partial dentures based upon anatomy and physiology. *J. pros. Dent.* **9,** 241.

3

AIMS IN PARTIAL DENTURE CONSTRUCTION AND A CONSIDERATION OF ALTERNATIVES

It may be necessary to make a partial denture for a patient for any one of the following reasons:
- to restore or improve the ability to masticate;
- to restore or improve appearance;
- to maintain the oral tissues in as healthy a condition as possible.

Obviously there will be many situations where a combination of two or all of these requirements are met by the provision of dentures.

The Necessity to Restore Mastication

It is a popular belief that food should be chewed to ensure that it is digested properly, and if it is not, indigestion leads to general ill-health. However, this is not necessarily true.

Farrell showed that although little more than 50 per cent of beef, bacon, chicken, lamb, pork, potatoes, peas and carrots, can be digested without chewing, such foods as fish, beef fat, eggs, cheese, bread and rice will be digested fully without any chewing at all. In addition, it has been shown that the amount of chewing required even for the least digestible foods is surprisingly small. Hence the ability to chew cannot be an essential prerequisite to good health. Consequently it may be asked: what is the use of partial dentures? Paradoxically the answer in many cases may be: they assist in chewing.

When a person becomes partially edentulous their chewing habits may change. If only a few natural teeth in both jaws oppose each other chewing will be carried out, as far as possible, with those teeth. This may well be so even if partial dentures are worn—and this person will claim that he chews better with the dentures than without them. This somewhat contradictory state of affairs can be explained by the fact that chewing requires the combined activity of both the teeth and the oral musculature. In the absence of a full complement of teeth it is not possible for the muscles of the tongue, cheeks and lips to control the food bolus since it will slip away and lodge in the edentulous areas. Hence in these circumstances, partial dentures may not contribute greatly to mastication simply by providing more teeth to take part in the act, but they will help to re-establish oral function as a whole by assisting the musculature to 'handle' the food bolus and keep it between the natural remaining teeth.

When the loss of natural teeth is much greater (for example, if a person is edentulous in the upper jaw and has only some natural anterior and two premolar teeth in the lower jaw and is supplied with a complete upper denture and a Class 1 partial lower denture) then hopefully the majority of chewing will be carried out on the artificial molars and premolars. In such a case the partial denture contributes directly to chewing. However the clinician must not presume that in such a case the patient will automatically revert to this natural and desirable masticatory pattern. How often have we all seen the resorption and fibrosis of the anterior maxillary alveolar ridges where an anterior chewing cycle has persisted over a period of years? (As an aside, this situation is always worse where anterior porcelain teeth have been preferred to acrylic resin teeth; in the latter much of the energy will cause a mutilation of the artificial teeth and spoil their appearance, rather than prejudice the edentulous alveolar ridge.) This persistent habit of using an anterior masticatory cycle also has a detrimental long term consequence on the natural teeth especially where the life of these teeth is threatened through progressive periodontal disease. If and when these teeth are lost the patient is just so much older and the less able mentally to cope with the considerable self-disciplinary learning process necessary to use complete dentures satisfactorily; in the latter eventuality the acquisition of the normal posterior chewing pattern is imperative to successful denture wearing. It would have been much more satisfactory to have acquired this masticatory habit at a younger age, as a result of the dentist's stimulation and the patient's application.

It is true that many people will suffer the loss of a considerable number of posterior teeth without complaining of inability to chew properly. Modern diet does not require a very efficient mechanism in order to convert it to a consistency acceptable for swallowing. Hence it is common for many people to accept without complaint the loss of posterior teeth provided several, in opposing jaws, remain in contact. Such persons, provided their oral health is satisfactory, should not be persuaded to wear partial dentures. Indeed, even following the loss of a tooth previously considered an indispensible unit in mastication, time should be allowed for healing before deciding that partial dentures are now needed. The exception described above remains; partial dentures should always be constructed to maintain or develop a posterior rather than an anterior masticatory cycle. Such an accomplishment will also add to the pleasure of eating by removing the sporadic painful traumatism of the palatal gingivae.

So far the debate has centred solely upon the decision whether or not to construct partial dentures to attain masticatory competence. However the distribution of periodontally sound teeth may well be such that the construction of fixed bridgework on a segmental or full mouth basis may be a feasible alternative. There can be no doubt that advances in dental technology have made the field of crown and bridgework a much more hopeful prospect than when the first edition of this textbook appeared (1954). More is now known about periodontal status and this should ensure a fortunate outcome to what will necessarily be expensive treatment. To many it is also a social embarrassment to have to decline food offered on the grounds of a crippled dental state. However the physical properties of the individual components and overall completed denture have been greatly improved so that the risk of these most embarrassing physical breakdowns have happily become rare rather than frequent. There are many people who gain great pleasure from eating good, sophisticatedly prepared food; to these the presence of an uncovered palate gives an undiminished appreciation of taste, temperature and consistency.

The Necessity to Restore Appearance

The student will not be in practice long before he receives a distraught telephone call from an anxious mother whose son has just suffered a traumatic injury involving the anterior teeth. Accidents commonly result from cycling, swimming and hard ball games such as cricket and hockey, rather than the apparently more robust physical contact sports such as association and rugby football. In these cases every effort must be made to retain the compromised tooth be it completely dislocated, displaced or fractured; it is always surprising how many such traumatized teeth fully recover with good treatment. However, some few will succumb and extraction will be necessary. Certainly the most commonly involved tooth is the upper central incisor especially where this has erupted into an extreme labial protrusion through failure to remove the deciduous lateral in good

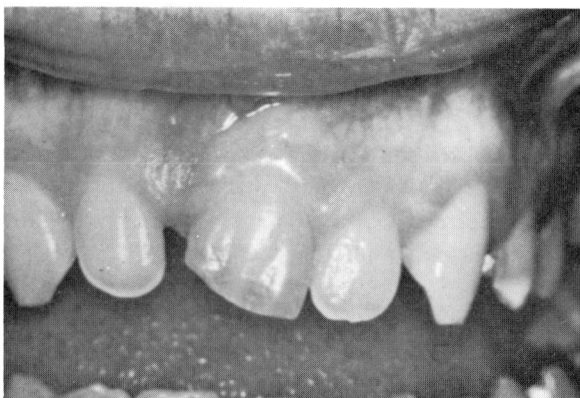

Fig. 3.1. The disastrous result following failure to replace a lost incisor in a child (by permission of Professor T.D. Foster).

time. It is imperative that in such cases a simple acrylic resin denture, possibly of spoon design if this gives satisfactory retention, should be constructed and inserted without delay. Its purpose is to retain the alveolar space without encroachment from the lateral incisor during the eruptive period. The disastrous aesthetic result of failing in this urgent treatment is well illustrated in Fig. 3.1. The components of poor aesthetics in this case are a mid-line shift of the central incisor and a lack of balancing symmetry in mesio-distal width of the middle tooth. This would be an unfavourable condition to correct by crowning as the midline shift is permanent and the slender lateral root would not be amenable to crowning with an artificial crown of the necessary mesio-distal dimension to obliterate the central diastema. But whereas there is no alternative in the foregoing case, if the traumatized tooth is a lower central incisor which has been dislodged completely or has had to be extracted because of extreme partial dislocation or severe fracture, then the position is very different. Such a tooth should not be routinely replaced by a partial denture. Here a mid-line shift invariably results but without significantly compromising the appearance. Since the width of the tooth is small, complete space closure takes place especially at a time when more posterior teeth are erupting and no diastema results in the late teens. Moreover the size of the lateral and central incisors is so similar as not to present an incongruity and the incisal edges of the lower front teeth come to lie as an even line. This is a fortunate chain of events since wearing a space-retaining denture in the lower jaw would be more deleterious to oral health than the equivalent in the upper. Moreover the smaller lower teeth would not be so amenable to supporting bridgework in the later teens.

Whereas it is conceivable that extraordinary circumstances may determine a course other than that advocated above in the case of the central incisors, the position is rather different when the only tooth lost is the upper lateral incisor, albeit this is a much rarer situation. Certainly no dentist could be reprimanded for electing to retain the space with a partial upper denture bearing the single lateral tooth. Such a condition would be expected to be one favourable to later bridging. But equally the writers are able to report a good aesthetic outcome when it was judged prudent to forego constructing a partial denture and leave the space available for mesial migration of the canine tooth which is generally at this stage unerupted. Needless to say decision as to whether decompressive extraction is indicated in the posterior segment is deferred until the permanent canine has fully erupted into approximation with the central incisor. The space generally closes completely, but the quality of the aesthetic result is largely determined by the form of the canine tooth. It might be anticipated that the sharpness of the pointed crown of this tooth would be the critical factor. However this is generally not the case as judicuous, continuous grinding in stages leaves an incisal edge form which is completely acceptable. The tooth form mesio-distally is another matter; here a pronounced bulbous convexity detracts from the result and a flatter form gives a much more desirable outcome. If a marked cingulum is present on the tooth and the overbite is marked an unattractive labial displacement of the tooth results but may be overcome by either timely grinding or placing a shallow palatal restoration. In any event resort to later crowning can often justify allowing space closure in this instance.

Probably the extensive consideration of the case of the lateral incisor is hardly justified on the grounds of the rareness of the traumatic event. However the same deliberation is appropriate in two other anomalies concerning this tooth. The upper lateral incisor is one of the commonest teeth to fail to develop; most often the predecessor in the deciduous dentition has developed and sometimes it is tempting to consider retention of this tooth on a permanent basis. Generally speaking, however, this approach is in long term the most unfavourable. The incongruous small size of the tooth alongside a large central incisor never looks becoming and with additional edge wear this effect is emphasized. Moreover its short root tends to loosen following gingival and bony atrophy and a periodontal abscess is likely in adult life. Again extraction and space retention by means of a partial denture is a possibility as is the hope of complete space closure by mesial movement of the permanent canine. Another exactly analogous situation is the presence of a peg-shaped lateral incisor. Very often this is a small conically shaped tooth with a poorly developed root. Retention of such a tooth should not be advised unless the root is well developed both in terms of length and circumference at the gingival level. In the latter situation the tooth should be retained and later crowned. Otherwise far superior aesthetic results are achieved by making the treatment choices open following early extraction of the traumatized tooth or its deciduous precursor in the event of its absence.

A somewhat analogous aesthetic problem deferred until young adult life is illustrated in Fig. 3.2. The marked diastema between the upper central incisors

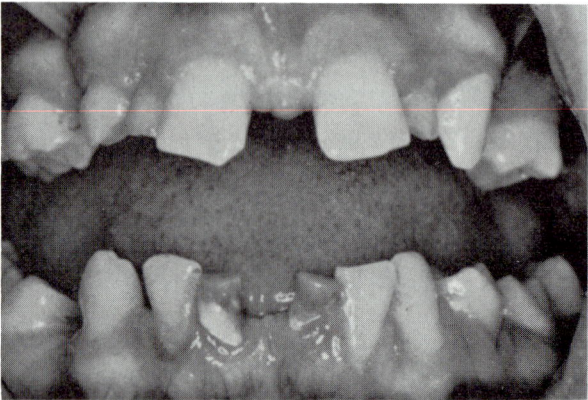

Fig. 3.2. Marked diastema between upper central incisors.

Aims in Partial Denture Construction and a Consideration of Alternatives 25

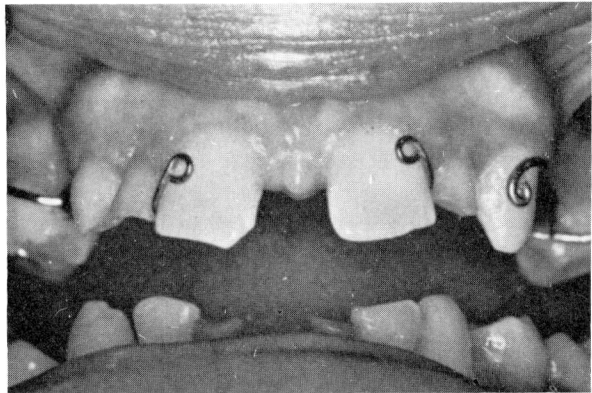

Fig. 3.3. Orthodontic appliance to close the diastema.

presented an unpleasant appearance in a girl aged 15. In addition there was congenital absence of both permanent upper lateral incisors and the right permanent upper canine. Orthodontic treatment with a removable appliance approximated the centrals (Fig. 3.3), after which the retained deciduous teeth were removed and a partial denture provided (Fig. 3.4).

A very different type of case with a quite specific appearance problem particularly amenable to treatment with a partial denture, presents for treatment at two very different ages. The first class of patient, more often a young lady in her late teens or early twenties, presents with an Angle Class II, division one malocclusion. The genesis is that large permanent upper incisor teeth have erupted into a protrusive position and the lower lip in repose, but especially on

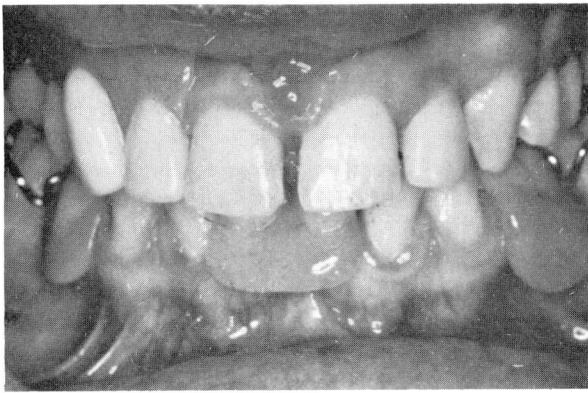

Fig. 3.4. The improved appearance following the combination of orthodontic and prosthetic treatment.

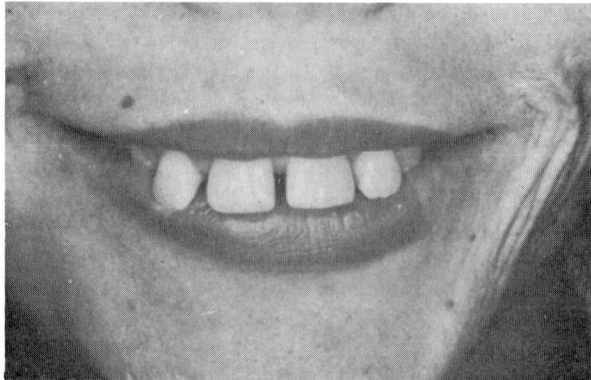

Fig. 3.5. Protrusion of upper incisors.

smiling, comes to be interposed between the opposing incisor teeth; there may or may not be an associated thumb sucking. Rather typically an associated exaggerated mandibular notch is palpable on the lower border of the mandible. Such cases generally respond very favourably to orthodontic treatment with an oral screen about the age of eight. Its effect is to retro-incline the permanent upper incisors while at the same time, through soft tissue drag, to stimulate condylar growth of the mandible and allow its forward development unhampered by the backward pressure from the lower lip now repositioned by the screen and not interposed between the two anterior dentitions. However very many cases do not present for treatment until later in life when the most successful orthodontic treatment can hardly be contemplated. Such a case is illustrated in Fig. 3.5. Following extraction of the offending teeth together with the appropriate degree of bone removal, an immediate Class IV partial upper denture was inserted with the fortunate aesthetic outcome depicted in Fig. 3.6. In this case and very many

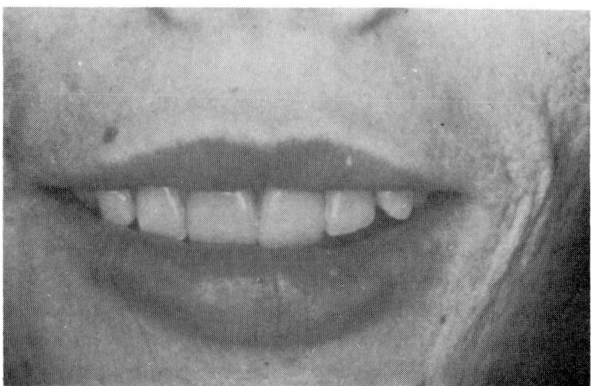

Fig. 3.6. Modified appearance following the insertion of a Class IV denture.

others similarly treated, it has been noted especially in young ladies how, along with their enhanced good looks, their whole outlook on life is elevated.

Another case presenting a similar appearance but in an older age group, generally in the forties or fifties, is well known to all dental practitioners. It is always associated with periodontal disease affecting the upper anterior periodontal status. In such a case there is over-eruption and elongation of the upper anterior teeth and spacing between these teeth becomes conspicuous. Mobility of these teeth can always be demonstrated in some degree. Often the low lip has come to lie behind the incisal edges of the elongated teeth and generates a more continuously acting labialward displacing force where none had acted previously; this provides a particularly noxious stress which results in rapid acceleration of the periodontal breakdown. The elongation of the teeth has, however, primarily resulted in a downward movement of the cingula of the anterior teeth and a traumatic premature occlusion comes to act as the lower incisors impact on jaw closure. The resulting movement of the upper anterior teeth can always be palpated on biting; in advanced cases it can easily be seen. Sometimes prior loss of posterior teeth has permitted closure of the bite with increased loading of the upper anteriors. Such a case is illustrated in Fig. 3.7. The treatment plan depends on the degree of periodontal involvement. In extreme cases, especially as assessed by tooth mobility, extraction and the construction of a complete upper denture can be the only reasonable treatment. When teeth have reached a certain degree of mobility (and this judgement can be learned only by clinical experience and not by description) it is futile to persist in attempts to retain the teeth. Too often the inexperienced dentist, especially when pressed by a not too intelligent patient, is tempted to conserve the situation; needless to say the outcome is satisfactory to neither patient nor dentist. Where the periodontal condition is less

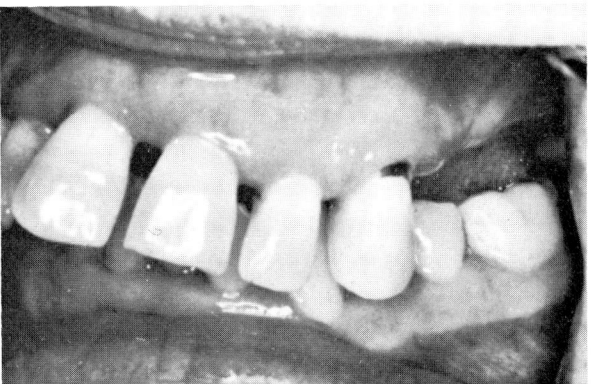

Fig. 3.7. Over-closure and protrusion of the mandible following the loss of the upper posterior teeth. The periodontally affected upper anterior teeth will not resist the resultant overloading.

severe conservative therapy should be embarked upon with the provision of a partial denture contributing in the overall treatment. Such a denture should in the first place aim to restore the posterior occlusal height if there has been overclosure due to the prior loss of the posterior teeth; it is necessary to motivate the patient sufficiently to master the use of the appliance as it presents a particularly difficult accommodative period. It is also imperative to appreciate that grinding of the anterior teeth is an essential adjuvant treatment. Grinding of the incisal edges should be extreme, so that the traumatic action of the lower lip behind the incisal edges is removed. As a rule such grinding greatly enhances the appearance and the patient will often comment gratefully on the fact that he or she looks much more youthful. Grinding of the cingula should also be effected. Early cases treated in this way often respond very favourably with considerable improvement in the periodontal condition of the anterior teeth.

Much less frequently a similar type of case is encountered in a patient in the same age group. This is characterized by loss of posterior teeth but here the periodontal status remains excellent and is often associated with considerable incisor abrasion (Fig. 3.8). With ageing the mandibular core straightens but the overbite mitigates against forward displacement of the mandible. In such cases there may be a resultant backwards, or backwards and upwards, displacement of the head of the mandibular condyle with a chronic traumatic arthrosis. Here successful treatment includes the provision of a partial denture.

Still considering the issue of appearance there can be little doubt that dental caries of the anterior teeth, particularly the uppers, may have a most unfortunate outcome. However the treatment position has radically changed since this textbook was first written in the mid fifties. Then the writers were regularly called upon to restore appearance by extracting grossly carious anterior teeth and replacing them with the relatively new immediate partial denture. This would be

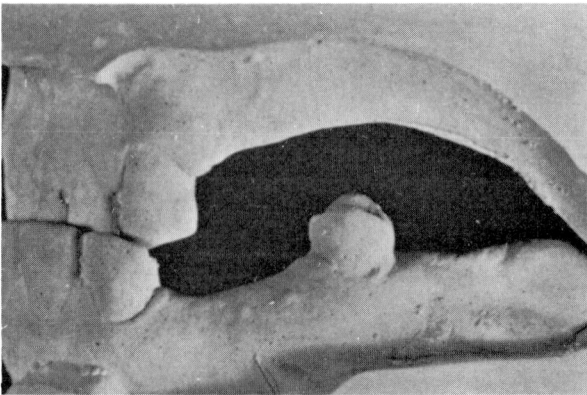

Fig. 3.8. Loss of posterior teeth, but the periodontal condition of the anterior teeth is good. Backward displacement of the mandible may occur.

a rare event today and the reasons for this are many. Socially speaking far greater stock is now placed on appearance than formerly. This is true of dress, deportment and features. The part a handsome smile contributes to good appearance is widely recognized and the way it is used is not lost on a conditioned public. Moreover, the condition and position of the upper anterior teeth is the central feature of a good smile. The presence of dental caries detracts largely from appearance but there is the added social stigma that unattended decay connotes unacceptable lack of concern with personal cleanliness and hygiene. It should, however, be recorded that whereas there have been advances in the field of dental materials, a first class aesthetic anterior restorative material has not yet been found. In many materials the coefficient of thermal contraction and expansion permits edge imbibition and results in a dark tell-tale marginal stain. Surface hardness is often such as to permit abrasion and staining in microscopic defects. Abrasion resistance of too low an order allows surface loss of filling material and loss of tooth contour. So even the well restored anterior region may well come to be aesthetically unacceptable. Fortunately the methods of crowning have greatly improved in the last two decades. Ceramics are stronger, greatly more life-like and can now be bonded to gold. It must be said that crowning of the upper anterior teeth is always a superior method to extraction and using a partial denture. Further the confidence with which endodontic treatment and apicectomy can justifiably be approached warrants the conclusion that partial dentures should only rarely have to be used to treat the aesthetic ravages of dental caries. The use of partial dentures in this area is most likely to have application in cases where there has been fracture of either root or post in failure of an existing crown.

An illustrative case depicted in Fig. 3.9 shows marked carious destruction of upper anterior incisors. It was decided that the best aesthetic result could be obtained in this case by providing porcelain jacket crowns (Fig. 3.10). However

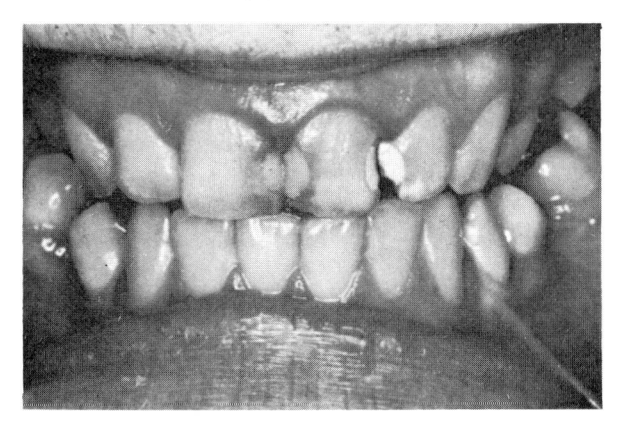

Fig. 3.9. Carious destruction of upper anterior teeth.

30   *Chapter 3*

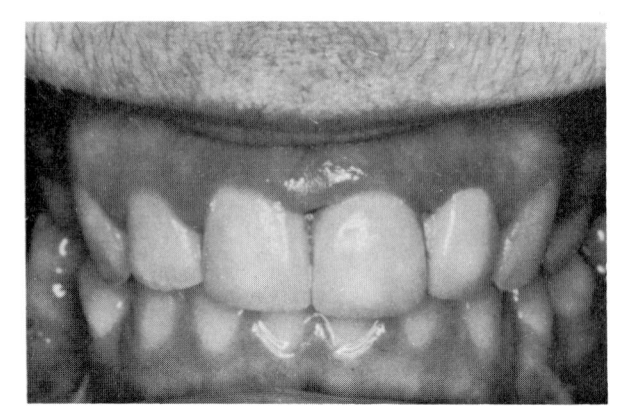

Fig. 3.10. Restoration by porcelain jacket crowns.

the posterior occlusion had been depleted previously and to avoid excess loading on the crowns which might have caused their fracture a partial upper denture was fitted to increase the potential masticatory efficiency of the posterior occlusion (Fig. 3.11).

Occasionally the aesthetic problem concerns the facial contour rather than the individual tooth. An example of such a condition is depicted in Fig. 3.12, where the loss of posterior teeth has resulted in overclosure of the occlusion accompanied by protrusion of the mandible (Fig. 3.13). Restoration of the posterior occlusion using partial upper and lower dentures corrects the inferior protrusion, restores normal face height and improves the appearance considerably (Fig. 3.14 & 3.15).

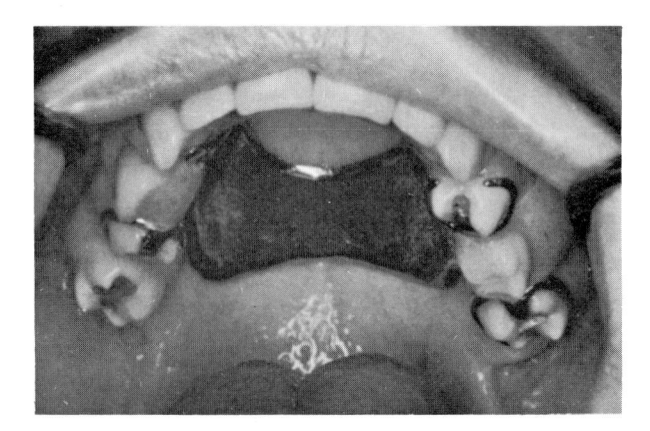

Fig. 3.11. Partial upper denture to complete the occlusal restoration.

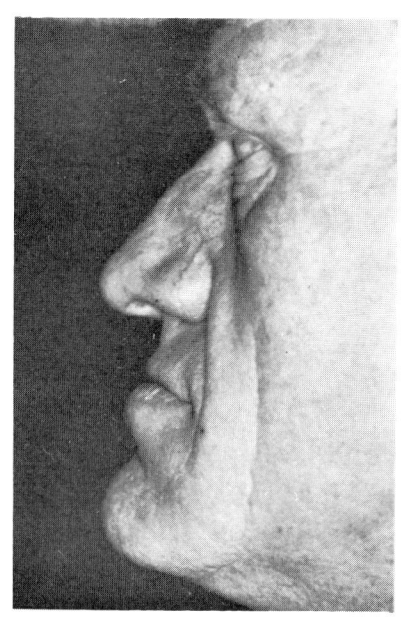

Fig. 3.12. Appearance following loss of posterior teeth.

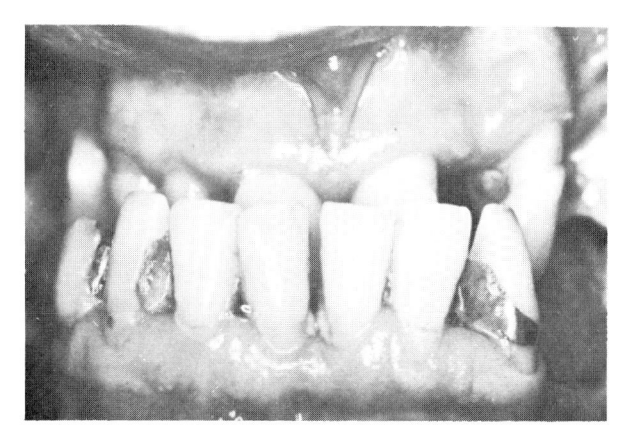

Fig. 3.13. Over-closure following loss of posterior teeth.

The Necessity to Maintain Healthy Oral Tissues

The teeth and their supporting structures, the oral mucosa, the temporomandibular joints and the muscles of mastication comprise the integrated masticatory apparatus. Loss of teeth and consequent occlusal derangement may

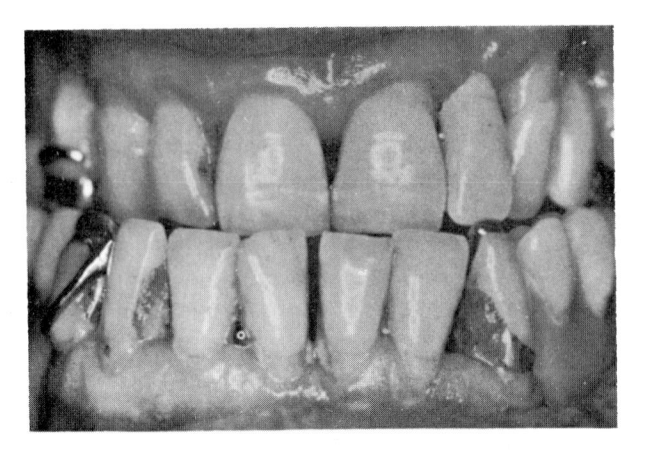

Fig. 3.14. Occlusion restored by partial dentures.

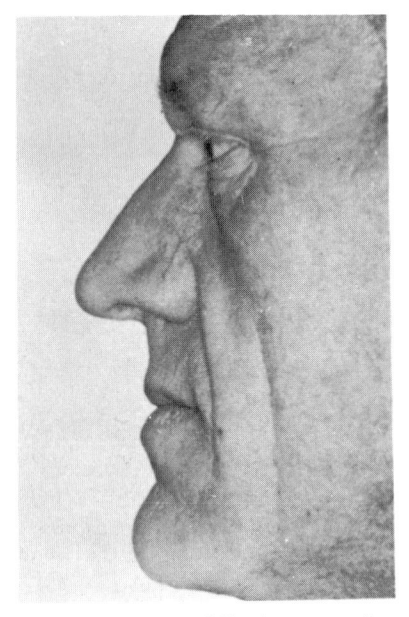

Fig. 3.15. Improved appearance following restoration of face height.

have deleterious effects on some or all of those components. The provision of a partial denture may do much to minimize retrograde and pathological changes in the oral structures, but because of the frequency of implication and the seriousness of the outcome, our main concern must be with the status of the periodontium.

Modern trends in partial denture concepts have tended to reduce a consideration of biological concepts and to overemphasize the importance of a mechanical analysis of the problem. Mechanical concepts of occlusion especially have relevance, but generally speaking changed occlusal form results from a change in biological status and is advantageously or deleteriously effective through biological reaction.

Central to the clinical problem is the aetiology of periodontal disease and partial denture prosthetics should, in considerable measure, be considered as a treatment method appropriately directed against this disease, rarely in preventive, often in therapeutic context.

Although at this stage it is not proposed to go into a deep analysis of the rather complex issues involved in the aetiology of periodontal disease, it is necessary to indicate trends of thought away from the rather too simple hypothesis that accumulation of dental plaque results in a gingivitis which extends deeply to involve the periodontal membrane and alveolar bone. That inflammation has a role in the aetiology of periodontal disease is not questioned. There can be little doubt that it contributes as one factor in an aetiological concatenation of pathological events important amongst which is degeneration or atrophy caused by a depleting circulation.

Loss of alveolar ridge volume is evident enough in the edentulous jaw, but this parameter is active in adult life even in the fully dentate state. As a result changes in tooth position give rise to traumatic occlusion which imposes a pathological stressor on the periodontium and more unusually on the temporomandibular joint.

Previously the accepted viewpoint was that tooth movement should be prevented to obviate the periodontal or joint insult imposed by the traumatic occlusion which would follow. However it is now appreciated that where tooth movement is associated with abrasion of the calcified tooth tissues, a compensatory mechanism operates which safeguards periodontal health. There are still a large number of cases where it is desirable and even essential to construct partial dentures, especially with a view to effecting a wide distribution of the occlusal load with the edentulous ridge sharing in this. It must, however, be appreciated that the partial denture should be constructed for a dental arch where controlled tooth movement has taken place after judicious grinding of the teeth. It is now felt that the earlier concept of preventing tooth movement by constructing partial dentures is ill-advised therapy as it perpetuates an ever augmenting demand on a failing blood circulation.

As long as the simple concept of periodontal disease being exclusively an extending inflammatory process held sway, the logically deduced corollary was that after the inflammation had been resolved and partial dentures constructed the pertaining healthy status would be perpetuated indefinitely given good oral hygiene. However as soon as atrophy is also implicated this situation is called to question and the need to compensate for further change rationalized.

It will become apparent when a detailed consideration of the aetiology of periodontal disease is considered that loss of bone interdentally and disintegration of the intact marginal ligament of the periodontium in this situation has several pathological sequelae, amongst which is significantly increased tooth mobility. It may even be that this is the single most important factor in facilitating the damaging action of the inflammation in periodontal disease. There are then rational grounds for splinting action, which may be regarded as replacing the interdental component of the composite marginal ligament with a supragingival metal connecter between adjacent teeth. Such a splinting action may be accomplished by appropriately designing a cast metal partial denture or by fixed bridgework. It is necessary to stress that bridgework is more effective, but is not so amenable to alteration under later tendancies for the teeth to move.

It remains to add that teeth are lost through caries and trauma before the onset of periodontal disease. Tooth movements follow extraction thus occasioned but the degree of movement is more restricted both immediately and following a period where there is adjustment for an overcrowded arch; a stable arch form results and is perpetrated on a long term basis. Here partial dentures may be constructed to increase the occlusal table and thus help mastication, and also to share the occlusal load between standing teeth and edentulous ridge. Such a denture too may provide a stimulatory occlusal contact with teeth on the opposing jaw and result in a beneficial hyperaemia of their periodontia.

The foregoing is a very general statement, which at this stage may well appear paradoxical. However forbearance is requested and some enlightenment will follow when the chapter on periodontal disease is studied; some paradox will, however, remain for atrophy unlike inflammation is a process which cannot be successfully treated although some of its effects can be mitigated.

Although not strictly a measure that can be said to be aimed at preserving the health of the oral tissues, the provision of partial dentures as a purely transitional treatment between the dentate state and total edentulousness, should be mentioned.

Many patients, particularly those in the older age groups, will find adapting to complete dentures a difficult and trying experience, especially so if they have never worn partial dentures. There are obvious advantages in ensuring that the patient is 'broken in' to denture wearing with partial dentures before trying to cope with complete dentures. Certainly it is undesirable to encourage the attitude that partial dentures inevitably lead to complete dentures; most partial dentures will be supplied with the expectancy that they will be worn for a long period before the remaining natural teeth are lost. However, when the prognosis for what natural teeth remain is undoubtedly poor, partial dentures may be provided merely to give the patient some experience of denture wearing in circumstances more favourable for stability and retention than in the edentulous state, with the hope that the acquired tolerance of these partial dentures will be beneficial when complete dentures become necessary. This principle is particularly applicable to the lower jaw.

The Possible Harmful Effects of Partial Dentures

The previous discussion has attempted to show some ways in which partial dentures may assist in preserving the health of the oral tissues. However, the good that they do must also be weighed against their harmful effects. In good partial denture work these can be minimized and hopefully controlled; however they can never be eradicated. No matter how carefully a partial denture may have been designed and constructed, it still remains a foreign body within the mouth and hence may cause damage to, (a) the remaining natural teeth, (b) the gingival and supporting structures of the teeth, (c) the oral mucosa, and (d) the alveolar bone.

The components of well-designed partial dentures should come into close physical contact with the standing teeth in order to distribute vertical and horizontal loads according to a preconceived plan. However coverage of mucosa, gingivae and teeth always increases the risk of inflammation of the soft tissues. The physiological action of the mucous barrier is always impaired when tissues are covered and accordingly bacteria, especially those living in the dental plaque, are not removed from the area of the gingival margin by the steady passage of mucus film as it courses backward to the fauces. Additionally the gingival fluid is not removed as it is extruded from the gingival crevice and becomes entirely available as a copious substrate source to the plaque bacteria. Plaque is therefore found in substantially increased amounts where it is covered by a component part of a partial denture. The need for more regular and more thorough oral hygiene measures is accordingly very obvious. But these are very often neither instituted nor promulgated. Coverage alone acts in this way but often this action is augmented by movement of the denture over the mucosa and gingivae. Obviously in a well constructed and well maintained denture this action should be restricted but it is never completely eliminated. Especially where the soft tissues are forcibly exposed to the action of a rough surface small, traumatic, epithelial lesions are regularly imposed; pathogenic bacteria are present and allowed a portal of entry with the result that the whole oral mucosa may become very inflamed. In this event what started as a gingival transudate of very modest volume has become a copious exudate deriving from gingival trough and mucosa alike. In this circumstance a substantial substrate containing high levels of blood sugar and free amino acids is available to the plaque acidogenic streptococci and caries is very liable to result. The clinical picture of denture caries is quite different to smooth surface caries commonly seen in the absence of an oral appliance. The lesion is much more extensive and is absolutely confined to the enamel and cementum which underly the denture. There is no local focal point in this initial decalcification; it is widely spread and rather slower in its penetrative action. The most extreme disease picture is seen where poor oral hygiene is associated with persistently wearing the partial denture when asleep; there is then no respite when the mucous barrier may return to physiological working over a protracted period. Even under these adverse circumstances the incidence of enamel caries is less than might have been anticipated; however with gingival recession in adult life the incidence of cemental caries is high. When partial dentures are required in childhood or adolescence strict attention must be paid to oral hygiene and very frequent examinations carried out; otherwise rampant caries may occur.

It was indicated above that a gingivitis and even a stomatitis were anticipated sequelae where poor oral hygiene and partial denture wearing co-existed. However the type of gingivitis encountered is often of a chronic confined type with little complicating oedema. Such a gingivitis may persist for many years without deep extension into a periodontal disease. However when periodontal disease is initially present the presence of inflamed tissues certainly enhances the rate of progress of the periodontal lesion. This seeming anomaly will be considered in a later chapter when the aetiology of periodontal disease is considered. In badly designed and ill maintained partial dentures rather than reducing the imposed load on an individual periodontally diseased tooth, the applied force may actually be increased and cause substantial tooth movement, a condition calculated to increase the rate of periodontal breakdown hugely.

The mucosa covering the edentulous ridges and hard palate is liable to retrograde change in partial denture wearers. Lytle has shown that lower free-end saddle dentures that were incorrectly designed in relation to extension, support or occlusion could cause gross displacement of the underlying soft tissues. Chronic denture hyperplasia, seen typically where a sharp denture margin impacts against moving tissue in the sulcar reflection, is less common with partial than with full dentures but may occasionally occur.

Alveolar bone reacts unfavourably to excessive pressure and resorbs, leading to sinking of mucosa supported saddles, instability of dentures and derangement of occlusion. The bone underlying free-end saddles in the lower jaw is particularly liable to resorption during the first few months of denture wearing and close observation must be maintained during this critical period. The effect is however, seen at its worst under a free-end anterior upper saddle especially where porcelain teeth have been used. Here the size of the alveolar process is greatly reduced and it becomes entirely fibrous and mobile; there is usually associated mucosal inflammation and flattening of the palatal rugae. Denture movement is marked, often leading to fracture of the appliance and a higher incidence of periodontal disease in clasped teeth. Such a condition presents a very considerable complication when the complete denture required sooner, rather than later, comes to be constructed.

The Influence of Personal Factors in Partial Denture Prognosis

It should be appreciated that the success or failure with dentures depends on many factors other than a careful and thorough clinical examination and diagnosis. Important as these are, before decisions regarding treatment plans are made the personality of the patient must be considered. Such factors as the patient's attitude to, and standard of, oral hygiene, the incentive to wear and look after a denture, the general health of the individual and their economic circumstances, must all be taken into consideration.

The development of a happy dentist–patient relationship will enable information on these significant factors to be obtained more readily.

Oral hygiene

When partial dentures are supplied to a person whose oral hygiene standards are poor the prognosis is extremely bad. In fact it can be said that there is no quicker way of ensuring that the person is rendered edentulous rapidly. It has already been stated that gingival coverage is likely to produce a degree of inflammation. This fact combined with poor oral hygiene is significant in the initiation of periodontal disease.

Gingival coverage, to some extent, is unavoidable, but is undesirable since it interferes with the physiological action of the mucous barrier and limits the natural cleansing action of the tongue. When the gingivae are covered by a partial denture that is entirely mucosa borne and is not regularly rebased then the effect can be particularly pernicious, especially in the lower jaw. Poor oral hygiene associated with these circumstances leads to a rapid deterioration in the periodontal condition.

It is likely that the initial lesion takes place in the vulnerable gingivae, but the inflammation spreads by continuity of mucous membrane over the whole of the covered mucosa. In severe cases this becomes dark red and oedematous, showing here and there small haemorrhagic points. Occasionally, too, small areas of leukoplakia develop on top of this gross picture. Always in these worst reactions there is proliferation of the underlying fibrous tissues and obliteration of the rugae, especially where pressure is heavy. This condition is not calculated to ease the task of the dentist who will be required to construct full dentures, at a date that is certainly going to be earlier than if the condition were left as it existed.

Even when partial dentures of the most hygienic design are supplied it is essential that the patient's standards of oral hygiene are of the highest. In fact, it is likely that they need to be even higher than they were prior to the fitting of the dentures if oral health is to be maintained.

A four-year follow-up study of patients wearing partial dentures, carried out by Carlsson *et al.*, verified the close correlation existing between oral hygiene and the presence of caries and periodontal disease. They concluded that 'the success of partial denture treatment would therefore seem to depend to a considerable extent on the patient's co-operation and regular and efficient oral hygiene'. It is reasonable to recommend that whenever the patient's standards of oral hygiene are suspect the condition is better left untreated by partial dentures.

Incentive

In the first few weeks following the insertion of partial dentures, the patient experiences some degree of inconvenience. This period is critical, since often the patient may be unprepared to persevere, and the dentures are relegated in the first instance to a convenient pocket or handbag, and finally to an inconspicuous place in a drawer at home. It is thus most important to judge whether the patient will make the necessary initial effort to overcome the inconvenience of wearing partial dentures for the first time.

The vanity of man is such that even the most badly designed dentures are worn when appearance is restored. When however, a restoration replaces posterior teeth only, the need for continuing to wear the appliance is not so obvious. In such a case the dentist must estimate whether or not he can so present the case for wearing the denture that the patient will find the necessary incentive to overcome the initial inconvenience.

The general disposition of the patient must also be considered when assessing the amount of incentive that will be required. Although it is many years since House classified the mental attitude of denture patients into the following four classes, his observations are still most practical and simple.

(i) *The philosophical mind.* This patient is generally phlegmatic in type, busy and able in his work, confident in the ability of the dentist who is treating him, and co-operative in overcoming difficulties which are never magnified; these are blamed rather upon himself than upon the workmanship of his practitioner.

(ii) *The exacting mind.* This patient is fussy in his work, in his relationship with other people, and about his dress. He demands perfection of service and tends to magnify difficulties. However, when satisfied such a patient is genuinely appreciative and acknowledges the skilled attention which has been given.

De Van described the above two classes as 'practice builders', but has rightly labelled House's remaining groups as 'practice destroyers'.

(iii) *The hysterical mind.* This patient is nervous in his disposition and mannerisms, generally relatively ineffective in his undertakings, difficult to reason with, and typified by an unco-operative attitude. In this case a great deal depends on the personality of the dentist and his ability to instil into his patient the necessary drive to persevere; 'when you can get them to admit they *can* and *will* wear them, half the battle is won'. In most cases success is only relative, the patient always tending to complain and to find fault with good work.

(iv) *The indifferent mind.* These patients often belong to an older age group, and are quite content to carry on without dentures. Their masticatory ability is adequate and they are not concerned about their appearance. Generally they do not come to the dentist of their own volition, but are driven by concerned relatives. The soundest approach to such a patient is to realize that dentures are not required, and not to be tempted to undertake to make appliances which will never be worn.

Nor is the problem a simple one when the type of appliance is considered. There can be little doubt that the simple mucosa-borne denture, whatever its faults in other directions, is the one that is most readily tolerated. At the other extreme, complex skeleton dentures, particularly those incorporating a continuous clasp, are notoriously difficult to tolerate.

In conclusion, the operator must decide, if, with suitable presentation of the case for wearing the denture, a high enough incentive exists in the patient for the proposed line of treatment; it is the personality of the operator versus that of the patient.

General health

When the general health of a patient is poor the dentist may be confronted with a problem in treatment planning which includes partial dentures. In a number of conditions of chronic ill health it is an essential part of the medical treatment that the patient has an efficient masticatory mechanism. Hence the dentist is frequently asked to provide partial dentures as a contribution to this end. When designing dentures for these patients it should be borne in mind that they will be less concerned with appearance than with function. Further, simple designs should be used since the level of tolerance will be low.

Female patients at the menopause or post-menopausal period often present difficult prosthetic problems. Complaints of discomfort, inability to tolerate dentures, burning or tingling sensations in the tongue or oral mucosa, are not uncommon at this difficult time of life. Certainly these persons may suffer from a desquamation of the oral epithelium and hence be unhappy with any appliance that covers the easily traumatized mucosa. However, many of the complaints will be directly unrelated to the dentures and will be manifestations of the general state. So far as it is practical it is undesirable to change the dental status of women during this period. Certainly it is always advisable to carry out temporizing treatment to avoid rendering such patients partially or totally edentulous at this time.

Economic status

Economic factors must, in many cases, discount the possibility of the ideal treatment. It is impossible, for example, to construct metal dentures for all those who would appreciate them. Although the line of treatment is often restricted, lack of money should never be made an excuse for falling below minimal standards. The ideal type of restoration should first be described to the patient, together with some illustrative material if this is possible. Obviously, the conception of what is the ideal will vary according to the experience and skill of the dentist, but a standard of treatment which can only be achieved by referring the patient to a specialist must occasionally be considered. It is only by telling patients of dentistry's highest potentials that increasingly discriminating demands will be made by them.

References

CARLSSON G.E., HEDEGARD B. and KOIVUMAA K.K. (1962) Studies in partial denture prosthesis. *Acta Odont. Scand.* **20**, 95.

DE VAN M.M. (1925) Prognosis in denture construction. *J. Amer. dent. Ass.* **12**, 960.

FARRELL J.H. (1956) The effects of mastication upon digestion. *Brit. dent. J.* **100**, 149.

FARRELL J.H. (1957) Partial dentures and the restoration of masticatory efficiency. *Dent. Pract.* **7**, 375.

LYTLE R.B. (1962) Soft tissue displacement beneath removable partial and complete dentures. *J. pros. Dent.* **12**, 34.

OSBORNE J., BRILL N. and HEDEGARD B. (1966) The nature of prosthetic dentistry. *Int. dent. J.* **16**, 509.

4

PHYSIOLOGY AND PATHOLOGY OF OCCLUSION

Historical Introduction

The earliest studies of the occlusion of the teeth were conducted by persons interested in either orthodontics or prosthetics. From the orthodontic aspect Angle formulated what was regarded as an ideal form of arch arrangement and an ideal inter-arch relationship, with two broad classifications of variation from this ideal. Prosthetic investigators were concerned mainly with the problem of restoring occlusion with complete dentures and in developing articulators which, it was hoped, would reproduce mandibular movements in the laboratory. It appears that there was insufficient concern with physiological functioning of the occlusion, be it natural or artificial, and too much concern with mechanical concepts.

By the middle of this century many workers, amongst whom may be mentioned Posselt, Thompson, Sicher, Schuyler, and others, realized that an understanding of occlusion must be based, not only upon knowledge of the anatomy involved, but upon physiology. The concept of a stomatognathic system comprising muscles, joints and teeth, became accepted and attention was given to study of the relevant neuro-anatomy and neurophysiology.

The modern trend is to substitute the neuromuscular mechanism for a purely local concept of muscular action, and to emphasize the overriding importance of control by the central nervous system over the stomatognathic system. This concept focuses attention on the physiology of the central nervous system and that field of psychology concerned with learning. In both these branches of science the critical student is immediately faced with the all too apparent gaps in our knowledge.

Basic Mandibular Positions

Although the most important consideration in a study of occlusion must be the functional movements of the mandible, it is first necessary to consider its basic positions, as their definition is of help in describing the more important functional movements. The head may be regarded as having three planes of refer-

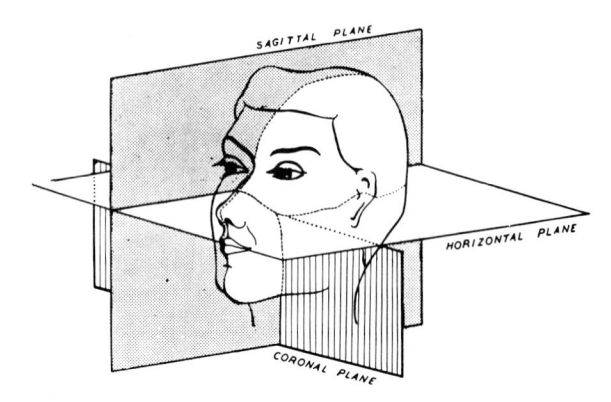

Fig. 4.1. The saggital, coronal and horizontal planes of reference.

Basic vertical positions of the mandible in the sagittal plane

Table 4.1. Nomenclature

Nomenclature of position	Synonyms used in dental literature	Definition
Rest position	Postural position	That vertical postural position of the mandible governed by muscle tonus
	Endogenous postural position	
Tooth position	Maximally intercuspidated position	That vertical and horizontal position of the mandible in which the cusps of the mandibular and maxillary teeth intercuspidate maximally
	Maximally interdigitated position	
	Cuspal position	
	Centric position	

ence; sagittal, coronal, and horizontal (Fig. 4.1). Viewed in the sagittal plane the mandible has vertical and horizontal axes of reference.

The most important vertical position of the mandible is the *rest position* (Fig. 4.2). This position is considered to have a constancy which makes it a reproducible position of reference. Thompson and Brodie stated that this constancy of the rest position was maintained by the tonus in a ring of muscles comprising the post-vertebral, masticatory, supra- and infra-hyoid groups. Ballard has stressed the limitations of this explanation and has suggested that the rest position is an 'endogenous postural position' dependent on an innate central nervous mechanism. Certainly the constancy of the rest position finds a simple physiological explanation in terms of the stretch reflex, which depends on the presence of a monosynaptic arc, demonstrated by Szentágothai and described later in this chapter. If the masticatory muscles are stretched, a contraction is reflexly induced to re-establish the *status quo.*

However, the constancy of the rest position is not strictly true, since there are variables affecting its position on both a long- and short-term basis.

The short-term variables act throughout the day and include such factors as posture, respiration, and stress. If the head of a relaxed patient is inclined backwards the mandible moves away from the maxilla and the free-way space or interocclusal clearance is increased; the reverse effect is noted when the head is bent forwards (Javois and Mullin). During inspiration there is a small increase of the interocclusal clearance but its magnitude is of no practical importance. In stress situations the free-way space may be obliterated by the teeth coming into occlusion. From a practical viewpoint these variables indicate that the recording of the rest position should be carried out on a relaxed patient, whose head is held vertically.

The long-term variables are seen in the edentulous patient when the rest position of the mandible approximates more closely towards the maxilla. Atwood accounts for this on the grounds that the afferent proprioceptive stimuli which result in efferent opening impulses and are carried in nerve fibres arising from the periodontal membrane and gingivae are lost when all the teeth are removed, and their lack is reflected in an increased tonus of the mandibular elevators. It has been shown by Jarabak that people who have worn dentures with an excessive freeway space show some activity in the temporalis muscles when at rest; this is in contrast to patients with a normal free-way space when there is no muscular activity when at rest.

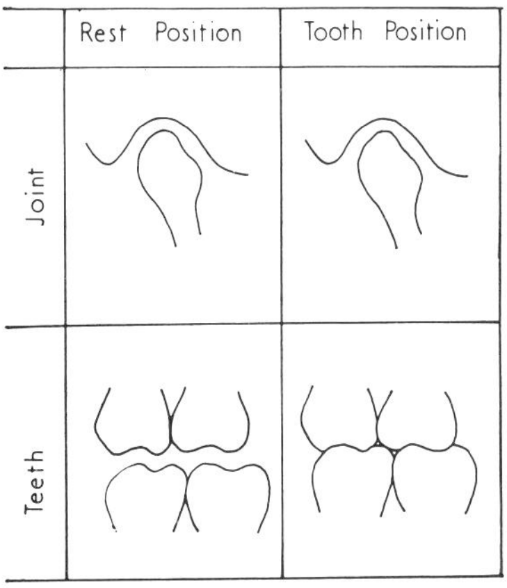

Fig. 4.2. Diagrammatic representation of joint and tooth relationships in the two basic vertical positions of the mandible.

It is generally considered that most older patients show a change in the rest position coincident with their general age atrophy, the mandible moving closer to the maxilla. In these older patients this is an irreversible change and attempts must not be made to revert to the original position by means of dentures with increased vertical dimension. Younger edentulous patients, although they may exhibit temporarily a changed rest position, can be restored to their original position.

The second basic vertical position of the mandible is the *tooth position* (Fig. 4.2). The authors consider that this term describes this position as defined in the table, better than either 'maximally intercuspidated' or 'maximally interdigitated position', since the curved form of the occlusal surfaces of the teeth in a dentition showing marked attrition still demarcates the horizontal jaw relationship although the cusps have been lost.

The nature of the movement of the mandible, with reference to the intercondylar axis, from the rest position to the maximally intercuspidated position has been the subject of investigation and dispute. Although earlier work indicated that the movement was a pure hinge rotation, concensus of opinion now favours the view that some small degree of translation of the condyles often takes place and that this is a physiological and not a pathological condition (Nevakari).

Basic horizontal positions of the mandible in the sagittal plane

Three horizontal positions of the mandible will be described, *the ligamentous position, the tooth position,* and *the muscular position* (Fig. 4.3) (Table 4.2).

The *ligamentous* is an *extreme* or *border* position; the mandible cannot be displaced more posteriorly than this position, the limiting factor to further retrusion being the lateral ligaments of the joints. This was shown by Posselt who

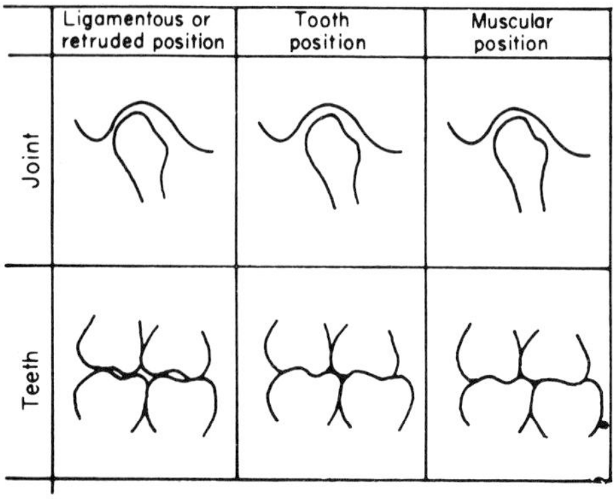

Fig. 4.3. Diagrammatic representation of joint and tooth relationships in the three basic horizontal positions of the mandible.

Table 4.2. Nomenclature

Nomenclature of position	Synonyms used in dental literature	Definition
Ligamentous position	Centric relation	That horizontal position of the mandible when further posterior displacement is restricted by both lateral ligaments of the temporo-mandibular joints
	Centric position	
	Forced retruded position	
	Hinge position	
Muscular position	Centric position	That horizontal contact position of the mandible defined by the reflex muscle pattern acting as the mandible closes from the rest position
Tooth position	Maximally intercuspidated position	That vertical and horizontal position of the mandible in which the cusps of the mandibular and maxillary teeth intercuspidate maximally
	Maximally interdigitated position	
	Cuspal position	
	Centric position	

was not able to retrude the mandible posterior to this position when curare, a muscle relaxant, was administered to a patient; he was, however, able to obtain a more backward displacement in the mandible of a cadaver after sectioning the lateral ligament of the joint capsule. Årstad, and Aprile and Saizar confirm this view, the former drawing attention to superficial vertical and deep oblique layers of fibres in this ligament and attributing the restrictive action to the deeper group of fibres. The mandible may be maximally retruded to this position, either by an active movement of the patient, or passively by the operator pressing on the symphysis menti when the patient is relaxed completely. Provided this relaxed condition is obtained there should be no difficulty in recording this position by means of a wax wafer and it is one which is repeatedly reproducible on account of the permanency of the limiting joint structures. As well as being recordable by a wax wafer this position may be located by the well-known Gothic arch tracing. Posselt has shown conclusively that the most retruded jaw position corresponds with the apex of the Gothic arch.

From this position the jaw may be opened, again either actively by the patient after training or passively by the operator, in such a way that there is no protrusive component to the movement. The jaw will describe a 'hinge movement', the

Chapter 4

condyles providing a 'hinge axis' for the movement which operates through an average opening distance of approximately 20 mm measured at the incisal region (Posselt). Further opening is accompanied by concomitant forward translation of the condyles in the glenoid fossae. The association of the ligamentous position with hinge opening has led to its being referred to alternatively as the hinge position.

Only in a few people does the ligamentous mandibular position coincide with the tooth position. In about 90% of adults the tooth position lies approximately 1 mm anterior to the ligmentous position (Posselt, Donovan). During all the different functional movements carried out by the mandible, only during mastication, and then only for a short time when chewing the hardest food, is this ligamentous position utilized.

The second position is the *tooth position*. It can be recorded by a wax wafer or by simply interdigitating upper and lower casts. However, it is only a basic position of the mandible when opposing posterior teeth are present. Naturally it is absent in the edentulous state. It is a position used recurrently in all categories of jaw movement.

It will be apparent that the ligamentous position of the mandible is defined by the joint ligament and the tooth position by the teeth. The third, or muscular position, is controlled by the musculature.

In the majority of patients with standing cusped teeth present, the *muscular position* is coincident with the tooth position. However, in an appreciable number it is not, and in such cases it may be more anteriorly or more posteriorly placed than the tooth position (Fig. 4.4). Minor lateral deviations between the two positions are also possible. It is postulated that the coincidence of the muscular and the tooth positions constitutes a physiological condition: where these two

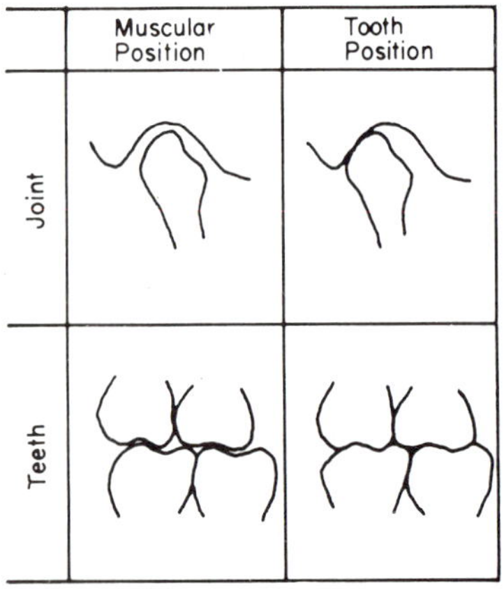

Fig. 4.4. Diagrammatic representation of joint and tooth relationships when the muscular tooth positions do not coincide.

positions do not coincide a pathological, or potentially pathological, condition results. In a very few patients all three mandibular positions—ligamentous, tooth, and muscular—coincide.

In some well co-ordinated patients the muscular position of the mandible can be reproduced with exactness from one day or even week to the next. However, in others it is not so exact and shows a very small variation antero-posteriorly when recorded at the same or successive sessions. There are some patients also in whom the muscular position cannot be demonstrated; this does not mean that it does not exist, but that a relaxed condition cannot be induced in that particular patient by that dentist.

Relevant Neuro-anatomy and Neurophysiology

All muscle movements are initiated by the reception of a nerve impulse at the motor end plate. All these impulses arise in nerve cells in the central nervous system and since they proceed peripherally from the centre they are known as *efferent* impulses. The ways in which the central nerve cells initiate an efferent impulse will be discussed later, but it always takes place with reference to *afferent* impulses of the immediate, or even long standing, past. Afferent impulses arise in receptors or nerve endings, either on an external body surface when they are known as *exteroceptors*, or from an internal receptive area from *interoceptors*. For our present purpose only exteroceptors responsive to touch and light pressure need be considered; nerve impulses resulting from stimulation of these nerve endings are transmitted in nerves of large diameter at high velocities. Of the interoceptors, only the *proprioceptors* require consideration here; these are described by Sherrington as those end organs that are stimulated by 'actions of the body itself'. It is necessary to describe the courses travelled by these different afferent and efferent impulses.

Afferent nerve impulses induced in receptors sensitive to touch, light pressure, and proprioception, are carried in the maxillary and mandibular divisions of the trigeminal ganglion. This ganglion is situated intracranially over the apex of the petrous bone but outside the brain. The impulses continue in the central process of the nerve cell to the pons where a synapse occurs with nerve cells in the main sensory nucleus of the trigeminal. From here processes of these nerve cells cross the mid-line and join the medial lemniscus on its medial aspect. These fibres then ascend through the mid-brain and end in the thalamus; thus representation of touch fibres in the mid-brain can only be indirect. From a final synapse in the thalamus, touch and light pressure impulses are carried in fibres traversing the thalamic radiation, which reach consciousness on the cerebral cortex in the post-central gyrus in its most lateral part. The main sensory nucleus maintains direct connection with the motor nuclei of the same nerve for short reflexes (Jamieson).

Proprioceptive receptors arise in three structures of the stomatognathic system—the capsules of the temporomandibular joints, the masticatory muscles and their tendons and the periodontal membranes of the teeth. Histologically, different structures are responsible for the initiation of these interoceptive impulses in the different tissues, but all are stimulated by change in tension. One pathway taken by impulses originating in these nerve fibres has been described by Corbin and Harrison and by Szentágothai (Fig. 4.5). Impulses again travel in nerves of the second and third divisions of the trigeminal nerve and ascend to the trigeminal ganglion. The nerves pass directly through this ganglion, however, and do not have their cell bodies in it. They enter the pons and ascend some way in the mesencephalic tract of the trigeminal before ending in cell bodies lying around the lateral side of the aqueduct. Collaterals from this mesencephalic root make two connections, the more important being with the adjacent masticatory nucleus of the trigeminal. Motor fibres arising from unipolar cells of this nucleus innervate the muscles of mastication. Some collateral fibres also descend to the nuclei

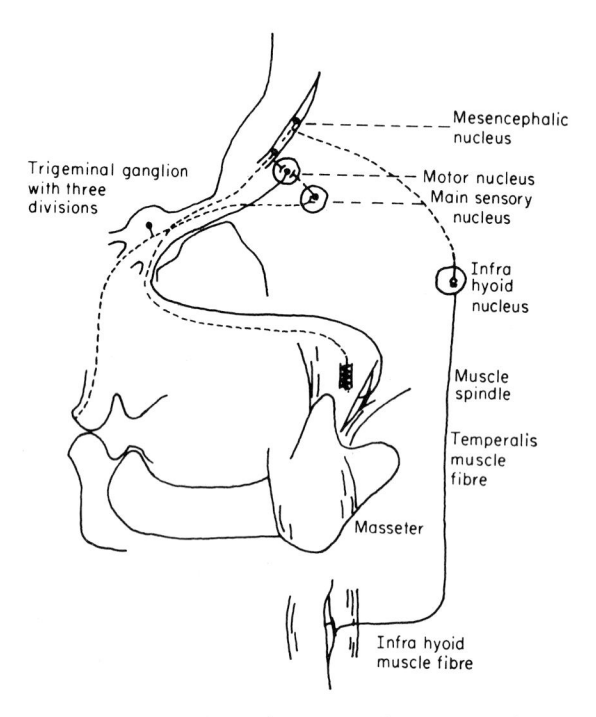

Fig. 4.5. Diagrammatic representation of mono- and bi-synaptic reflex arcs controlling mandibular movements in the new born. Afferent pathways are indicated by broken lines and efferent pathways by solid lines.

of the infrahyoid muscles. It should be noted that the pathway described by Szentágothai forms a simple monosynaptic reflex arc, and an unusual situation exists in that the cell bodies of the nerves lie within the central nervous system. The discovery of the collaterals making connection with the nuclei of the infrahyoid musculature suggests direct inhibition as a feature of this monosynaptic reflex.

As already described some proprioceptive impulses gain cortical representation and, although afferent pathways are not described, connection must exist with the cerebellum.

On the effector, or motor, side impulses arise in the pre-central or motor gyrus of the cerebral cortex in its most lateral part and belong to the pyramidal system. These nerve fibres pass down in the corona radiata to the internal capsule at about the genu. They then pass down through the cerebral peduncles to the pons, where they cross the mid-line and synapse in the masticatory nucleus of the trigeminal. It will be recalled that the proprioceptive fibres made direct contact with this nucleus. The efferent fibres then leave the brain in the motor root of the trigeminal and proceed to end plates on the various masticatory muscles.

The extrapyramidal system is centred in the basal ganglia and is mainly concerned with postural adjustments and automatic movement patterns; in general it may be said to exert an inhibitory effect on movements including those of mastication. The extrapyramidal cortical projection concerned with mastication is situated in Broadman's area 6 of the pre-central gyrus, and nerve fibres from it connect with the globus pallidus, a component of the corpus striatum, one of the basal ganglia which lie between the cerebral cortex and the diencephalon. One of the connections of the globus pallidus is to the masticatory nucleus from whence, as already described, the efferent motor nerves to the muscles of mastication take origin (Fulton).

Although the cerebellum plays no direct part in the initiation of voluntary movements it is concerned with the synergism of the various muscles taking part in a functional movement. An animal deprived of its cerebellum shows no paralysis, but its movements are shaky, jerky, and ill-controlled, this being referred to as cerebellar ataxia. Anatomical pathways for this function as it affects mastication have not been demonstrated but are known to exist since in disease of the cerebellum, ataxic symptoms are seen. Presumably just as the cerebellum acts to synergize muscle actions in movements, it synergizes the same actions at rest to produce the postural tone.

All muscular activity whether reflex, automatic, or purposive depends for its efficiency on a background of tone; this has been succinctly described by Sherrington when he stated that 'All movement begins and ends in tonus'. The resting tonus in a muscle is variable in health and disease (Elliott, Hughes and Turner), and it is suggested that a control of this exists between excitor and suppressor mechanisms. For instance, cerebellar activity causes a hypertonicity, whereas cortical suppressor bands and the globus pallidus through separate mechanisms, when stimulated, cause a hypotonicity. It is well known that tonus is increased by excitement and decreased by apathy.

To summarize (Fig. 4.6), it has been shown that proprioceptive fibres form a monosynaptic arc with the neurones of the masticatory nucleus and direct connection to it exists from the main sensory nucleus of the trigeminal nerve; descending fibres from the cortex (pyramidal system), and basal ganglia (extrapyramidal system), also synapse in this nucleus. Connection with the cerebellum is postulated to account for synergism in masticatory movements.

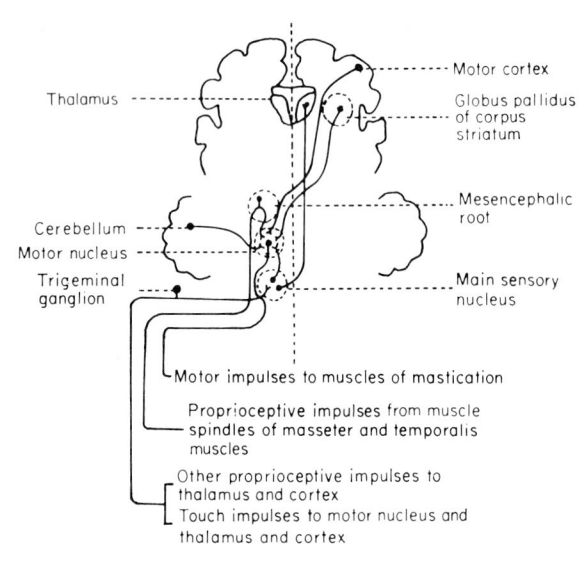

Fig. 4.6. Diagrammatic representation of nerve pathways impinging on the motor nucleus of the trigeminal nerve.

A monosynaptic pathway would appear to be the simplest reflex pathway concerned with the masticatory act. This lies at the mesencephalic level and Sherrington showed that it was an effective circuit when he produced successive opening and closing jaw movements by pressing on the teeth and gingivae of the decerebrate cat. The proprioceptive gingival or periodontal fibres carry the stimulus which is effective in inducing this reflex and jaw opening results. Opening ends and closure is initiated after a certain threshold stimulus has been reached in the proprioceptive receptors of the stretched masticatory muscles. This is a basic mesencephalic reflex and results in a simple open-close movement of the jaw. Another simple afferent pathway is described through the touch receptors and it is probable that this is the circuit effective in producing the familiar sucking reflex before the teeth erupt in the infant (Brain).

Unconditioned reflex actions are characterized by their innate quality and by the fact that they are carried out below the conscious level. Two such unconditioned reflexes are described above, and initiate simple open-close jaw movements in the newly born child, whose very survival depends on such movements. It is difficult to trace these movements but observation suggests that sucking includes simple open-close movements. All joints operating at this level tend to work at the lowest possible equalized internal pressure, a fact which tends to give the movement a constant pattern. *It is suggested that the muscular jaw position already described is positioned on this reflex muscular pathway;* this would account for its lack of absolute precision in some cases and for its presence in the periods both before and after tooth eruption, and when the teeth are lost in later life. Whilst such a surmise is speculative, it would account for the fact that the muscular mandibular position can only be demonstrated in the relaxed state, when cortical effects are removed from active participation. The fact that it is impossible to record this position in some individuals can be accounted for by the fact that they continue to exert cortical activity; this may be due to their resistance to suggestion or the inability of the operator to induce relaxation.

Main act and acquired movement patterns

Man's mind at any one time can be concerned with only one conscious act; Sherrington called this the *main* or *focal act*. For instance, a dentist concerned with judging the position of an incisor tooth cannot, at the same time, be reasoning the correctness of the vertical dimension or be contemplating his prospects on the golf course at the week-end. But so that life may go on, other essential human activities must continue; the reflex act of breathing is an obvious example. However, there is another large group of organized acts which may be described as *acquired* or *automatic patterns:* walking and writing are examples. The conscious mind is not concerned with the act of walking; the dentist may walk away from the patient and still be concerned with the main act of judging the position of the patient's tooth.

Thus an acquired pattern may be regarded as an intermediate act between the main act and the pure reflex. Sherrington suggests that 'the transition from reflex action to volitional is not abrupt and sharp. Familiar instances of individual acquisition of motor co-ordination are furnished by the cases in which short simple movements, whether reflex or not, are by practice under volition combined into new sequences and become in time habitual in the sense that though able to be directed they no longer require concentration of attention upon them for their execution.'

After infancy the process of learning movements depends to a high degree upon an interplay between the cortex and the extra-pyramidal system, which comprises the corpus striatum, nucleus hypothalamicus, nucleus niger, nucleus ruber, and the structurally more loose grey substance of the mesencephalon known as the formatio reticularis grisea, which may be regarded as a widespread field of association (Benninghoff). Initially the learning process is directed by the cortex, where an evaluation of impulses takes place, and this is followed by their co-ordination and concatenation. From the cortex the impulses are conveyed to the extrapyramidal system, where an automization takes place and through this process suitable perfection is conveyed to movements. As the extrapyramidal system takes over the responsibility for the performance of movements, the cortex is relieved of its participation and will only occasionally dominate these acquired patterns.

On eruption of the permanent teeth, change of tooth position, and when dentures are inserted, masticatory patterns are *learned* or *acquired*. At these times mastication is the main act and demands the whole conscious attention of the individual.

When the deciduous teeth erupt the simple jaw movements associated with sucking are replaced by more complex movements which will be described in detail later. At this stage new proprioceptive impulses make their impact on the central nervous system, and conditioned reflexes results in response to these new afferent stimuli. At the same time the motor response is expanded through a myelination of developing neural pathways and a larger range of movements results. Facilitation and inhibition takes place at synapses and modifies the nature of the resulting motor act. These muscle patterns are very stable since they are based on the simple mesencephalic reflex and acquired in infancy when nerve conductivity displays its highest velocity and when synaptic delay is shortest.

Importance has been given to conditioning and brain development in the infant and to cortical action in the more mature person. It must, however, be appreciated that the neurological processes involved are essentially the same. At some developmental stage the new afferent stimuli reach a conscious level and the cerebral cortex becomes the important relay centre; such events as the eruption of the permanent dentition, tooth movement or the acquiring of dentures, result in afferent stimuli being perceived at a cortical level. When, to take two extreme examples, new dentures have been inserted or the preferred masticatory side is changed due to a tender extraction wound, the masticatory act becomes the focal act; this can be established by investigation of the patient by subjective observation and by the study of electromyographs. The facilitation of acceptable movement forms and the inhibition of those less favourable continues until new nervous pathways are developed to propagate the changed masticatory act as a learned pattern. This solidified pattern will then proceed without cortical direction, but at any time it may be immediately directed to conscious control upon the receipt of any unusual sensory impulse, such as biting on a hard object.

The central neural pathways for all these acts can only be speculative. The monosynaptic mesencephalic reflex route of the newly born child can, however, be accepted. The acquisition of more complex movements most certainly involves the myelination of multisynaptic pathways. Whether or not in the developing child the masticatory act is directed at the level of the basal ganglia is uncertain; this is a phylogenetically old part of the brain and its connection with the lower motor neurone is established. The direction of a new pattern during the phase of learning in the adult certainly stems from the motor area of the cortex along the pathway described.

Mandibular Movements

The whole emphasis in a study of mandibular movements must be on *function*. Extreme or border movements are seldom used during function even as short-acting components. Moreover, to reproduce extreme positions during the occlusion of teeth and to assume that straight line paths between these positions resemble function in the mouth, is not necessarily correct. The starting point for an understanding of the occlusal problem is a thorough study and understanding of functional mandibular movements. These may be divided into:
1   Masticatory movements,
2   Swallowing movements,
3   Empty movements.

1   Masticatory movements

The descriptions to be given of the manner in which mastication takes place are based on evidence obtained from the following methods of investigation.

(a) *Direct examination.* Subjective visual observation should not be considered so inferior to objective study as to be of little value, and much can be learned from a critical examination of the manner in which different people eat, especially when independent observations are made by several investigators. Direct examination in the mouth will also reveal the presence of facets on natural teeth, giving an indication of habitual tooth contacts and movement patterns.

(b) *Electromyographic studies.* Much can be learned by the interpretation of myographs obtained when subjects chew different types of food, particularly information regarding the power of muscle contraction and the synchronization of muscle components, and hence the mandibular positions at different stages of mastication.

(c) *Cine-radiological studies.* By this means it is possible to observe the manner in which different types of food bolus are chewed by different types of occlusions, either natural, artificial, or combinations of both. By serial tracings of successive frames of the film, movements of the mandible or the temporomandibular joints may be plotted.

(d) *Gnathosonics.* Interesting information regarding tooth contacts in occlusion can be obtained by recording the sounds of tooth contact graphically (Watt). By this means it is possible to detect the presence of hypercontacts that may be responsible for deviating the mandible from its correct path of closure.

(e) *Examination of the temporo-mandibular joint.* The sequence of jaw movements during mastication has been reconstructed by Murphy as a result of examining pressure areas where the condyle acts under pressure on the surface of the glenoid fossa.

(f) *Miniaturized electronic devices.* Aerospace research has resulted in miniaturization of electronic devices, and Brewer and Hudson, Neill and others have incorporated miniature transmitters in dentures and have been able to record tooth contacts during mastication, working periods, and sleep.

The first important fact to emerge from a correlation of the information made available by all the above methods is that the pattern of mastication varies with the particular type of food being chewed; this applies more to the physical characteristics of the food than the particular article of diet. For instance, fresh raw carrot is harder than raw carrot that has softened on standing whilst after it is cooked it is quite different again. For descriptive purposes food can be divided into three categories:

i   Liquid or semi-solid food,
ii Solid food which is comminuted by heavy masticatory force,
iii Solid food which flows or is comminuted by light masticatory force.

i   Liquid or semi-solid food such as soups or custards are mixed with saliva and prepared for swallowing by the action of the tongue against the hard palate and the teeth are not used. The beneficial stimulus to the supporting tissues of the teeth which results from using the teeth in mastication is lost when this type of food is eaten.

ii The classes of food that call for the greatest masticatory effort are some raw fruits and vegetables, hard breads and fibrous meats. The acts of incising a piece of fresh raw carrot and then masticating it will be described as typical in this class. In incision the mandible is protruded and often swings laterally, and the lower and upper incisors, canines, and sometimes premolars, penetrate the carrot. As the jaws approximate there is some retrusive mandibular movement. Just short of tooth contact the incisive act is halted and with the jaws slightly open a series of intermittent muscular contractions are noted (Jankelson, Hofman, and

Hendron). This stage is accompanied by a fixation of the head, neck, and even shoulders, while the hand executes a twisting motion on the carrot and effects its cleavage. The incised piece is then transferred by the tongue to the molar area of the side preferred for mastication. It is held between the molars by cheek and tongue action and is subjected to a series of a few heavy masticatory strokes which effect a gross comminution. During these strokes, which may be referred to as 'power strokes', Osborne has shown that on the working side there is a distraction of joint surfaces and the whole contractive load of the elevator muscles is concentrated on the bolus. As a result of heavy contraction in the posterior temporalis muscle this initial penetration of the carrot is followed by a retrusive movement of the mandible as further penetration is made. At this stage the mandible is momentarily in the ligamentous position. The condyle is restrained from further retrusive movement by the deeper fibres of the lateral ligament of the joint capsule. Thus the masticatory load is shared at this stage between the joint ligaments and the molar teeth, and with the bolus situated, in part at least, posterior to the anterior edge of the masseter muscle it is placed in the position of greatest mechanical advantage when the joint is considered the fulcrum of the jaw movement.

The first power stroke resembles the incisive act in that there may be a terminal intermittent muscular contraction and there is no inter-occlusal contact. In the succeeding strokes a close approximation of the teeth takes place with the mandibular teeth distal to the position of maximal intercuspidation. Thereafter there is a forward slide to that position and this movement is one in which fibrous structures are broken down. It is this movement which is responsible for the formation of retrusive facets on the posterior teeth. As this forward slide takes place the posterior temporalis fibres have been shown electromyographically to decrease in contractile power. After the gross comminution has been effected by a small number of these power cycles, smaller particles of food track forward and the whole of the molar and premolar occlusal areas take part in mastication, which proceeds until the carrot is reduced to such a state that it can be swallowed. The masticatory stroke at this time takes place in a more anterior position and the joint ceases to be weight bearing. However, a large number of teeth are now accepting the load and accordingly there is a shift of pressure distribution. The stroke at this time becomes more vertical and may or may not have a lateral component.

Many writers have described mandibular movement when viewed in the coronal plane and the cycle that each has described has reference to the second stage of mastication described above. All have observed a cyclic motion in which a straight opening jaw movement is followed by a deviation towards the working side. This is followed by an oblique path of closure the direction of which is directed towards a point a short distance lateral to the tooth position. Jankelson maintains that no actual interocclusal contact takes place before the opening phase of the cycle recurs. If contact does take place the distance of the lateral slide to the tooth position is very small.

Controversy has arisen over whether or not the opposing teeth actually meet in mastication. Jankelson and co-workers maintain that the teeth do not occlude, whereas Yurkstas and Emerson, Anderson and others take the opposite point of view. By the use of miniature radio transmitters incorporated into dentures, Brewer showed that denture teeth contact during chewing, and that the amount and character of the contact varies with the type of patient, the jaw relations, the cusp form, the occlusion and, by no means least, the type of food being eaten.

So far the description has referred to the working side on which mastication is taking place. Two comments will be made concerning the balancing side. First, the amplitude of myographic recordings from the masseter and temporalis muscles suggest that similar degrees of muscular force are developed on both working and balancing sides during closure (Perry). This increases the amount of energy available for breaking down the food, adds precision to positioning the mandible, and protects the ipsilateral joint capsule. Second, Murphy has shown that a pressure area exists on the anterior slope of the glenoid fossa and speculates that this bears the condylar load on the balancing side during that phase of the power closure when the condyle of the working side is being braced both by the lateral ligaments, and by a second pressure area which is situated posteriorly in the articulatory compartment of the fossa. Thus when the working side condyle is retruded, the balancing condyle is anteriorly and slightly medially displaced. Osborne has observed by cine-radiographs that in chewing, the condylar head of the balancing side maintains approximation with the glenoid fossa and that there is no distraction of these opposing surfaces.

This description of the masticatory sequence of incision, power comminution, finer comminution and finally swallowing may be considered a basic sequence since in the mastication of a hard food such as raw carrot all possible phases are demonstrated.

iii   The third group, which regrettably constitutes such a large part of the modern diet, is the softer food. A piece of boiled potato is a good example of a bolus which fragments easily under light load; some fruits also come into this category. Foods which flow rather than fragment come into this class and examples are the softer toffees and candies as well as many foods which are prepared by mincing, e.g. sausage and minced meats of all kinds. These are all masticated in the same way as the harder foods after the latter have been grossly broken down; in other words there is no power stroke and retrusive phase and molar and premolar areas are used immediately.

Thus the masticatory pattern is seen to vary with the type of food being consumed. Only during incision is there any anterior displacement of the mandible from the tooth position. During one phase, when heavy muscular effort is made, there is a posterior displacement. It would therefore seem that from the prosthetic viewpoint of mastication a balanced occlusal contact *posterior* to the tooth position is desirable to ensure denture stability when cusp contact is made in the power strokes.

2 Swallowing movements

Swallowing takes place both at meal times and between meal times, and in both cases two types of swallow can be differentiated; in one the opposing teeth do not make an occlusal contact, whilst in the other they do. When the subject is in repose and a small amount of saliva accumulates in the mouth it is swallowed without any marked muscular effort in a 'teeth open' swallow. However, when the person is talking or is faced with a situation producing sympathetic stimulation, the mouth dries and a forceful 'teeth shut' swallow is used, occlusion occurring in the tooth position. The mandible does not go through any searching activity to find this position; it moves directly into it as would be expected considering it is a perpetually reinforced learned pattern. The purpose of this mandibular fixation is to provide a static origin for the mylohyoid and superior constrictor muscles which make a considerable contractile effort. This 'teeth shut' swallow lubricates the dry oral mucosa more than it removes saliva from the mouth.

During eating, as between meals, swallowing may be of the 'teeth open' or 'teeth shut' variety depending on the viscosity and flow of the bolus as well as its size. The greater the viscosity of a liquid bolus the greater the contractile effort required whereas an easily deformed bolus, or one that flows readily, will necessitate a smaller contraction of the muscles. A bolus such as a ripe pear will be swallowed by the 'teeth open' method but most boli will necessitate the 'teeth shut' swallow and varying degrees of interocclusal force will result. Any large bolus, even if soft or liquid, will require contact of the opposing teeth.

To summarize, in the lubrication swallow and the swallowing of hard and large boli significant interocclusal pressure is developed in the tooth position.

3 Empty movements

Empty movements comprise all occlusions other than those taking place in mastication or swallowing. They are observed in some conditions of mental stress and in some cases of periodontal disease. As distinct from the occlusions of mastication and swallowing which are always intermittent, the occlusions occurring in stress situations may be either intermittent or continuous. Empty movements are characteristically horizontal in nature, whereas those of mastication and swallowing are mainly vertical. They may all be regarded as action patterns, characterized by an overflow of efferent impulses which originate centrally in some particular states of mind. Continuous clenching may be regarded as an abortive action pattern. In order to describe these occlusions it is necessary to differentiate between those occurring during the day and those when the subject is asleep:

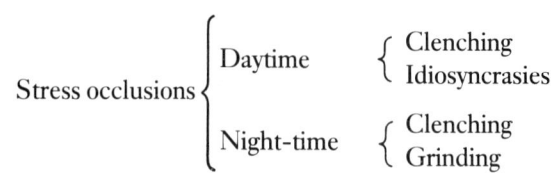

$$\text{Stress occlusions} \begin{cases} \text{Daytime} & \begin{cases} \text{Clenching} \\ \text{Idiosyncrasies} \end{cases} \\ \text{Night-time} & \begin{cases} \text{Clenching} \\ \text{Grinding} \end{cases} \end{cases}$$

Perry, Lammie and Main devised a series of experiments to demonstrate that when subjects were confronted with a stress situation there was considerably increased activity of the masseter muscles but comparatively little concurrent activity in the temporalis muscles. Continuous occlusion was noted in the tooth position, whilst in some subjects there was concomitant increased pulse rate in the carotids. Not all subjects showed stress occlusion and different magnitudes of resultant muscle force were noted: less muscular contraction was observed in the well adapted, plethoric individuals and a high degree was seen in more highly strung persons. It will be appreciated that the mandibular elevators are much stronger muscles than are the depressors, a situation also pertaining in the fingers where the flexor muscles form a stronger group than the extensors. A commonly observed associated stress reaction is clenching of the fist; the fingers nails may dig into the palms of the hand and blanching of the knuckles is often seen. Certainly, in both jaw and palm clenching, excessive stimulation of touch and pressure receptors must be induced, even if actual pain is not perceived. It is felt that clenching is more than a hypertonicity already described as being evident in states of excitement; however, the mechanism by which it takes place is not known. As well as a nervous factor it may be that a hormonal factor is involved. Such an explanation might account for the more gradual onset and increasing contracture noticed in this condition.

Somewhat different from clenching, and taking place in situations characterized by concentration rather than actual stress, are a group of occlusions or articulations peculiar to the individual; they may be referred to as idiosyncrasies. (Idiosyncrasy is used in the sense of 'a habit or quality of body or mind peculiar to any individual' (Dorland).) In these circumstances the occlusion is never in the tooth position, is of short duration, and generally has protrusive and lateral components. For instance, subjects may be observed who grind their canines and incisors when concentrating; biting of the tongue or on the end of a pencil for short periods are similar acts, when, although no occlusion results, certainly interocclusal force is developed. The duration of non-masticatory tooth contacts with full denture wearers has been recorded by Brewer, and varied from 150 per hour in some persons to as much as 1,500 per hour in others.

Stress occlusion is not confined to the daytime; it has been observed at night

Physiology and Pathology of Occlusion

following a day when the subject has been exposed to stress (Bundgaard-Jorgensen). It may even be noted during sleep when the moderating influence of the suppressor band of the cerebrum is reduced. It may be static in the tooth position and may be continued over a period of several hours. Brewer's recordings for full denture wearers indicated that contacts during sleep might vary in total duration from 3 to 15 minutes with one person to 1½ to 2½ hours with another. There is no reason to believe that the duration of contact of natural occlusions is less, and in fact it may well be greater.

Grinding of the teeth at night is also common, and is characterized by varying degrees of protrusive and lateral movement. Judged by the facets produced the lateral displacement of the mandible is marked; certainly it is often much greater than that used in daytime mandibular excursions. Two different mechanisms may cause this type of grinding:
i Initiated peripherally by the discharge of unusual concentrations of proprioceptive impulses.
ii Initiated centrally in a tense emotional state.

i *Peripheral initiation.* If there is disharmony between the muscular and the tooth positions, premature contacts result with high rates of impulse discharge from afferent nerve endings in the traumatized periodontal membrane. Similarly if some external force acts on the mandible causing a deviation from its reflex path of closure and causing the mandibular teeth to contact those of the maxilla eccentrically, then premature contacts are liable to result.

A similar mechanism is probably involved when grinding is associated with periodontal disease (Eschler). When a chronic or sub-acute inflammatory process is present there may be an increased internal pressure within the periodontal membrane of one or more teeth and proprioceptive stimuli result.

ii *Central initiation.* In emotional stress, impulses arise in the hypothalamus and are impressed on the extra-pyramidal system through fibres impacting on the globus pallidus, where efferent grinding impulses are initiated.

Grinding at night may be considered purposive when it results in the wearing away of some small hypercontact. The release of pent-up central nervous energy may also be considered beneficial. On the other hand if the periodontal response is poor and loosening of teeth in premature occlusion results, the outcome will be detrimental. Treatment will be indicated by the aetiology; occlusal grinding, treatment of periodontal disease and sedation have appropriate indications.

The reaction of the supporting structures of the teeth to occlusal loading

Occlusal stresses are resisted by the supporting structures of the teeth, these being the periodontal membrane and the alveolar ridge bone. The stresses are, however, resisted differently in each structure.

The periodontal membrane resists stress because of two physical characteristics. First, its collagenous fibres, which are inserted into both the cementum of the tooth and the lamina dura of the bony alveolar wall, are strained when load is applied to the teeth. The degree of load acceptable physiologically by this element of the periodontal tissue depends on the number and arrangement of the fibres as well as the physical (and hence chemical) characters of the collagen. Second, it has been suggested (Synge) that the extracellular tissue fluid of the periodontal membrane, being substantially enclosed, will not find easy egress into adjoining tissue planes, and consequently any force on the tooth tending to reduce the volume of the fluid will be resisted by a hydraulic action. In periodontal disease both these mechanisms are reduced in their ability to resist load without harmful deformation. In this disease the number of periodontal fibres is reduced, partly as a result of the action of bacterial toxins, and it is also possible that the molecular weight of their constituent collagen molecules is reduced, as it is in some disturbed hormonal conditions such as pregnancy. Also, since the lamina dura is broken down, the tissue fluid has a freer escape route and the hydraulic resistance is lowered. It must be realized that no sharp demarcation can be made between the healthy and the diseased periodontal membrane; the so-called healthy membrane may vary greatly from person to person and also in the same mouth. Genetic inheritance is an important factor in the make up of the periodontal tissue, as also are hormonal imbalances and inadequate vitamin absorption.

Ageing, also, affects the reaction of the periodontal membrane to stress. In youth when anabolic processes are in the ascendancy, high local forces, even with a marked horizontal component due to steep cusps, can be resisted adequately; in these circumstances the potentiality to rebuild damaged tissues is generally sufficient to ensure a healthy state. As age advances repair of the collagen fibres cannot balance the destructive action of the imposed stress; consequently the periodontium begins to fail as an adequate tooth support. Radiographically the periodontal membrane widens, especially towards the gingival margin, and an osteolytic action occurs in the lamina dura of the alveolus. Clinically these changes are evidenced by increased tooth mobility, especially in the direction of the offending stress. It should be remembered that ageing must be viewed from a biological rather than a chronological standpoint; one man of fifty may have a lower biological age than another of forty. Again, in ageing, the hormonal background is of supreme importance.

The most important local factor is use; the periodontal membrane of a tooth which has lost its opponent or is not used in mastication, atrophies, becoming thinner in section and showing sparser fibres. A diseased periodontal membrane shows various grades of breakdown.

The resistance to occlusal load is shared between the periodontal membrane and the supporting bone. In the past more attention has been given to the bone than the periodontal membrane, and certain biological facts regarding its reaction to loading are known. Like the periodontal membrane it is under the influence of genetic, general, and local conditions. The important general conditions are hormonal and dietary, while the local are the degree of usage stimulation and the presence or absence of disease. Alveolar bone which has to resist force normally reacts favourably by laying down extra bony trabeculae. The bone supporting a tooth continually subjected to functional and physiological loading, shows an increased number of coarser trabeculae in its cancellous component, and a thicker compact layer in the lamina dura. When bone reacts to loading in this way it shows a favourable or physiological adaptation.

However, with further increase in load, osteolysis occurs and the reaction becomes unfavourable and pathological. The cancellous bone shows sparse, finely calcified trabeculae and the lamina dura becomes thin. Consequently it is possible to imagine a 'physiological limit' of force beyond which osteolysis and not osteosclerosis takes place. This is not a fixed and finite value for every person but varies from one individual to another and in any one person at different times.

One obvious point regarding occlusal loading requires to be made. The greater the number of teeth resisting the various muscular contractions the less is the pressure falling on any one, and accordingly the better are the chances of its supporting structures reacting favourably.

It is necessary, when considering the occlusal load, to refer to its direction as well as its magnitude. Clinical observation supports the contention that the supporting tissues of the teeth can withstand vertical loading better than horizontal loading. If one reasons purely on the relative numbers of periodontal fibres stressed in horizontal loading as compared to vertical, this observation is readily accounted for. However, from the practical viewpoint, the magnitudes of the horizontal and vertical components are determined by the nature of the muscle patterns during mastication, swallowing, and stress situations; these patterns, and hence the directions of the muscular components of force, are not readily amenable to change. The only possible way of securing more vertical stress is to change the occlusal form, and this may be done by grinding or by onlay appliances or fixed full-mouth reconstructions.

The occlusal load may be either intermittent or continuous. For any particular value of load an intermittent force is more likely to produce a favourable reaction in the supporting tissues, whereas a continuous force will be more likely to result in osteolysis. Although mastication and swallowing are intermittent, some stress occlusions are continuous and claimed by many to be the most damaging.

Pathological Reactions in the Stomatognathic Tissues in Different Occlusal Conditions

It is necessary to discuss the effects of different occlusal conditions upon the different tissues of the stomatognathic system—the muscles, the joints, the teeth, the periodontal membranes and the bony support. The following occlusal conditions must be considered:
1 Normal occlusal formation
2 Lack of balanced occlusion
3 Non-coincidence of the tooth position with the muscular position
4 Loss of posterior occlusal stop.

Normal occlusal formation

Normal occlusal formation refers to a relationship of the teeth to the other components of the stomatognathic system which is in harmony with innate and learned muscle patterns. In no sense does it refer to the morphological characteristics of the teeth and their arrangement into any idealistic arch pattern. Certainly in this group are conditions such as irregular arch arrangements, and missing teeth. Nor does it imply that dental disease is absent; conditions in which both caries and periodontal disease are present are included in this group.

In this occlusal condition the muscles of mastication, the teeth, and the periodontal membrane may be affected by the occlusion.

Possibly as a result of circulatory insufficiency the masticatory muscles of some patients appear to be predisposed to a clonic contracture or spasm. Pain in relation to the joint and restriction of movement occurs on awakening or after keeping the jaw open continuously as during a dental appointment (Schwartz). The onset of symptoms on awakening suggests that a continuous occlusion has been operative during sleep and that metabolites collecting in the muscles have not been adequately removed by the lymphatic and venous drainage; the local accumulation of these products causes the muscle spasm. Especially when this occurs in the external pterygoid muscle unilaterally there is a disturbed occlusion, as the normal pattern of closure is complicated by a lateral mandibular displacement brought about by the continuous pterygoid action. The perpetuation of this situation may result much later in pathological change in the musculature (contracture causing restricted opening) and in the temporomandibular joint (osteo-arthritis).

The result of night time occlusal contacts and grinding may be abrasion of the teeth, which may be beneficial for the following reasons:
1 Small movements of the teeth are compensated, the changed occlusal surface maintaining a form in harmony with the prevailing functional muscle pattern and vice versa.

2   The horizontal component of force acting on the periodontal membranes is reduced in magnitude.

Even abrasion resulting in loss of enamel and dentine cannot be considered unusual. Only failure of the pulp to lay down secondary dentine can be considered a deleterious outcome.

The supporting tissues of the teeth may also be affected adversely. In the majority of cases occlusal loading accelerates the advance of existing periodontal disease and this is most noticeable when the total number of teeth in contact has been reduced. It is difficult to assess the pathological potentialities of force developed during mastication and empty movements. When the latter are active articulations, the horizontal muscular component is more harmful than the vertical muscular action used in mastication. However, especially in established periodontal disease, masticatory forces hasten periodontal breakdown.

The horizontal component of force during incision, mastication, and eccentric stress occlusions is an important factor in causing the infra-bony pocket. The protrusive movement of incision causes the incisor teeth to suffer a breakdown of their labial and palatal supporting tissues and hence the mobility is antero-posterior, as also is that of the most posterior teeth, especially if they are short-rooted second or third molars. This is due to the inclined plane action of the cusps as the mandible moves from the retruded (ligamentous) to the tooth position. The small lateral component that accompanies this movement is resisted by the strong lateral bony plate in the lower jaw and in the bone inferior to the zygomatic processes in the maxilla. In the premolar area, if there is also molar contact, the mobility is lateral; in such cases there is no retrusive masticatory component and during the second phase of mastication lateral deviation of the mandible towards the working side occurs. When there are no teeth in contact distal to the premolars, increased mobility in all directions occurs. These variations in the mobility of periodontally diseased teeth arise from the variations in the pattern of mastication already described.

The power stroke of mastication is a cause of very deep pocketing sometimes seen between the molar teeth, especially in the maxillae. As periodontal disease advances, the resistance of the teeth to loading is reduced and the first signs of antero-posterior mobility are noted. This means that during the power stroke a space is opened up between the molar teeth which allows the ingress of relatively large food particles, this being the area where the gross communution is effected. Food packing of this kind has three effects, all of which lead to a speedy and localized periodontal breakdown. The first is the mechanical trauma of the impacting food particle; the second is the provision of a food pabulum from which bacteria can gain nourishment, and thirdly, food wedged between the teeth sets up a continuous antero-posterior force which is more likely to accelerate breakdown than the previously existing intermittent force.

Eccentric stress occlusions occurring either by day as idiosyncrasies or by night as grinding, are liable to concentrate excessive horizontal force over a few teeth, whose periodontia are prone to infra-bony pocketing. Since the direction of these occlusal contacts is often protrusive and lateral, it is the lateral incisors, canines and first premolars of the working side that are most affected; hyper-contacts on the balancing side during these movements are often seen in the molar area and account for the familiar gingival recession seen over the palatal roots of upper molars. The extent and frequency of such occlusions in the particular patient may be judged by an examination of the facets and by compiling a careful case history.

Lack of balanced occlusion

The term balanced occlusion as applied to full dentures requires continuous cuspal contacts in all segments of the opposing arches during protrusive or lateral movements. The object of such an occlusal arrangement of the teeth is to attempt to maintain the bases of the dentures in static relationship to their supporting tissues. During the third decade of this century the term balanced occlusion was extended to apply to the natural dentition; the term remains in popular use. However, the purpose of attempting to develop such a condition in the natural dentition is to distribute the interocclusal load widely over the opposing teeth.

A completely balanced occlusion in the natural dentition is so seldom seen that it cannot be regarded as the usual condition. It may be regarded as an *ideal* condition but certainly it is very far from being normal. Consequently it does not mean that any occlusion which is not ideal should be regarded as abnormal. Replacement of the ideal of complete balance by a more practically attainable partial balance is not only justified in theory but is a considerable clinical advantage; the desirable degree of this partial balance should be indicated from an examination of the faceting present and an examination of the gingivae and periodontium (Maunsbach and Posselt).

Clinically, the desirable extent of the balance depends on whether or not a particular patient indulges in day or night grinding; this diagnostic point is decided after questioning the patient. Facets which can only have been caused by excessive lateral movements of the mandible are positive evidence of bruxism and indicate that a more extensively balanced occlusion is required where periodontal disease is evident. The traumatic effect of bruxism is often marked and measures should be taken when indicated to obtain appropriate distribution of the load.

In patients who do not show evidence of empty grinding movements a lesser degree of balance is required, the extent of which should be designed to effect a sufficiently wide distribution of the load when the teeth make protrusive, lateral and retrusive contacts during incision and the two stages of mastication. It is suggested that the minimal requirement is a balanced occlusion in anterior, right and left segments of the arch. Since the need for a segmental balance is universal its development will be treated first.

The idea is that instead of protrusive balance requiring simultaneous contact of all posterior teeth, only four or six anterior teeth are required to maintain contact as the jaw is moved anteriorly from the tooth position to the edge to edge position. Likewise, lateral balance only demands simultaneous tooth contact in posterior teeth of the same side, canine, premolar and first molar balance being an acceptable condition. Nor is it necessary that these balancing contacts are maintained during extreme lateral deviation; an acceptable degree is half the length of the cuspal slope, since segmental balance generally serves to distribute the load during mastication. As well as these conventionally accepted protrusive and lateral balances, the desirability of distributing the load in the power stroke when masticating hard boli necessitates a posterior balance on the molar teeth of each side.

Lack of segmental balance is commonest in the anterior region, as it is here that irregular tooth arrangements are most common. The reaction to lack of segmental balance can be seen both in the teeth and their supporting structures. Teeth which make premature contact during a protrusive movement will be more abraded and the gingivae associated with them may show the classical signs of inflammation and sometimes cleft formation. Gingival and periodontal reactions are more noticeable in the lower than the upper teeth and are worst when the interference is located at either the mesial or distal corners of the incisal edge rather than distributed over its entire width. It is obvious that this causes a damaging torque to act at a maximal distance from the vertical axis of the root, which has a comparatively small lateral dimension.

As well as protrusive balance, retrusive balance is necessary to avoid traumatic occlusion as a complicating factor in established cases of periodontal disease. It is especially necessary where the first molars are missing and only the second and third molars remain in the upper jaw. In this situation the third molar is called upon to accept masticatory load in the power strokes. It is generally a short, conically rooted tooth and, if subjected to a premature contact in retrusion, a pathological stress may be produced. As previously described, a space is created between the molars into which food is packed, with its attendant sequelae. It is advisable in these cases to ensure that the second as well as the third molar accepts a proportion of the load by balancing the retrusive occlusion on these teeth.

Where grinding movements are prevalent either by day or night, two additional criteria should be met with regard to obtaining balance. First, in the lateral excursion a segmental balance should be obtained over an increased range of movement and, second, a diagonal balance should be obtained on the balancing side. Above all, an occlusal contact occurring on the balancing side which prevents teeth contacting on the working side must be avoided. This is often the result of tooth loss and subsequent overeruption. Levene cites two particular instances:

1   The loss of the mandibular first molar with the subsequent mesial and lingual tilting of the remaining molars and the extrusion of the upper molar.
2   The extraction of the upper third molar, followed by the overeruption of the lower third molar.

The extent of the diagonal balance need not be great; it is suggested it should be gradually developed over a few years. For example, a second molar contact on the balancing side should be extended to include a first molar balance. Moreover, its development should not be delayed after the *first* signs of trauma in the gingival margin or periodontium.

The development of segmentally or diagonally balanced occlusion can be achieved by grinding the natural teeth. Two practical points with regard to this procedure should be stressed. The first concerns timing; occlusal grinding should always be carried out in easy stages (Maunsbach and Posselt) and it may well take a few years, in the case of diagonal balance, to obtain the desired working and simultaneous balancing contacts. Such grinding should, however, be complete by the age of thirty-five when catabolic processes start to predominate and when a less favourable reaction can be expected in the periodontium. The second point concerns those patients who grind their teeth; it has been found clinically that it is best to delay grinding in these cases until the patient has come through a period of particular anxiety. The satisfaction achieved as a result of the grinding habit, although causing detriment to the supporting tissues of the teeth has the advantage of averting a psychological breakdown by providing an exit for pent-up nervous energy.

Non-coincidence of the muscular and tooth positions of the mandible

The teeth erupt into an intercuspidated position which, in most cases, is coincident with the muscular position of the mandible. This fortunate relationship may be lost later in life so that there is a greater or lesser deviation between the two positions. It will be recalled that the muscular position may have a small degree of deviation when viewed in the horizontal plane and accordingly, small deviations of the tooth position are likely to be accommodated within this range. When the tooth position moves outside this area a potentially pathological condition results. Actual pathology may or may not follow; fortunately, it usually does not.

Several mechanisms may cause a change in the tooth position. In each there is a relatively rapid change in the occlusal position of one tooth, or a small group of teeth. Two conditions may then develop. First, the tooth may be loosened to accommodate to the pattern of closure, this being most likely when the periodontium is either poorly developed or when periodontal disease is present. Second, an alternative position of the mandible may result, which is more acceptable and more interdigitated, and is found by a trial and error learning process. This new position is reinforced as a main act and is perpetuated as a

learned pattern in functional movements. The tendency is for this newly acquired position to become stabilized by further movement of teeth establishing a greater interdigitation. Such changes of position occur more commonly when some teeth have been lost previously and accordingly there is less definition of the original position of maximal intercuspidation. The following are the causes for the initial tooth movement:
1 Ill-advised orthodontic treatment
2 Badly contoured occlusal restorations
3 Tilting and eruption of teeth following extraction.

Orthodontic treatment aims to move teeth and then secure them in their new positions by retention appliances so that they cannot again be deflected. Especially when the upper anterior teeth have been retruded a new tooth position may be acquired with the mandible in a position distal to the muscular position. Where extensive occlusal restorations are made with amalgam or gold inlays, altered cuspal inclines may initiate a mandibular deviation. The tilting of lower second or third molars following the extraction of more anteriorly placed teeth is the most common cause of a deviation of mandibular position; in particular, sharply inclined lower third molars should always be viewed with suspicion. In these cases the displacement of the mandible is usually posterior.

Non-coincidence of the tooth and muscular positions may lead to pathological changes in any of the tissue of the stomatognathic system. In these circumstances there will be a conflict between the innate muscle pattern and the acquired learned pattern, which may lead to a continuous muscular contraction which can be demonstrated electromyographically. Perry showed that the minimal electrical activity which characterizes resting muscular tonus is replaced by increased contraction potential. It is postulated that this continuous muscular contraction results in the accumulation of metabolites with which the circulation cannot deal and these cause typical pain, each muscle having a particular area of pain reference. The commonest pains are pre-auricular from the masseter, supra-auricular from the temporalis, and zygomatic and intra-oral caused by external pterygoid spasm. More remote pain, dull and aching in nature, is sometimes located in the dorsum of the neck and on the posterior aspect of the shoulder, and has been observed to be associated with increased electrical activity in the post-cervical muscles. It is supposed that the normal functioning of these more remote muscle groups has also been affected.

A displacement of the muscular position of the mandible is necessarily associated with a displacement of the position of the condyle within the glenoid fossa. Many clinicians rely on the radiographic demonstration of this shift as evidence of the presence of a temporomandibular joint arthrosis; others content that the variables involved are so great as to negate the significance of small displacements seen on the film. Such displacements may be posterior or anterior, but the majority are backwards and upwards and it is with these that pain is most common. Further, it has been suggested that some of the pain felt in these cases might arise from the posterior displacement of the condylar head on to a vascular pad of tissue, rich in nerve endings, which normally occupies the posterior non-articular part of the glenoid fossa. It can readily be appreciated that if any rheumatic arthritic tendency is present this can only be aggravated by forcing the ligaments of the joint into a strained position.

Excessive loading of teeth which make premature contact as the mandible closes along its innate reflex path will act as an aggravating aetiological factor when periodontal disease is present.

Loss of posterior occlusal stop

A common example of this condition is an edentulous maxilla opposing a mandible carrying the six lower natural anterior teeth only. Often the full upper denture is worn successfully but the partial lower denture is not; this concentrates the occlusal contact on to the anterior jaw segment. The condition is found also where only the natural anterior teeth are in occlusion, possibly augmented by a premolar contact.

Loss of posterior occlusal stop may affect the musculature, temporomandibular joints, teeth, and periodontium; the most constant effect is on the muscular pattern and is one which may cause difficulty when dentures are first worn.

When mastication is carried out with anterior teeth only, the sequences of mastication described previously do not occur. In the absence of a posterior occlusal stop all mastication must be carried out with a basic incisive pattern in which tooth contact takes place in a protruded mandibular position, followed by a retrusive movement. This is not an efficient system, especially with those boli that require prior power comminution, since the incisal edge replaces the occlusal table and is in a postion of relative mechanical disadvantage, being far anterior to the fulcrum and elevators of the mandible. The other muscular sequences normally used in mastication are not reinforced during this period, and, when such a patient commences wearing dentures, this necessitates some re-education before these sequences are re-established as learned muscular patterns. This is one reason why such people may have difficulty when they come to wear either partial or full dentures.

The temporomandibular joint may also suffer in these circumstances. It necessarily becomes more weight-bearing than previously since the posterior occlusal stop cannot accept its usual large share of the energy released by contraction of the mandibular elevators. Further, as there is now no position of intercuspidation, the lower incisor teeth are free to slide back over the palatal surfaces of the uppers. On functional mandibular closure they may continue to do this until the ultimate resistance to the movement comes from the joint structures, by which time the condyle head is in an abnormally posterior and superior position. This strained condition of the joint often leads to pain.

However, in this situation it is possible that the periodontium may suffer rather than the joint. If the upper anterior teeth are periodontally involved, their overloading will result in their labial migration with resultant diastema. This forward displacement of these teeth allows the mandible to move upwards without, at the same time, being displaced backwards. Hence, if the periodontal condition of the upper teeth is not good they will suffer, but the joint will not be affected. If their periodontal condition is good and they remain firm in the alveolar bone, then joint arthroses are more likely to ensue.

When there is occlusion between the premolars the situation may be modified in varying degrees. When all the premolar teeth are present and have a sound periodontium it is unusual to find any pathological change occurring. When, however, only one pair of opposing premolars is present together with some degree of periodontal disease, tilting takes place and a condition results very similar to that described where only anterior teeth oppose each other. Varying resistance to backward displacement of the mandible is seen and, rather than a backward movement of the condyle occurring, a rotation takes place about the most posteriorly placed anteriorly facing cusp inclines. This produces displacement of the condyle in an anterior and superior direction and displacement of the anterior part of the mandible in a downwards direction. Hence over-eruption of anterior teeth may be allowed (Applegate, Sears).

In the absence of a posterior occlusal stop the anterior teeth become abraded quickly as mastication is sometimes a prolonged procedure requiring an excessive number of short strokes. The rate of loss of tooth substance is increased when the intact enamel caps over the incisal edges of the teeth are lost.

Since decreased magnitudes of muscular force are used by patients wearing dentures (Yurkstas and Curby) it is not surprising to find, where lower natural teeth oppose a full upper denture, that pathological reaction to force is uncommon in the lower teeth. On the contrary, unfavourable sequelae are commoner in the upper jaw which bears the denture. Unless retention is positive, difficulty is experienced in retaining the appliance during mastication. When, however, there is good retention, two possible deleterious results may occur depending on the type of anterior teeth on the denture. If porcelain teeth are used the occlusal load is directed on to the premaxilla which undergoes an osteolysis, fibrous tissue replacing the bone and creating the familiar 'flabby' ridge. When acrylic anterior teeth are used the ridge is sometimes better preserved, some of the interocclusal force being dissipated in abrading the teeth. These are often reduced substantially in length, giving a poor appearance and reduction of vertical dimension. Since there is often an associated lack of horizontal denture stability, the resultant forward movement of the denture over the mucosal surface accounts for the frequency of denture stomatitis in this type of case (Nyquist).

Fewer joint arthroses are seen where an upper denture rather than natural teeth is present; this is doubtless due to lack of retention and stability. Some patients, however, have been seen where a well retained and stabilized upper denture has been associated with a temporomandibular joint disturbance.

Summary

In this chapter the basic positions of the mandible have been demarcated and its functional movements have been classified and described. In addition an attempt has been made to provide a neurophysiological explanation for these movements. The reaction of the teeth and their supporting tissues to load has been considered and the possible pathological reactions in the stomatognathic tissues have been described.

When the aetiology of periodontal disease is considered (Chapter 6) the importance of failure of the periosteal and endosteal circulation will be emphasized. Such failure may be aided by traumatic occlusion which has a deleterious effect upon the terminal vascular bed, damage to capillaries and fine lymphatics resulting in a depleted blood supply.

References

ANDERSON D.J. (1955) Physiology of mastication. *Dent. Pract.* 5, 389.
APPLEGATE O.C. (1954) Loss of posterior occlusion. *J. pros. Dent.* 4, 197.
APRILE H. and SAIZAR P. (1947) Gothic arch tracing and temporo-mandibular anatomy. *J. Amer. dent. Ass.* 35, 256.
ÅRSTAD. T. (1954) The capsular ligaments of the temporo-mandibular joint and retrusion facets of the dentition in relationship to mandibular movements. Akademish Forlag, Oslo.
ATWOOD D.A. (1956) A cephalometric study of the clinical rest position of the mandible; part 1, the variability of the clinical rest position following the removal of occlusal contacts. *J. pros. Dent.* 6, 504.
BALLARD C.F. (1955) A consideration of the physiological background of mandibular posture and movement. *Dent. Practit.* 6, 80.
BRAIN W.K. (1951) *Diseases of the nervous system.* 42, Oxford University Press, London.
BREWER A.A. (1963) Prosthodontic research in progress at the School of Aerospace Medicine. *J. pros. Dent.* 13, 49.
BREWER A.A. and HUDSON D.C. (1961) Application of miniaturized electronic devices to the study of tooth contact in complete dentures. *J. pros. Dent.* 11, 62.
BUNDGAARD-JØRGENSEN F. (1952) Iagttagelser af underkaebens forhold hos et barn under sovnen samt hos nogle patienter. *Odont. Tidskr.* 60, 397.
CORBIN K.B. and HARRISON F. (1940) Function of the mesencephalic root of the fifth cranial nerve. *J. Neurophysiol.* 6, 163, 3, 423.
DONOVAN R.W. (1953) A cephalometric and temporo-mandibular joint radiographic

study of normal and abnormal function of the temporo-mandibular joint. *Ph.D. Thesis*, Northwestern University Dental School.
ELLIOTT F.A., HUGHES B. and TURNER J.W.A. (1952) *Clinical Neurology*, 9–10, Cassell and Co., London.
ESCHLER J. (1955) *Die functionelle Orthopadie des Kausystems.* Carl Hanser Verlag, München.
FULTON J.F. (1949) *Physiology of the nervous system,* 488, Oxford University Press, London.
GELLHORN, C. (1953) *Physiological foundations of neurology and psychiatry,* 1st Ed. The University of Minnesota Press, Minneapolis, Minn.
JANKELSON B., HOFMAN G.M. and HENDRON J.A. (1953) The physiology of the stomatognathic system. *J. Amer. dent. Ass.* **46**, 375.
JARABAK J.K. (1957) An electromyographic analysis of muscular behaviour in mandibular movements from rest position. *J. pros. Dent.* **7**, 682.
JAVOIS J.A. (1956) An electromyographical and cephalometric roentgenographic study of rest position of the mandible and the interocclusal clearance. *M.S.D. Thesis*, Northwestern University Dental School.
KAIRES A.K. (1957) A study of occlusal surface contacts in artificial dentures. *J. pros. Dent.* **7**, 553.
LAMMIE G.A., PERRY H.T. and CRUMM B. (1958) Certain observations on a complete denture patient. *J. pros. Dent.* **8**, 786.
LEVENE B.F. (1957) Occlusion in general dental practice. *J. pros. Dent.* **7**, 650.
LINDBLOM G. (1957) Cineradiographic study of the temporo-mandibular joint. *Acta Odont. Scand.* **15**, 141.
MCCOLLUM B.B. (1939) Fundamentals involved in prescribing restorative dental remedies. *Dent. Items Interest* **61**, 522, 641, 724, 852, 942.
MAUNSBACH O. and POSSELT U. (1955) Bettslipning som funktionskorrigerande hjälpmedel. *Odont. Rev.* **6**, 163.
MULLIN R.P. (1956) An electromyographic investigation of the postural position of the mandible. *M.S.D. Thesis*, Northwestern University Dental School.
MURPHY T. (1956) Control of the pressure strokes at the temporo-mandibular joint. *Aus. dent. J.* **1**, 276.
NEILL D.J. (1967) Studies of tooth contact in complete dentures. *Brit. dent. J.* **123**, 369.
NEVAKARI K. (1956) An analysis of the mandibular movement from rest to occlusal position. *Acta Odont. Scand.* **14**, suppl. 19.
NYQUIST G. (1952) A study of denture sore mouth. *Acta Odont. Scand.* **10**, Suppl. 9.
OSBORNE J. (1957) *Abstracts of I.A.D.R.* Atlantic City, March 1957.
PERRY H.T. (1955) Functional electromyography of the temporal and masseter muscles in class II, division 1 malocclusion and excellent occlusion. *Angle Orth.* **25**, 49.
PERRY H.T., LAMMIE G.A., MAIN J.H.P. and TEUSCHER G.W. (1960) Occlusion in a stress situation. **60**, 626.
PERRY H.T. (1957) Muscular changes associated with temporo-mandibular joint dysfunction. *J. Amer. dent. Ass.* **54**, 644.
POSSELT U. (1952) Studies in the mobility of the human mandible. *Acta Odont. Scand.* **10**, Suppl. 10.
POSSELT U. (1957) An analyser for mandibular positions. *J. pros. Dent.* **7**, 368.
POSSELT U. (1957) Movement areas of the mandible. *J. pros. Dent.* **7**, 375.
POSSELT U. (1958) Range of movement of the mandible. *J. Amer. dent. Ass.* **56**, 10.
SCHUYLER C.H. (1929) Principles employed in full denture prosthesis which may be applied in other fields of dentistry. *J. Amer. dent. Ass.* **16**, 2045.
SCHWARTZ L.L. (1957) Temporo-mandibular joint syndromes. *J. pros. Dent.* **7**, 489.

SCHWARTZ L.L. and TAUSIG, D.P. (1954) Temporo-mandibular joint pain treatment with intramuscular infiltration of tetracaine hydrochloride; a preliminary report. *New York dent. J.* **20**, 219.

SEARS V.H. (1956) Occlusal pivots. *J. pros. Dent.* **6**, 332.

SICHER H. (1952) Functional anatomy of the temporo-mandibular articulation. *Dent. J. Australia* **24**, 1.

STUART C.E. (1939–40) Articulation of human teeth. *Dent. Items Interest* **61**, 1029, 1147, **62**, 8, 106.

SYNGE J.L. (1933) The tightness of the teeth, considered as a problem concerning the equilibrium of a thin incompressible elastic mambrane. *Phil. Trans. Roy. Soc. London*, Series A, **231**, 435.

SZENTAGOTHAI J. (1948) Anatomical considerations of monosynaptic reflex arcs. *J. Neurophysiol.* **11**, 445.

THOMPSON J.R. (1954) Concepts regarding function of the stomatognathic system. *J. Amer. dent. Ass.* **48**, 626.

THOMPSON J.R. and BRODIE A.G. (1942) Factors in the position of the mandible. *J. Amer. dent. Ass.* **29**, 925.

THOMPSON J.R. (1946) The rest position of the mandible and its significance to dental science. *J. Amer. dent. Ass.* **33**, 151.

WATT D.M. (1968) Gnathosonics in occlusal evaluation. *J. pros. Dent.* **19**, 133.

WATT D.M. (1969) Recording the sounds of tooth contact. *Int. dent. J.* **19**, 221.

YEMM R. (1968) Irrelevant muscle activity. *Proc. Brit. Soc. pros. Dent.* 1968.

YURKSTAS A.A. and EMERSON W.H. (1954) A study of tooth contact during mastication with artificial dentures. *J. pros. Dent.* **4**, 168.

YURKSTAS A.A. and CURBY W.A. (1953) Force analysis of prosthetic appliances during function. *J. pros. Dent.* **3**, 82.

5

THE REACTION OF THE DENTAL APPARATUS TO LOADING

The dental apparatus in this context is taken to include the tooth, the periodontal membrane, the alveolar bone and the mucosa. All independently behave differently to imposed load although in general terms the tooth and alveolar bone behave elastically in that they return immediately to their previous form after removal of the load. Mucosa and periodontal membrane, however, react viscoelastically and do not regain their original form immediately after removal of the applied load, but tend to do so after a lapse of time.

Since this behaviour and other changes which will be discussed later reflect the macroscopic and microscopic structure of these separate organs or tissues it is relevant to consider their anatomy and histology from a functional viewpoint.

1 The teeth

In general terms the teeth behave as elastic bodies. However it is necessary to emphasize change in physical qualities with ageing. The dentine becomes less porous and its tubules calcify from the periphery; deposition of secondary dentine progressively obliterates pulp chamber and canals. This structure shows a reduced elastic limit, modulus of elasticity and ultimate strength; it is accordingly prone to fracture. It should also be noted that its vitality is meanwhile reduced and ultimately it becomes a bioacceptable dead mass. However, by dint of its being incorporated in the alveolar process via a living periodontal membrane its attachment is assured through deposition of incremental layers of living cementum. Cemental apposition is specially noted in the apical area often resulting in a terminal globular mass.

2 The bone

Bone is a living tissue and is subject to continuous anabolic and catabolic change. In the first two decades of life especially during the period when the dental arch is being developed, growth is evident as a series of sporadic anabolic events. However, during the early years of adult life, the jaws and especially their alveolar processes, maintain a constant shape and their microscopic morphology, in terms of lamellar bone thickness and trabecular size and distribution, show remarkable stability. This suggests a complex environmental control of the anabolic and

catabolic processes, and the following factors are influential in this connection:
(i)   hereditary factors
(ii) general factors
(iii) local factors.

This stability of the bony pattern is not permanent since at different times new bone may be laid down, when an osteosclerosis occurs, whilst at other times local resorbtion of bone, known as osteolysis, takes place. Which of these conditions occurs depends on the relative anabolic or catabolic activity, and also upon changes in the local and general factors influencing bone biology.

(i)   *Hereditary factors.* Of the three influences, hereditary factors are least understood. However, their importance must be recognized since they impose severe limitations on the anabolic potentialities of the local factors. However it must still be recognized that the young men and women of today are taller and physically better developed than their counterparts a generation ago; but the enigma remains that the jaws have not shown commensurate development. One extreme viewpoint has been expressed that jaw growth is entirely a response to forces such as soft tissue growth, acting upon it, but it must be pointed out that a mandible always retains the shape of a mandible and familial resemblance is not least obvious in facial form.

(ii) *General factors.* Bone physiology requires hormonal balance, vitamin sufficiency and the availability of necessary mineral ions. It is known that disease of bone can result from either hormonal disturbances or dietary insufficiency. However our concern is not with rare bone pathology, but with altered bone physiology. For example, vitamin and mineral intake are important after multiple extractions as during this period a blood clot must become organized and later converted into bone. Vitamin C sufficiency is necessary for collagen formation and vitamin D for the calcification process. Sex hormones are also important especially in climacteric osteoporosis caused by a decreased oestrogen level.

(iii) *Local factors.* Pressure is of the utmost importance as a local factor in bone metabolism. Weinnmann and Sicher state that 'As long as pressure does not interfere with the blood supply and drainage of the bone tissue, it is resisted and, if increased within the limits of tolerance, will even lead to formation of new bone'. This concept substantiates the idea that a physiological limit exists in bone above which further increase in applied force results in osteolysis; it also highlights the dependence of bone on an adequate blood supply.

3   The periodontal membrane

It is not proposed to describe the histological structure of the periodontal ligament in detail, but since the ability of the periodontium to resist loads imposed on the crown of the tooth is intimately related to some structural features it is pertinent to call special attention to these.

Collagen fibres form 75% of the dry volume of the periodontal ligament; in repose these consist of wavy bundles which straighten out on loading. The insertion of these fibres into the cementum is evenly distributed whereas in bone the insertions are concentrated into more dispersed areas of connection. Within the periodontal membrane the collagen fibres have an intermediate, interwoven plexus of fibres, so that there is no continuity of the individual fibres across the periodontal space. This arrangement permits change in tooth position and width of the periodontal membrane with sustained functional potential.

The periodontal membrane is a vascular tissue when compared with other densely collagenous tissues; however the blood vessels occupy only 3% volume of the tissues and the diameter of the vessels is conspicuously small. The indications are that the rate of turnover of collagen in the periodontal membrane is high and therefore a critical regulation of the available blood supply is necessary. This concept is supported by the demonstration of pre-capillary sphincters which control the flow of plasma and blood and of glomera which may shunt blood from arteries to veins bypassing the capillary bed. The small blood vessels enter the periodontal membrane in two particular locations, apically and marginally; because of this distribution the vessels are not required to run through the length of the periodontal membrane when they would be unnecessarily exposed to trauma; moreover some are accommodated in protective grooves in the bone.

Fibroblasts are few in relation to the number of collagen fibres and lie in longitudinal relationship to them. They are capable of changing shape under imposed load without being damaged. Under load fibroblasts, ground substance and tissue fluid may all change position within the periodontal membrane and the fluid constituents are free to be expressed from the periodontal membrane through the Volkmann's canals. Normally the marginal ligament of the periodontal membrane is resistive to such movement but when depleted loses this potential in some degree.

Changes Following Tooth Extraction

Where there is no complicating infection extraction of a tooth is followed by a predictable series of events. Immediately following extraction there is some inversion of the marginal gingiva into the wound space; this fills to its surface limit with blood clot. Progressively thereafter an immature epithelial surface comes to cover the blood clot, which is gradually replaced by granulation tissue. With these events there is some contraction of tissue in the healing wound and a surface depression is noted. Thereafter gradual change of shape occurs which is continuous over a period of about a year. During this time an undulated form of the alveolar process is replaced by a smoothly confluent tissue form. This necessarily involves bone remodelling. However there is always associated loss of ridge dimension during this period, loss in height and width of the edentulous ridge are consistent as is also loss in mesio-distal dimension where tooth movement permits. But the degree to which loss of alveolar ridge volume takes place is variable and it is dependent on the local availability of a sustaining blood supply. Where the blood supply is good preservation of a well formed ridge is evident; following upon periodontal disease and in old age the edentulous alveolar ridge is much more atrophied. Even after a year a static position cannot be considered to have been established; every dentist is aware that in the ageing process to variable degree there is progressive further loss of alveolar bone as ridge dimensions are further reduced. Again it is suggested that this is an atrophy in response to a failing peripheral blood supply. Characteristically, as in growth, this is not a continuous gradual process but is characterized by periods of depletion followed by long intervals of consolidation.

The net result of the bone remodelling is an inversion of the vestibular and oral plates of the alveolar process; these processes approximate but never fuse. On the crest of the alveolar ridge there is always a small bony area where the surface is rough, nodular and permeated by numerous pores. This type of bone is very different in appearance from that of the proximate alveolar plates the smooth dense surface of which is derived from a covering periosteum, which must be regarded as a tissue with low regenerative potential. But some areas of this cancellous type of bone are consistently of greater area; thus in the mandible the molar and incisor areas are more conspicuous than the premolar area where approximation of the plates may be almost complete. In the maxillae the whole alveolar process is covered by a less dense, more porous bone than in mandible but again in molar and anterior areas the more cancellous types of bone are evident. Two reasons for the failure of the alveolar plates to invert in these areas are the immediate peripheral presence of muscle attachments and heavy buttresses of bone. These crestal bony areas are more liable to further loss of tissue, and the mucosa covering them, especially when atrophic, is liable to inflammation and pain when covered by a partial denture saddle.

Change in the form of the alveolar ridge implies the action of some externally derived moulding force. This surmise is confirmed by the not uncommon clinical appearance of a mobile fibrous ridge. Typically this is seen in the maxilla where upper anterior teeth have been replaced by a denture covering a large palatal area and where mastication is carried on entirely with natural lower anterior teeth; the alveolar bone has resorbed under the influence of heavy load but loss of ridge dimension has not been commensurate. It is noted that well developed alveolar ridges are generally associated with a covering mucosa of substantial thickness and that the lining of the cheek invaginates into the oral cavity with an undulating surface (Fig. 5.1). Where the loss of alveolar ridge is extreme the covering

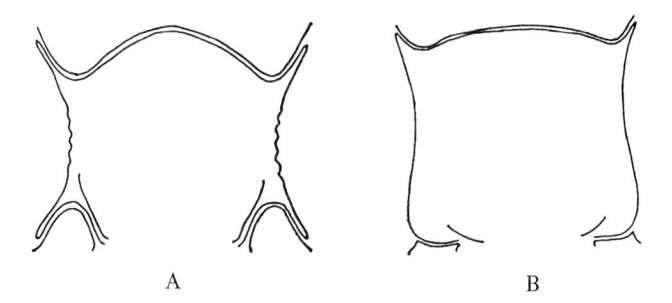

Fig. 5.1. Diagrammatic representation of coronal sections of the mouth in edentulous subjects. A shows the conditions pertaining in a young subject; the ridges are well developed and are covered by soft tissue of substantial thickness. The cheek tissue invaginates into the oral cavity. B shows the condition in atrophy when there is marked ridge reduction and atrophy of the overlying soft tissue. The cheek invaginates into the oral cavity to lesser degree. It will be noted that in the atrophic case the outline of the tissues has become more spheroidal.

mucosa is always thin as is that of the cheek, which invaginates less into the oral cavity and appears more taut. In cross section there has been a change in oral form from an involuting surface to a more circular surface as if an economy of surface epithelium were being effected. Such an atrophying mucosa is considered to be the moulding force which acts to give a smooth ridge contour. A second externally applied force which acts to mould an edentulous section of the alveolar ridge is the application of a denture saddle under occlusal load; Newton (1964) demonstrated histologically that the mucosa underlying denture saddles was liable to degenerative change in the collagen component of the submucosa.

A final, consistent clinical appearance following extraction deserves comment. When a standing tooth abuts on an edentulous space the buccal marginal gingiva courses diagonally across the tooth (Fig. 5.2). On that surface where there is a contacting tooth the gingival margin is higher, and on the other cemental exposure is always seen. This appearance is constantly seen in the

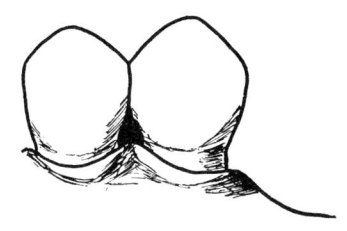

Fig. 5.2. Shows the line of the marginal gingiva as it courses buccally from mesial to distal across a premolar tooth which abuts on to an edentulous section of the ridge. Distally the marginal gingiva is apical to its mesial position.

physiological condition and is more exaggerated where periodontal disease coexists. Moreover the shape of the edentulous ridge is not uniform; it is highest in relation to the abutment tooth and dips to a maximal low in the centre of the edentulous space; the presence of a tooth would seem to stimulate the production or maintenance of alveolar bone.

Hyperplasia and Atrophy of the Dental Apparatus

When a tooth is subjected to increased loads certain hyperplasias may occur. The periodontal membrane may increase in width up to 50% while the thickness of the principal fibre bundles increases commensurately. The thickness of the lamina dura of the tooth socket increases as does the number and thickness of the supporting trabeculae of the cancellous bone. The marginal ligament may also show a favourable reaction, its integrity being preserved by hyperplasia of its various fibre components. This favourable response is conditional upon the causative change of load being gradually imposed and upon its limitation in magnitude. Moreover the reaction applies only in the case of 'young' tissues suggesting again that the reaction is ordained by the availability of a sufficient blood supply. When these conditions are not met, degenerative rather than hyperplastic changes ensues.

When a group of teeth loose their opponents an atrophic condition exactly opposite to that described above is noted. The periodontal membrane becomes thinner; in fact in very special circumstances it may be obliterated with ankylosis of the tooth. The constituent principal fibres become less numerous and thinner. The lamina dura, too becomes thinner and is supported by fewer and finer trabeculae. The narrow spaces, little in evidence in the hypertrophied condition, now become conspicuous. The histological or radiographic appearance of the atrophic condition indicates that increased load would need to be small not to enter the traumatic range.

An Analysis of Forces Acting on Teeth through Occlusal Contacts

It is generally accepted that vertical loading is well resisted by the periodontium of the tooth, which comprises periodontal membrane, alveolar bone and marginal ligament. It should also be appreciated that the application of a horizontal force, either lateral or antero-posterior, does not cause bodily movement of the tooth but a rotation of its long axis. The centre of this rotation lies in the middle vertical third of the tooth somewhat more apically than coronally. Confirmatory evidence of this is the fact that the periodontal membrane has its minimum width in this region and widens towards its apex and gingival margin.

However, this discrimination between vertical and horizontal force is of more theoretical interest than practical application, since it is seldom that an uncomplicated vertical force acts on a tooth; usually there is some degree of horizontal force present, the magnitude of which cannot be assessed clinically other than very approximately. The first important factor which determines the degree of horizontal force acting on a tooth is the direction of the applied muscle force. During mastication, swallowing and empty movements, anterior, posterior and lateral muscle pulls act at different times, consequently uncomplicated vertical resultants of muscular force must be rare. In addition the arrangement and form of the teeth themselves make uncomplicated vertical force unlikely, since the following factors tend to produce horizontal components:
(i) degree of inclination of the cusps
(ii) the arrangement of the long axes of the teeth.

(i) The degree of inclination of the cusps

When a tooth is loaded vertically, at its greatest the horizontal components of force can never be more than half the applied load and this maximum occurs at an angle of 45°. However horizontal components of force may well cancel out, when equal and opposite forces arise from reciprocally sloping inclines. For instance, a premolar may have occlusal contacts on the mesial and distal aspect of the buccal cusp and consequently anterior and posterior components would nullify each other (Fig. 5.3). Ideally, when viewed in sagittal section, equal and opposite anterior and posterior components should act along the line of premolar and molar teeth. However, irregular occlusal arrangements or loss of teeth are so common as to make this more of an ideal than a normal situation (Figs 5.4 & 5.5). A partial denture provides occlusal contact with natural teeth so that the latter are loaded on opposing inclines; this does not assure uncomplicated vertical force but is more likely to reduce the horizontal force.

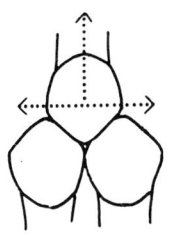

Fig. 5.3. Upper premolar with mesial and distal contacts.

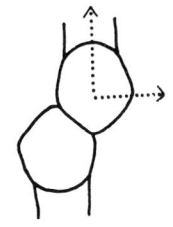

Fig. 5.4. Upper premolar with mesial contact only.

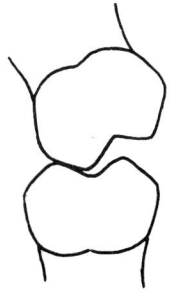

Fig. 5.5. Molars in irregular occlusal contact.

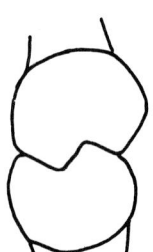

Fig. 5.6. Ideal cuspal arrangement in the tooth position.

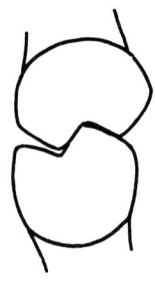

Fig. 5.7. Opposing facing cuspal inclines occluding.

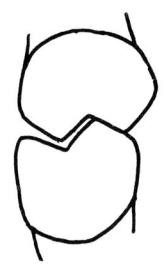

Fig. 5.8. Only one inclined cuspal surface.

When viewed from the coronal aspect the ideal configuration of upper and lower cusps is three pairs of opposing inclines in contact in the tooth position (Fig. 5.6). This relationship, and also the condition where the oppositely facing inclines occlude (Fig. 5.7) results in a purely vertical force. However, when only one inclined surface occludes (Fig. 5.8) a horizontal component of force results. When vertical load is applied with the mandible displaced to the working side in the first of these conditions (Fig. 5.8) a downward rotation of the lingual cusp of the upper molar may be prevented (Fig. 5.9). In the remaining conditions a lateral component of force must result from the single opposing inclines in occlusion (Fig. 5.10).

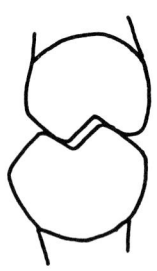

Fig. 5.9. The condition in Fig. 5.6 when a lateral excursion to the working side is made.

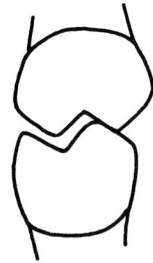

Fig. 5.10. The condition in Figs 5.7 and 5.8. when a lateral excursion to the working side is made.

Practically speaking, the reduction of cusp inclines by grinding, onlays or fixed occlusal reconstructions will reduce the horizontal component of force when uncomplicated vertical loading is considered. Grinding or placing artificial teeth to give reciprocal contact on the opposing cuspal inclines is another helpful measure.

The Reaction of the Dental Apparatus to Loading 81

This detailed consideration of the mechanical conditions prevailing under vertical load is justified because the very powerful muscles of mastication develop almost purely vertical force and it is likely that the damaging action of the horizontal component of force is maximal under the condition of heavy loading. When lateral jaw movements are considered the muscular action is less powerful, but horizontal displacing forces on the dental apparatus are inevitable.

(ii) The arrangement of the long axes of the teeth

Clinical examination reveals that few teeth are vertically placed and even in the 'ideal' dentition only the upper premolar and first molars may be in this position. Upper and lower anterior teeth generally show an anterior tilt, the upper second and third molars a posterior tilt, and the lower posterior teeth varying degrees of anterior and lingual tilt, this being most marked in the more distal teeth. In a tilted tooth, if the whole occlusal surface is evenly loaded, the line of action of the vertical component of force will lie some distance anterior or posterior to the rotational axis of the tooth and a damaging torque will result (Fig. 5.11). The greater the degree of tilting of the tooth the greater will be the moment of this force, and accordingly the greater its pathological potential.

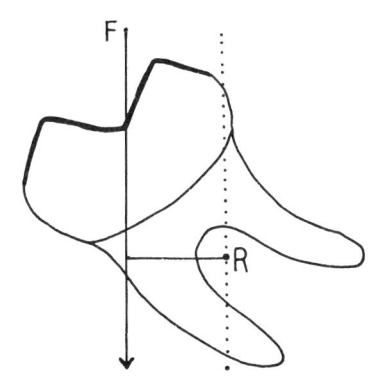

Fig. 5.11. Line of action of the load applied (F) over the whole occlusal area of a tilted lower molar and the resultant torque action about the fulcrum of rotation (R).

When viewed in coronal section the upper posterior teeth have a buccal, and the lowers a lingual tilt. Opposite torques are accordingly liable to result.

When the complete natural dentition is accommodated in well developed jaw bones the degree of tilting of the teeth is not marked. But with good preventive and restorative dentistry the number of complete or nearly complete dentitions is much more frequently seen than formerly. Unfortunately these are all too frequently accommodated in inadequately developed jaws and a crowded state results; this always results in exaggerated tilting especially in the most posterior segments of the mouth. When this crowded condition is relieved by extractions usually necessitated by caries rather than as a planned preventive measure, exaggerated tilting is again liable to result in teeth adjoining an edentulous space.

In the posterior segments antero-posterior force may be transmitted through interstitial tooth contact; contiguous teeth thus accept a share of this force and a favourable result is more likely. However, in the same region lateral force cannot be distributed through tooth contact. But some distribution to adjacent teeth still takes place and this is effected through the action of the transeptal fibres of the marginal ligament and the alveolar plate of bone, an effect Picton (1985) has referred to as strapping action. In the anterior segment of the arch an antero-posterior component of force is resisted by the same action, whereas a lateral force may be resisted by contacting teeth. Thus the preservation of interstitial tooth contacts and the development of light contacts between abutment teeth and denture saddles will reduce some of the horizontal forces acting on the teeth and accordingly enhance their preservation.

To summarize, whereas it is doubtful if, in function, purely vertical forces can be applied, the incidence of more damaging horizontal forces and torques may be reduced by:
(i) Reduction of cusp inclines by grinding, onlays or fixed restorations.
(ii) Provision of occlusal contacts on reciprocal cusp inclines by grinding and careful placement of artificial teeth.
(iii) Extraction of seriously tilted teeth.
(iv) Preservation of interstitial contacts in the natural teeth by well contoured fillings and by saddles adapted to give interstitial contact with abutment teeth.

Experimental Findings on Loading of the Natural Teeth

For an understanding of the behaviour of teeth under load we are indebted almost entirely to the careful work of Picton and his collaborators. Short term effects of imposed loads on the teeth will only be considered here, as it is more appropriate to consider the long term reactions when periodontal disease and traumatism are considered. However it should be appreciated that the long term outcome may well result from the repetition of short term forces.

With the application of simple horizontal or axial loads in the range 0.1–4.0 N there is first an instantaneous relatively free movement followed by a period of progressive but decreasing creep. Complete recovery to the resting position of the tooth is only accomplished after 1½ minutes and again an instantaneous substantial recovery is followed by a longer period of more restricted movement.

In this action and reaction tooth, alveolar bone and periodontal membrane are all involved. The tooth and alveolar bone are distorted elastically and both action and reaction are immediate, but the magnitude of tooth deformation is much less than that occurring in the alveolar bone. The distortion of the bone is greatest relative to the loaded tooth but displacement of the bone related to contiguous teeth is also noted and this feature is more marked when the applied load is horizontal rather than axial.

The phenomenon of creep in both the displacement and recovery of the loaded tooth is ascribed to the visco-elastic property of the periodontal membrane. 'When force is applied to an elastic material there is an immediate displacement or distortion until the force is removed, and then recovery is immediate and complete. If a viscous substance, such as oil, is subjected to load, time becomes a factor in the response as the material is gradually displaced to the equilibrium state. When the force is removed however, there is no tendency for the material to return to the original condition. Viscoelastic materials display a combination of these effects'.

At different times three different concepts of periodontal tooth support have been advanced, and it is certain that all make simultaneous contribution in resisting imposed load on a tooth within the alveolar socket.

(i) *Simple tension theory.* In the oldest and most obvious concept load is resisted by straightening then lengthening of the principal fibres of the periodontal membrane and more especially those of the marginal ligament. The presence of the intermediate fibre plexus allows some movement of the fibres over each other and preserves the integrity of the longitudinally coursing blood vessels.

(ii) *Support due to compression alone.* Two premises are the incompressibility of the tissue fluid and its confinement within a rigid compartment sealed crestally by the marginal ligament. However, it is found that apicectomy, naturally occurring fenestrations and incomplete sockets during eruption only somewhat increase mobility. Again periodontal disease substantially increases tooth mobility but is associated with depletion of the marginal ligament (Smyd, 1958).

(iii) *Hydrodynamic damping.* This effect is ascribed to progressive squeezing of blood within the deformed vessels of the periodontal membrane.

Since the periodontal membrane is viscoelastic, its response to loading depends on several inter-related factors. These include: the magnitude of the load, the loading rate, the duration of action of the load, the frequency of serial loads, and the previous loading history. In addition physiological factors within the periodontium, such as blood pressure and the state of hydration of the ground substance and pathological conditions will mediate the response of the periodontium to loading.

Perhaps of special importance is the case where the tooth is loaded repetitively. High rates of loading cause:
(i) Less deformation and displacement of the tissues.

(ii) A more nearly elastic character to the dimensional changes.
(iii) A relatively rapid recovery of the tissues to the resting condition .
Particularly it has been shown that the elastic recoil of the teeth and bone is complete before the next load in a chewing sequence can be expected.

The Effects of Pressure on the Edentulous Alveolar Ridge

The soft tissues covering the alveolar processes consist of three layers, a mucosa, a submucosa and a periosteum. The mucosa consists of a stratified squamous epithelium and a fibrous lamina propria with papillary and reticular layers; the epithelium is differentiated into an outer stratum corneum, a middle stratum medium and a basal stratum germinativum. This stratified epithelium is thin although its dimension varies greatly. The submucosa consists of connective tissue and carries the blood vessels, lymphatics and nerves. The collagen fibres of this tissue merge into those of the thinner periosteal layer which covers the bone except on the crestal area where the periosteal layer is absent. The submucosa in particular contains much extracellular fluid.

If pressure is applied over part of the surface of this soft tissue, the tissue fluid is expelled laterally into the adjoining tissues. Thus the structure affecting the pressure, often a partial denture saddle, is depressed into the soft tissue while the adjoining uncompressed tissue accommodates the expelled tissue fluid. The compression of the tissue which is stressed ceases when the hydrostatic pressure immediately peripheral to the compressed area becomes equal to the pressure in the tissue fluid under the compressed area. The amount of compression effected is greater in those tissues that display a deep submucous layer and where this contains a diminished number of collagen fibres. The amount of compression depends also on the nature of the immediately peripheral tissues. Lax tissues, such as those present in the vestibular sulcus, accommodate the displaced tissue fluid without marked increase in hydrostatic pressure and therefore allow a larger amount of compression in the stressed tissue. With increased pressure, too, there is a tendency for the veins and lymphatics to be drained of their fluid contents, and, if the increase in pressure is high, for a reduction in blood flow to the part through compression of the arterial vessels.

It is well to assess the comparative compressibilities of the different areas having pressure applied by partial dentures. The most revealing case to consider is the mandibular free-end saddle (Fig. 5.12). Looked at sagittally at the mesial end is the abutment tooth. This suffers little displacement under vertical load because of the suspensory nature of the periodontal membrane. The soft tissue over the ridge is more compressible but is not nearly so compressible as the retromolar tissue; anteriorly, the corium contains less tissue fluid the displacement of which is resisted by the more densely packed fibres in the neighbouring tissues. Taking a coronal section of the mandibular ridge it is seen that the tissues merging into the buccal sulcus are lax and compressible. The buccal incline of the ridge has a thin fibrous submucosa and is not as readily distorted as the alveolar crest area where after healing of the extraction wounds, a deeper corium exists which overlies a bone with many pores which may accept expressed tissue fluid. The lingual alveolar slope is covered by a very thin mucous membrane which is not readily displaced.

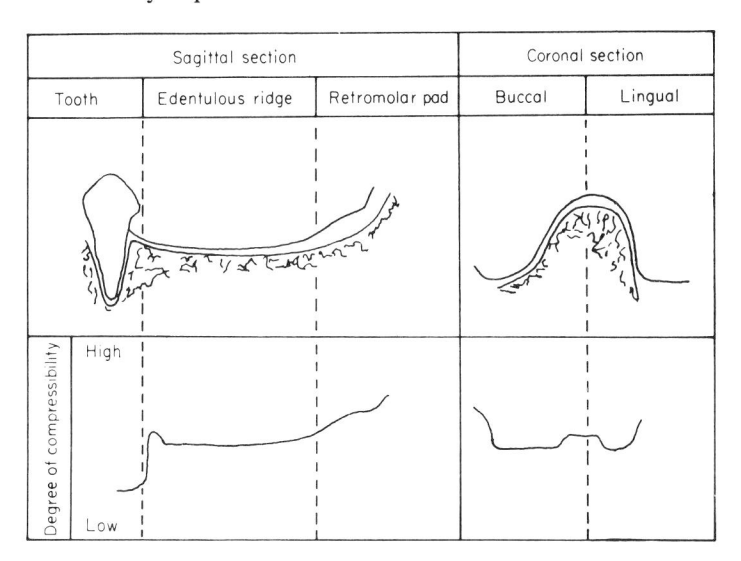

Fig. 5.12. Diagrammatic representation of the relative tissue compressibilities found in various areas of the lower free-end saddle case.

A similar situation exists in the maxilla (Fig. 5.13). Here, however, the tuberosity region although more fibrous than the remainder of the alveolar crest, is not so compressible as the corresponding retromolar area in the mandible. The slopes of the hard palate are covered bilaterally by the palatal glands which are compressible in varying degrees. In the area of the median raphe there is virtually no submucosa and the mucosa lies in direct contact with the periosteum; this area is the least compressible of all the soft tissue denture-bearing surfaces.

The above descriptions are based upon normal conditions when no dentures have been worn and hence there has been no fibrous tissue proliferation. Tomlin et al. (1968) measured, by means of a force–distance probe, the thickness and hardness of the soft tissues overlying edentulous ridge areas and found wide variations not only between different persons but between different areas within the same mouth. In general the soft tissues had an average thickness of 1.5 mm and a Young's modulus of 2.0 N/mm but the thickness tended to be greatest in the retromolar areas of the lower jaw.

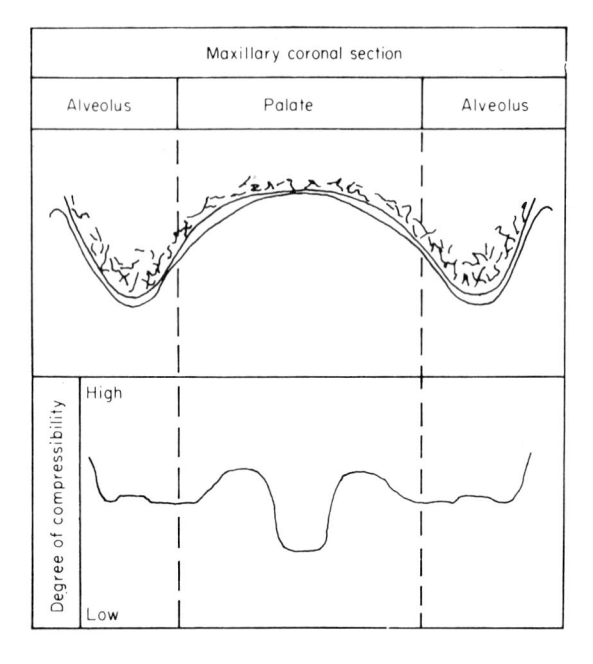

Fig. 5.13. Diagrammatic representation of the relative tissue compressibilities found in a coronal section through an edentulous maxilla.

As in the case of tooth reaction to loading the experimental work of Picton has given more detailed appreciation of the conditions resulting from the loading of the mucosa covering the alveolar ridges taking special cognizance of the rate of application of repetitive loads and the time factor. These findings are specially pertinent in the construction of partial dentures:

(i) When chewing is considered the soft tissues do not recover their resting form before the next masticatory stroke is applied; this is progressively incomplete at least for a series of 20–30 loadings.

(ii) The magnitude of mucosal deformation is substantially greater than the intrusion of a tooth or small groups of teeth under the same load.

(iii) Reducing the number of teeth which support a tooth-borne plate increases (though not in simple proportion) the amount of displacement of the plate.

(iv) Reducing the load-bearing area of a mucosal bone plate increases the displacement of the plate, though not in simple proportion; this effect was specially noted when the mid-line area of the hard palate was not covered by the plate.

It will be appreciated that depending on the viscosity of the impression material used and the duration and magnitude of the pressure imposed, the denture bearing bone may be represented in varying degrees of tissue compression. When an impression material such as alginate is used correctly the resting state of the mucosa is faithfully recorded. When a viscous material, such as compound or some of the zinc oxide-eugenol pastes or some rubbers is used the soft tissue form is represented in a more compressed state after expression of tissue fluid. The first class of impression material is known as mucostatic. In function if the denture is heavily tooth supported, quick and considerable tissue fluid displacement gives rise to a condition where the alveolar ridge makes little contribution to load bearing. When such an impression material is used and the denture is entirely mucosal borne, loading of the underlying bone is uneven and the contours of the underlying mucosa are changed within a few hours. On the other hand a 'mucocompressive saddle' which is firmly attached to abutment teeth provides greater support under vertical chewing loads than a 'mucostatic saddle', or from the abutment teeth alone. In this connection it should be pointed out that the mucocompressive impression represents the teeth in a position very near to their resting position. When heavier pressure is used in impression taking with a viscous medium, a mucodisplacive condition is recorded. Here there is little further displacement of tissue fluid but the teeth are intruded into their sockets. Such a condition necessarily induces a permanent tissue change and should always be avoided.

It will be appreciated that it is very difficult to take the view of a permanent mucosal form in function and this has its important implications in partial denture construction. When it is desired to take a mucostatic impression it is necessary to avoid wearing any denture or engage in chewing for two hours before taking the impression. When a mucosal borne plate is constructed to a mucostatic impression different areas of the supporting tissues are stressed in varying degrees. When the overlying submucosa is thin increased load is committed to this area. The mildest possible and even desirable reaction in this event is confined to the ground substance of the fibrous tissue; this moves from a more colloidal to a more sol condition a shift which is followed by hydration of the ground substance and an increase in its volume. This results in the establishment of a thicker corium but one still lacking in fibres and unlikely to be supportive. However in the longer term a local hyperaemia may be established through the action of chemical mediators and this followed by the generation of fibrous tissue. Such an action must be considered advantageous to the denture wearer as a more even layer of submucosa is established over the denture bearing area and a denser fibrous tissue results making the tissue less compressible and therefore more capable of bearing an evenly distributed load. It must be emphasized, however, that this favourable reaction is entirely dependent on the ability of the blood supply to respond.

At the other extreme an unfavourable sequence of events is liable to be encountered, and is typically seen in the case of a free-end saddle covering an atrophic alveolar ridge. In this condition the mucosa and submucosa are specially thin and have no capacity to absorb energy when load is applied to the saddle. Trauma is liable to concentrate over the mylo-hyoid ridge which forms a sharp superficial edge of cortical bone and painful ulceration of the overlying mucosa develops. But the crestal area of bone by dint of its spicular surface is another area where inflammation and ulceration rather than regeneration are liable to appear, and make initial denture wearing a particularly painful matter.

In addition to the overlying soft tissues of the alveolar ridge imposing particular problems so also does the underlying bone. The bone of the edentulous alveolar ridge responds to pressure change according to the general principles already discussed. In the absence of pressure, or upon its reduction, the lamellae of the cortical bone and the trabeculae of the medullary bone are decreased in number and in size. When pressure is increased but is still below the physiological limit, according to Wolff's law, an osteosclerotic reaction occurs. However Wolff's law refers to both the magnitude and *direction* of the applied force. If the direction of the applied force is changed this necessitates a rearrangement of the trabeculae, an initial osteolysis being followed by a reconstructive phase. The direction of the force applied to the alveolar ridge is entirely different when a denture saddle is placed over it from when the natural teeth are standing. Certainly load is not applied over the cortical plates when natural teeth are standing and the fact that these plates are not naturally weight bearing is confirmed by the vascular condition of the periosteum. Thus, although the edentulous ridge may react by laying down favourably orientated trabeculae, this is secondary to an osteolytic phase, which is often predominant, due to the age of the patient. Practically speaking, therefore, the edentulous ridge is more predisposed to catabolic than anabolic change and is not so favourably disposed to load bearing as it was when teeth were present.

Wolff's law refers to the structure rather than the form of the bone and the above discussion takes no account of the predisposition of the edentulous ridge to lose height and undergo 'resorption'. Change in form implies the application of some external moulding force and as already stated two such forces may act on the edentulous ridge. The first is the healing or atrophying mucosa and the second is that imposed by a denture saddle. In the latter the moulding force is more intermittent but its higher magnitude may make it of greater significance. That such a force causes resorption of the alveolar ridge is confirmed by the need for rebasing free-end saddles after a short period of wear. The structure of the bone itself offers varying resistance to these moulding forces. The well developed ridge stands up well; the atrophic ridge is prone to further resorption. In the end it is again the potential of the blood supply that would appear to be the critical factor. But an atrophic alveolar ridge may result from either disuse such as is the case when opposing teeth are lost or deficient endosteal blood supply generally through arteriosclerosis but also resulting from several other conditions listed later. The potential in disuse to respond favourably may well be better than when basic arterial insufficiency pertains. However, in both cases which are very difficult to differentiate, it is essential that increased loading be applied gradually. The method by which this may be accomplished is known as conditioning.

Clinical Assessment of Probable Bone Reaction to Increased Pressure

Whether a partial denture is mucosa supported or tooth supported, the ultimate structure that receives the load is bone. The periodontal membrane of the abutment teeth or the mucosal tissues covering the ridge are merely fibrous connective tissues via which the load is conveyed to the bone. Hence, an accurate assessment of the condition of the bone is the most important diagnostic procedure to be carried out before deciding upon any treatment plan involving partial dentures. Unfortunately no scientifically accurate method of making such an assessment exists. Two approaches, the anatomical and the radiographical, are, however, clinically useful.

1 Anatomical

An examination of the macroscopic anatomy of the edentulous alveolar ridges can be of some help. In cases where extractions have been carried out six months or more previously, a well-developed alveolar ridge, showing slow and minimal resorption after extraction, indicates that a high physiological limit exists and that the bone will stand up favourably to increased pressure. Such bone is often associated with a somewhat incompressible covering mucosa and is characteristically hard on palpation. The ridge crest, rather than feeling smooth is slightly undulating due to the slower resorption of the interdental septae. Whilst such a ridge stands up well to the pressure of a saddle by reason of its increased surface area, it also shows a resistance to osteolytic action. On the other hand, where there has been considerable resorption of the alveolar bone following extraction it is often found that further osteolysis follows the application of increased load.

An examination of the ridge form can be even more useful when the patient has been wearing a partial denture since its design will give an indication of the load placed on the ridge. If a well-preserved ridge form is found after a considerable period of wear, it can be assumed that the physiological limit of the individual is high. On the contrary, a discrepancy between the ridge form and shape of the fitting surface of the denture, coupled with some fibrous proliferation over the ridge crest, suggests a low tolerance to increased load, or a load greatly in excess of that which any bone could tolerate.

2 Radiographical

Two radiographical methods, not always completely corroborative, can be used to assess the probable reaction to pressure on alveolar bone.

The first method is to gauge the density of bone by a 'reasonably standardized X-ray exposure and processing technique'. Wilson has drawn attention to variation in osseous structure and describes dense, cancellous, and non-cortical types:

(i) *Dense.* Compact trabeculae. Medullary spaces are in the minority and the overall picture is one of opacity. The cortex is solid and well defined (Fig. 5.14). Such structure gives proportionately slow or little absorption, all other factors being constant. Providing the mucosa covering is of medium density this bone constitutes the optimum foundation for partial denture support.

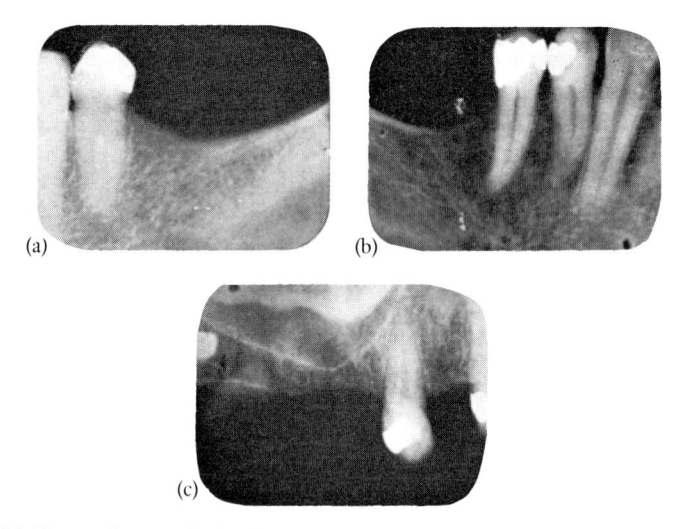

Fig. 5.14. X-rays showing Wilson's three classes of bone density. *a* Dense, *b* cancellous, *c* non-cortical.

(ii) *Cancellous.* Much lighter in structure. Trabeculae and medullary spaces more evenly balanced. The film appearance has more contrast. Cortex is defined but lighter in character (Fig. 5.14). When attention is given to occlusal and horizontal loading within the tolerance of such bone it supports the restoration very well, but, generally will not suffer abuses.

(iii) *Non-cortical.* This is one of the prosthetist's greatest problems. The bone is thin and radiolucent, poor in organic salts. There is no defined cortex the margin being feathery, thin, and often spiculated giving poor support for a denture (Fig.

5.14). Unless loading is strictly reduced there follows an endless history of discomfort and resorption.

A difficulty with this method is that even with apparent standardization of technique, films of the same area taken at different times give a variation in shadow density. This point made, however, it must be said that it is usually possible to decide into which of Wilson's three groups the bone falls, but regard must be paid to its location. For instance, the upper ridge does not normally show such a thick cortical plate as the mandible. The upper trabeculae, too, are finer than those in the lower jaw. Even in the lower jaw itself different normal appearances are obtained in different situations. The ridge in the region of the lower second and third molars is very wide, giving a dense radiographic appearance; this effect is intensified by the cortical bony plate being extremely thick in this region.

There is little doubt that dense bone structure in general stands up well to the demands of denture support. Since this bony structure has been built up under the influence of the three factors listed at the beginning of the chapter (and important among these is the influence of pressure) it must be assumed that this bone has demonstrated an osteosclerosis. It is logical to assume that this will continue.

Applegate has suggested a second radiographical method of assessing the tolerance of alveolar bone to increased load. In the partly edentulous jaw it often happens that certain teeth bear more of the masticatory stress than their neighbours. Applegate describes three such classes:

1 Those that have been subjected to more than normal stress by having to assume the functional load of missing adjacent teeth.
2 Those teeth that have been overloaded by stresses arising from occlusal interferences or traumatic occlusion.
3 Those teeth having increased stress loads due to the tooth being tipped (migrated) out of regular vertical positions, so that the normal occlusal forces are magnified by the factor of leverage.

Such teeth are readily recognized clinically and the reaction in their supporting bone can be used as an index of the expected change under the stress of a partial denture. Typical areas and situations which may give significant information by this method are (a) bone that has already had to support the abutment tooth of a partial denture, (b) bone supporting teeth adjacent to a posterior edentulous area, and (c) bone adjacent to a posterior tooth which is tilted mesially. In each of these situations the bone will have been subjected to loads in excess of normal. Where the reaction has been osteosclerotic it can be assumed that a favourable prognosis can be expected, when well-designed partial dentures are constructed. On the other hand, where the bone shows osteolysis in these areas it can only be inferred that the physiological limit is low and the prognosis unfavourable. Longitudinal radiographic studies have shown that a considerable proportion of abutment teeth will, after supporting a partial denture for four years, show a reduction of the level of the alveolar bone margin, both mesially and distally (Carlsson *et al.*).

This method probably gives the best index of the bone tolerance to increased load. The reaction to increased load in the patient's present condition is clearly represented as radiopacity or radiolucency. Further, no standardization of radiographic technique is required as a comparison is being made between two areas on the one film.

It is wise when assessing the 'bone factor' to take into account the patient's age and general health. Individual ability to meet environmental changes decreases with advancing age. It may be expected, therefore, that a more favourable tissue response would be met in the young adult than the older patient. In particular, the liability of bone to resorb under pressure at the menopause must be mentioned. This is caused by the hormonal imbalance at this period, particularly in respect of oestrogen. When a balanced hormonal state returns, the potentiality of the bone to react physiologically increases and a better prognosis exists for the partial denture.

Again, where the general health of the patient is not good, the ability to lay down extra bone is reduced. Diseases displaying a disturbance of protein metabolism particularly show an osteolytic tendency; among these are diabetes, the nephritides, duodenal ulcer, and tuberculosis.

Load Applied to a Denture Saddle

Load applied to a partial denture may be either vertical, lateral or anteroposterior, and any single saddle may, at different times, be called upon to resist loading in each of these different directions. To illustrate this point a lower posterior saddle carrying premolar and molar teeth may be taken as an example. In the power and second phases of mastication, before the teeth come into occlusion, an essentially vertical force acts on the saddle and this also applies when occlusion takes place in the tooth position in swallowing and empty occlusions. If the teeth come into occlusion (or near occlusion when a very resistant mass intervenes) during the later power strokes, a complicating anterior component of force is added to the vertical component, as a result of only the posteriorly facing inclines making contact with opposing upper teeth. In the second stage of mastication when contact of the buccally facing cusp inclines takes place prior to a slide into the tooth position, there is a lingually directed force acting on the saddle. In addition if the denture is rigidly constructed and has a posterior saddle on the other side of the mandible, stress in a buccal direction will be transferred to the saddle under consideration. Posterior movement of the saddle may be caused by rigid connection with an anterior saddle which is used during incision, or in day-time idiosyncratic movements, or in night-time grinding movements that involve an anterior displacement of the mandible with the opposing teeth in contact. It will be appreciated that had an upper posterior saddle been taken as the example the forces would have been opposite in direction. Finally it must be stressed that the above analysis is a simplification of the functional activity of the mouth, where inclined ridges and varying soft tissue displacements complicate the situation.

Traditionally, application of load to a denture saddle has been confined to load applied in the direction of the alveolus. However forces do act which tend to displace the denture saddle away from the covering alveolar ridge. In mastication an adhesive food bolus may drag the saddle away from its supporting tissue with considerable force. Again especially in wide opening of the mouth, facial and lingual muscles acting at the denture periphery often tend to unseat the dentures. A displacing force may also be generated from a taut inelastic mucosa in an old, atrophied mouth in extreme opening. In practical terms when determining the extension of the denture saddle it is wise to seek for a retentive denture when the mouth is held in a half open position. This compromised approach necessitates patient co-operation in limiting functional jaw movements to achieve comfort. If there is saddle displacement in function uneven occlusal contact takes place on the following mandibular closure and the denture is reseated dynamically rather than statically into a displaced position on the ridge; this may well be both damaging and painful. At the same time food may be allowed to move under the saddle and if this is hard (the seed of a raspberry is often cited by the patient) pain is experienced, which cannot be relieved without taking out the denture.

From a practical point of view all dentures should be designed to resist vertical and horizontal force on the saddles in all directions. This is necessary when it is remembered that the form of the residual ridge, because of its various alternatives, may convert a purely vertical load into horizontal components initiating saddle movement. Whereas the lower edentulous ridge may be horizontal in the premolar area, in the molar and retromolar area it slopes upwards and backwards to the mandibular ramus. In the upper jaw less constancy is noted in the antero-posterior inclination of the posterior ridge, sometimes it slopes upwards sometimes downwards, and sometimes parts of it may even show each of those contours. Looked at in coronal section, the palate is often seen to lie obliquely to the horizontal plane.

It has been pointed out that the magnitude of muscular load applied to the natural teeth may be assessed as approximately proportional to the degree of development of the muscles of mastication. When, however, a denture saddle is considered other limiting factors apply:

(i) *Pain limitation*. When load is applied by the saddle to the underlying ridge, nerve endings receptive to pain may be stimulated by being compressed against bone. Since this effect is increased as the load applied to the saddle is increased, the patient, consciously in the first instance and later as a learned pattern, comes to use a range of muscular force below the pain threshold. This predisposition to pain depends on the area of the saddle and the mucosal and bony conditions of the underlying tissues.

(ii) *Location of the saddle.* Different degrees of load are applied in the comminution of different types of food, and at the different stages of mastication. Since the power strokes invoke the strongest muscular effort a saddle carrying molar teeth is certainly going to be subjected, in the early stages of mastication of tough foods, to higher loading than one carrying premolars, which are concerned in the mastication of softer foods and only in the later stages in the mastication of harder and tougher foods. Generally the incisive function does not call for large muscular forces, but the small size of such saddles, may mean a large force is applied.

(iii) *Length of saddle.* Generally speaking the larger the number of teeth on a saddle the greater will be the total load applied to it; this factor should be related to the area of the fitting surface of the saddle.

(iv) *Size of the occlusal table.* By reducing the size of the occlusal surface on a saddle, a reduction is effected in the size of the bolus that can be comminuted between the opposing surfaces of the teeth. Since less food requires less masticatory force to effect its breakdown after the teeth come into occlusion, the amount of force exerted by the saddle on the ridge is reduced with a smaller occlusal table. The patient, however, takes a longer time to chew a fixed amount of any type of food.

(v) *Degree of food comminution acceptable.* The food is swallowed when it has been reduced to a state acceptable for swallowing by the individual. The degree of comminution required varies for different kinds of foods. It has been noticed that denture wearers accept a less well chewed bolus for swallowing than those who have maintained their natural dentition. The acceptance of this reduced degree of comminution preparatory to swallowing results in a reduction of the number of masticatory cycles used in the preparation of a given bolus.

As a corollary to this finding it has also been found that patients come to regulate the consistency of their diet to meet the limitations of their masticatory ability. This is wholly desirable and the attitude should be encouraged by the dentist. The point should even be extended to the giving of advice on the nature of the diet, assuming that the patient receives adequate nutritional components and sufficient roughage in appropriately reduced form. This is of course in accord with good medical advice directed at maintaining a healthy condition throughout the whole of the alimentary canal; old people especially are advised to take smaller, appropriately prepared meals more often.

Load Distribution in Partial Dentures

The source of energy acting on food being masticated, the partial denture and the dental apparatus, which includes the teeth, periodontium and supporting bone is dynamic, in other words it generates force by dint of motion and acceleration. The impact force in mastication is intended to deform the food bolus and eventually bring about its comminution. Unfortunately the energy cannot be centred on this action and the impact force is resisted both by the denture and the living tissue. The energy imparted through the bolus to the denture is partially absorbed by the appliance but this must always be restrained within its elastic limit otherwise unacceptable permanent deformation would result. The amount of energy absorbed by the denture depends on its modulus of resilience. The more rigid the appliance the greater is the energy imparted to the tissues which they are then called upon to accept (but within the elastic limit). Elastic deformation of a particular component of a denture may be arranged for in its design; for instance an acrylic resin tooth will be deformed more than a porcelain tooth, a special kind of metal connector known as a stress breaker may absorb considerable energy in being deformed elastically, or a resilient saddle lining may be stressed in the same way. The behaviour of such components is to absorb dynamic forces and to disperse less energy to the supporting living tissues; they also permit more or less load to be directed to different tissue structures—the alveolar bone or the teeth may be accorded a greater or lesser role in finally absorbing the imposed impact force, but it must be understood that this can only be an approximate matter. As well as reacting physically the tissues react biologically and although the physical reaction may be considered favourable from the restricted viewpoint of the force having acted within the elastic limit of the tissues, it may still be unacceptable biologically. For instance the patient may experience pain in the short term or the blood vessels may be damaged causing longer term tissue breakdown. Such biological reactions have their mental counterparts; if a patient finds excessive tissue deformation unacceptable confidence in his ability to use the denture will be eroded.

As a general rule it is wise to distribute the load applied to saddles as widely as possible. This is justified on the grounds that the pressure applied to a unit volume of bone will be reduced and therefore the physiological limit is less likely to be exceeded. Where a considerable number of teeth share the vertical and horizontal loads, the principle of splinting is employed. Wide distribution of load also demand maximal coverage of the edentulous ridges by the saddles and in some cases wide palatal coverage.

The principle of discriminative distribution of load should be practised in addition to that of wide distribution. It is possible to distribute the load applied to a saddle on the one hand between the periodontium of the teeth and on the other to the ridge and palate. In cases where the anabolic potential of the bone is high a successful result is obtained regardless of how the load is shared between these tissues. In other cases, again regardless of load distribution, an unfavourable result follows; such cases must be considered diagnostic and prognostic mistakes which require further mouth preparation perhaps including further or total extractions. In some cases, however, the tissue with the stronger anabolic potential may carry some additional load with advantage. For instance where the remaining teeth show advanced periodontal disease and for some reason are to be retained, as much as possible of the load may be placed on to the edentulous ridge. Alternatively where the ridge is atrophic it is sometimes good therapy to load as many standing teeth as possible and with bounded saddles not to use saddle contact with the ridge at all.

References

APPLEGATE O.C. (1959) *Essentials of removable partial denture prosthesis.* 2nd edition. W.B. Saunders Co., Philadelphia.

APPLEGATE O.C. (1961) Evaluating oral structures for removable partial dentures. *J. pros. Dent.* 11, 882.

CARLSSON G.E., HEDEGARD B., and KOIVUMAA K.K. (1965) Studies in partial denture prosthesis. *Acta Odont. Scand.* 23, 443.

LAMMIE G.A. (1960) The reduction of the edentulous ridges. *J. pros. Dent.* 10, 605.

MANLY R.S. and BRALEY L.C. (1950) Masticatory performance and efficiency. *J. dent. Res.*, 29, 448.

NEWTON A.V. (1964) A factor affecting the resilience of connective tissue. *Dent. Pract.* 14, 289.

PICTON D.C.A. (1963) The effect on normal vertical tooth mobility of the rate of thrust and time between thrusts. *Arch. oral Biol.* 8, 291.

PICTON D.C.A. (1969) The effects of external forces on the periodontium. *In*: Melcher A.H. and Bowen W.H. *Biology of the periodontium.* Academic Press, London: 363–419.

PICTON D.C.A. and DAVIES W.I.R. (1967) Dimensional changes in the periodontal membrane of monkeys due to horizontal thrusts applied to the tooth. *Arch. oral Biol.* 12, 1635.

PICTON D.C.A. and DAVIES W.I.R. (1976) A study of the fluid systems of the periodontium of macaque monkeys. *Arch. oral Biol.* 21, 1976.

PICTON D.C.A. and MANDERSON R.D. (1984) On the biomechanics of complete and partial dentures. *In*: Bates J.F., Neil D.J. and Preiskel I.W. *Restoration of the partially dentate mouth.* Quintessence Books, London.

PICTON D.C.A. and WILLS D.J. (1976) Viscoelastic properties of the periodontal ligament and mucous membrane. *J. pros. Dent.* 40, 263.

SMYD E.S. (1958) Role of mechanical stress in dentistry. *New York Dent. J.* 28, 227.

TOMLIN H.R., WILSON H.J., and OSBORNE J. (1968) The thickness and hardness of soft tissues. *Brit. dent. J.* **124**, 223.

WEINMANN J.F. and SICHER H. (1950) *Bone and bones, fundamentals of bone biology.* p. 137. C.V. Mosby Co., St. Louis.

WELLS D.J. and MANDERSON R.D. (1977) Biomechanical aspects of the support of partial dentures. *J. Dent.* **5**, 310.

6

A PERSPECTIVE ON PERIODONTAL DISEASE

The current paradigm on periodontal disease is that chronic marginal gingivitis extends by tissue continuity into a chronic periodontitis. Inflammation is considered to be the essential aetiological process, but those who advocate the mechanism are always careful to point out that a balance exists between the invasive nature of the disease and the containing action of what is always referred to as the host response. Especially during the last two decades, and probably because of the great advances made in the study of immunology, emphasis has centred on the destructive mechanisms involved in inflammation and emphasis on the concept of host response has been neglected. Possibly sight has been lost of the fact that primarily inflammation serves to contain a bacterial antigen.

In very recent times however, there has been a marked reaction emphasizing the critical role of the host response in the aetiology of periodontal disease, especially when this concerns the blood supply to the periodontium. It is felt that a balance of emphasis should now be restored and this brief conceptual presentation should seek to widen the paradigm even at the expense of making it more complex. Atrophy and traumatic occlusion must be accorded some significance in the aetiological complex of periodontal disease; however the contribution of inflammation must be preserved. This would necessarily make the hypothesis more tenuous and call for a tolerance of viewpoint characteristic of the noblest scientific attitudes, in the confident hope that real progress to understanding might be achieved. Truth can be approached but never reached and it would augur well to recall Claude Bernard's view that hypotheses are not right or wrong but productive or unproductive.

In this presentation it is proposed to consider the aetiology of periodontal disease in three temporal stages:
1 chronic marginal gingivitis
2 the breakdown of the marginal ligament and crestal alveolar bone
3 the extension of periodontal disease into the periodontal membrane.

1 Chronic Marginal Gingivitis

The critical observation upon which the inflammatory concept of periodontal disease is based is that if oral hygiene measures are suspended a chronic marginal gingivitis will ensue. This is true but it is necessary to add the rider that in some subjects the response is considerable and quick whereas in others it is much less in evidence and presents only after a time interval of a few weeks rather than a few days.

It is also necessary to differentiate two types of chronic marginal gingivitis which really represent two extreme conditions in a continuum of graded response. The first of these is chronic confined marginal gingivitis, well illustrated by the inflammatory reaction seen in the lingual gingiva where this is covered by a plate connector of a partial lower denture in the presence of substandard oral hygiene. Here the gingival margin has a continuous and uniformly red coloration. It bleeds easily when touched and is not accompanied by any oedema or fibrosis. The inflammation is contained and shows no tendency to spread into either the attached gingiva or periodontal membrane. The condition is essentially reversible and simply be re-instituting good oral hygiene it is resolved. Chronic confined marginal gingivitis must be differentiated from chronic oedematous marginal gingivitis which has a different clinical appearance. Here the affected gingival margin has a more purplish hue and is not affected uniformly. The interdental papilla is more critically involved with the intervening gingiva less influenced. Again the gingiva bleeds easily, but here there is associated oedema and swelling with these characters most noticeable in the interdental papilla. In this gingivitis spread is more noticeable first to involve the whole length of the gingival margin and then the attached gingiva where the characteristic stippling is lost. Spread of the inflammation into the periodontal membrane is more common than in the former case but still the gingivitis may exist without deeper extension for many years. Typically this type of gingivitis is seen in the twenties when the third molar attempts to erupt into an overcrowded arch. It is important to note that this gingivitis arises without any change in oral hygiene habit and cannot be resolved by attention to that matter. Because it arises in conditions of increased pressure on the tissues, amongst them the terminal vasculature of the gingiva, it became clear that the inflammation might be trophic in nature and indeed resolution can be attained by releasing the imposed pressure on the small vessels supplying the interdental papilla either by extraction or interstitial grinding of the teeth. The papilla is selectively involved since as distinct from the rest of the gingival margin, it derives more of its blood supply through endosteal vessels arising interdentally; the rest of the gingival margin receives significantly more of its blood supply via periosteal vessels.

In the genesis of chronic marginal gingivitis it is helpful to consider the tissue as being protected by a series of four barriers:
(a) the mucous barrier
(b) the crevicular transudate
(c) the bacterial plaque
(d) the epithelial barrier.

(a) *The mucous barrier* and (b) *The crevicular transudate.* In health a sheet of mucus is constantly drawn backwards across the oral mucosa towards the pharynx. Mucus is secreted by the numerous discrete glands of the oral mucous membrane and, being a lyophilic sol, it adsorbs the watery secretion of the salivary glands to form a mobile but viscous film which courses back over all the oral tissues. In moving back it picks up bacteria which are eventually transported to the stomach after swallowing where the hydrochloric acid secretion kills them. As well as transporting viable bacteria, in a physiological state the mucus should also adsorb the crevicular fluid which is either a transudate or an exudate transversing the gingival trough. This fluid is a derivative of tissue fluid and contains antibodies and leucocytes which have a defensive action. However, the crevicular fluid is a copious source of free amino acids required by many pathogenic bacteria. It is also a viable source of glucose and at different times may even provide the major source of soluble carbohydrate to the plaque organisms.

It is the availability of crevicular fluid at the gingival margin that localizes plaque formation in the gingival area. If plaque is allowed to accumulate the mucous barrier is prevented from adsorbing the crevicular fluid which becomes available *in toto* as a substrate source for bacterial growth. Production of exotoxins and endotoxins then takes place at an increased level and their concentrated action is directed at the marginal gingiva, in which inflammation is liable to ensue. In fact when good oral hygiene is not practised some gingivitis invariably results; upon its re-institution the mucous barrier may resume acting competitively with the developed plaque as an imbiber of crevicular fluid.

(c) *The bacterial plaque.* Thoughts on the action of plaque have centred on its action as a bacterial stressor and have disregarded an important concomitant barrier action centred in the plaque itself. Attempts to innoculate plaque successfully with a specific extraneous organism are generally unsuccessful. Plaque is a symbiotic complex of many different organisms whose mutual existence depends on the products of the others. In this circumstance it is not surprising that the introduction of a new organism is unlikely to find a niche in the chain of biological dependencies, long established, which provides a stable viable environment for the established zooglia. In this way the plaque itself displays a constancy and protects the underlying epithelium from the insult of some new potentially harmful pathogen.

(d) *The epithelial barrier.* Formerly as a result of Fish's analysis it was believed that the condition of the gingival epithelium was the critical factor in protecting the gingiva from bacterial insult. It must be appreciated that the surface layer of the epithelium is in a constant state of desquamation and as successive layers of squames are shed, so also are contaminating surface bacteria. However it must be appreciated that the junctional epithelium is only a few cell layers deep; it is, in fact, this very structure that permits the egress of tissue fluid or exudate. But there is no doubt that the action of toxins can further reduce the number of cell layers and affect unfavourably the nature and number of the intercellular bridges. In this condition the epithelium allows the easier ingress of toxins and egress of tissue fluid in increased amount. The depletion of the epithelial barrier constitutes a vicious circle which augments the gingivitis.

In general terms there are many chronic non-specific inflammatory processes which may persist for a long period of time but they are not deeply destructive, especially to the extent of involving bone. When chronic inflammation and deep destruction co-exist, either malignancy, as in the case of rodent ulcer, or a specific chronic infective process such as leprosy or tuberculosis where specific organisms can readily be demonstrated in the inflamed tissue, should be suspected.

However there are just a few acute surface inflammatory lesions which are deeply invasive and destructive. Cancrum oris is such a disease, but it has been suggested that the critical factor in the necrosis is a resistive incompetence due to an acute and complete vascular failure. A similar deeply destructive ulceration may be seen in the leg of a person suffering from vascular insufficiency secondary to varicose veins or diabetes. Such an ulceration is described as trophic and little importance is attached to the pathogenicity of the concerned organisms. Even acute ulcero-membranous gingivitis may damage tissue moderately deeply, but here again vascular compromise has been demonstrated associated with mental stress and cigarette smoking.

The initiation of any inflammatory process may be due to an increase in the pathogenicity of the external antigen or to a decrease in the resistive capacity of the host. This suggested that chronic oedematous marginal gingivitis may be trophic in nature and that both types of chronic marginal gingivitis are associated with the same mixed bacteria which do not invade the tissue.

2 The Marginal Ligament and Crestal Alveolar Bone

The term marginal ligament is used to describe the dense accumulation of collagen fibres that separates the periodontal membrane from the marginal gingiva. The term ligament is suggested by the very dense and orderly arrangement of the fibres and their relation to the periodontal membrane which is correctly classified as a joint; the suggestion is made that the marginal ligament is analogous to the capsular ligament of a limb joint. When the continuous figure-of-eight structure which surrounds all the teeth of the arch is considered as a single organ, the term composite marginal ligament is applied.

Arnim (1953) and others have described the microstructure of the marginal ligament which interdentally comprises the axial gingivae fibres originating both from the cementum of the tooth and the interdental bony septum; these include the transverse interdental or transeptal fibres which run from tooth to tooth above the crest of the septal bone and the alveolar crest fibres lying more apically which attack cementum to alveolar crest bone. Free gingival and circular fibres also are present in an integrated structure. Vestibularly and orally the structure of the marginal ligament is similar but interdental fibres are absent.

The marginal ligament is not in itself a vascular tissue, the capillary bed of the tissue not being extensive. Its metabolism appears to depend more on eddying movements of tissue fluid. However, the marginal ligament is permeated by vessels arising in, and draining to, the periodontal membrane. These vessels often enter the periodontal membrane through Volkmann's canals in the interradicular bone just apical to the marginal ligament, so that they course through the periodontal membrane for a short distance only. These are the important vessels which carry blood to and from the col and interdental papillae, and to a considerably lesser degree, to the marginal gingivae.

It must be appreciated that bone has both an endosteal and a periosteal blood supply. The endosteal supply derives from a nutrient artery which enters the bone through a nutrient canal, moves centripedally to the body of the bone where it courses to its extremity. Small vessels radiate off at intervals to move centrifugally and such vessels supply the interdental bone and periodontal membrane. The periosteal supply derives from different arteries and supplies the outer part of the cortical bone. The inner cortex has an endosteal supply as does all the cancellous bone. However it is important to appreciate that generically the lamina dura of the socket of the tooth is a condensation of cancellous bone and has only an endosteal blood supply. Only where the vestibular and oral alveolar plates are thin and this bone approximates to the lamina dura of the socket at the crestal edge does a dual blood supply exist with the advantage of a collateral circulation. The interdental septum and the col above it have an endarterial supply with no collateral circulation.

The marginal ligament serves these important functions:
(i) It is responsible for holding the marginal gingiva in close relation to the tooth and for maintaining a healthy gingival cuff; this action is calculated to minimize the subgingival extension of plaque.
(ii) The presence of a complete and dense marginal ligament prevents the extension of a marginal gingivitis into a periodontitis. The mechanical action of a dense fibrous tissue limits the spread of bacterial toxins and this is the explanation of the fact that both types of marginal gingivitis may exist for years without extending into a periodontitis. This is a special case of an observation made in the war before antibiotics became available that septic wounds hardly ever spread to involve joints.
(iii) It serves to distribute horizontal load to contiguous teeth and thereby preserve the supporting tooth tissues. The transeptal group of fibres are specially important in this function, which is often referred to as splinting action.

(iv) It resists the hypereruption of a single tooth and therefore preserves the occlusal pattern of the segment or arch; in this way the development of hyper-contacts is resisted.

(v) The transeptal fibres by dint of the contractile character of their fibroblasts serve to maintain firm contact between contiguous teeth. Loss of tooth substance interdentally as in filling and abrasion is compensated spontaneously and immediately as long as these fibres are intact.

If for any reason the marginal ligament is depleted on a coronal level it *tends* to regenerate at a more apical level. Within certain limitations which will be described later it has a potential to repair and reconstitute its integrity. In this way all of the actions of the marginal ligament are preserved. Especially important amongst these is the role of the transeptal fibres in maintaining a barrier interdentally between the gingival and periodontal compartments; their loss is the key to understanding the pathology of periodontal disease.

The breakdown of the marginal ligament and crestal alveolar bone

It therefore becomes necessary to study critically mechanisms which might cause a breakdown of the critical marginal ligament; three possible mechanisms are listed:
(i) the extension of the inflammatory process
(ii) ischaemia
(iii) traumatism.

The point must also be made that all three processes are not mutually exclusive; in fact the probability is that all three act conjointly. Certainly as periodontal disease progresses traumatism becomes a pervading and increasingly important complication. However there may be some prior importance of ischaemia over the ever present inflammatory condition, but it would be completely impossible to ascribe exclusive roles to either.

(i) The extension of the inflammatory process

It was formerly accepted that the existence of a chronic gingival inflammation exerted a continuous damaging action on the underlying periodontal membrane and that the inflammatory extension, postulated as the basic pathogenic process involved was a continuous and slow one. An edited report of an FDI/WHO Scientific Workshop (1980) discussed the pathology in these terms:

'The mechanism by which plaque organisms destroy gingival tissues, periodontal fibres and alveolar bone and cause changes in the cementum cannot be specified as yet. However, several direct and indirect mechanisms can be invoked to explain the initial changes in the superficial tissues and the progressive destruction of connective tissues and bone.

Direct mechanisms involve the production of histolytic enzymes (hyaluronidase, chondroitin sulphatase, collagenase and other proteinases) by several of the plaque bacteria. Cytotoxic agents like endotoxin are released during distintegration of Gram negative organisms and tissue metabolites (ammonia, organic acids, hydrogen sulphide) are regularly produced by plaque bacteria. All of these substances may singly or collectively have an adverse effect on normal tissue metabolism and produce inflammatory responses, some of which are themselves destructive. In addition agents produced by the plaque organisms indirectly stimulate host mediated responses, some of which are themselves destructive. Prominent amongst these individual mechanisms are the release of endogenous enzymes and immunopathological responses.

Recent studies of immunological responses have indicated the involvement of cellular and humoral mechanisms (leucocytes, lymphocytes, plasma cells, complement, etc.) in defence against bacterial antigens. There is also some evidence that some of these reactions may be detrimental to the periodontal tissues.

The presence, action and target tissues of each one of these mechanisms in the destruction of the periodontium have been reasonably well documented; however the relative importance of these factors and their combination in the periodontal destruction are not well understood'.

It must be appreciated that this represents a more or less complete catalogue of processes inherent in inflammation. Nobody would deny that inflammation has some role in periodontal disease and it would be surprising indeed if all of these mechanisms had not been demonstrated. But to infer that a unique causal relationship between these processes and periodontal destruction has been demonstrated is unsound. It must be appreciated that in the evolution of the inflammatory process a uniquely efficient process has not been developed; destruction of some tissue including collagen fibres and their immediately environmental ground substance invariably takes place alongside the wholesale destruction of the invading stressor. What really matters is the qualitative and quantitative balance which exists between tissue destruction and tissue repair, which continuously proceeds even in the physiological state. The remarkable overriding fact is the continuing preservation of a structural unity of the marginal ligament in the face of both superficial inflammation and persistent traumatic insult.

A specific inflammatory response may occur at any time. On immunological grounds it should be anticipated, however, that the incidence of these processes should decrease following exposure to a whole spectrum of organisms in younger years. Yet contrary to logical anticipation, periodontal disease is not seen commonly until middle adult life. At this stage too its incidence is widespread, the number of people entirely escaping the disease in later life being very small indeed. These parameters are not consistent with a simple inflammatory concept of the breakdown of the marginal ligament and the inception of periodontal disease.

In recent times two separate concepts of the inflammatory scheme have been put forward and it must be said that their acceptance goes at least some way towards better explaining the clinical signs and symptoms.

The first was put forward by Socransky *et al.* (1984) when it was demonstrated that the tissue destruction was not a continuous process but consisted of localized destructive episodes of short duration followed by much longer periods when the status quo was preserved. But this would put the inflammatory episode in either the acute or sub-acute category when it would be reasonable to expect evidence of clinical symptoms; however these are not usually evident. This approach would open the possibility of some specific organism especially of a Gram negative kind being effective over a short time. Again, however, it is difficult without some complementary change to account for the infection with such an organism.

The second inflammatory variation advanced especially in the last decade is the viewpoint that autoimmune disease has an important aetiological role. On the credit side, this hypothesis is theoretically, qualitatively and quantitatively capable of accounting for the speedy breakdown of the dense collagenous marginal ligament. It is, however, unable to account for the later containment of the lesion. Moreover any autoimmune disease is a relative rarity. True joints are involved in such a process in rheumatoid arthritis, but the incidence of this disease is 3% of the population and it can be seen in patients of all ages, but generally younger than is the case in periodontal disease.

(ii) **Ischaemia**

When a soft tissue is considered atrophy is associated with a reduction in volume of the organ concerned. It is also implied that the viability and metabolism of the organ are not changed. As the volume of the organ is diminished, however, so also is its potential to function at its former capacity. It is suggested that atrophy is a response to a depleting blood supply aimed at maintaining an effective, functional organ uncomplicated by degenerative change.

However when atrophy of bone is considered the freedom of the organ to contract does not exist to the same degree. Considering a long bone, its length and external form do not alter significantly, however, its diameter does show some reduction but not in the area of muscle attachments. Nevertheless atrophy does take place within the internal bony structure. The medullary cavity increases in size and loses its haemopoietic function. The cancellous bone comes to consist of this trabeculae, branching and with smooth surfaces mostly devoid of osteoblasts. The cortical bone too becomes thinned on its medullary surface.

However the architecture of the bone is preserved by the cortical bone and cancellous bone maintaining an integrated structure, since the endosteal blood supply is responsible for the metabolism of not only the cancellous bone but also the medullary aspect of the cortical bone; the periosteal component of the cortical bone is supplied by the periosteal vasculature, with an anastamosis between the two systems. These general principles of bone atrophy illustrated in the case of a long bone apply equally in the case of the jaw bones but some special additional features warrant description. Change with age in the mandible occurs with bone apposition on the posterior and superior surfaces of the condyle and a straightening out of the mandibular core (Murphy, 1964). The muscular processes decrease in size, and the core of the mandible straightens out becoming if anything longer with age. In the maxillae the size of the sinuses increases and loculi become less prominent.

However the most marked change is the reduction in length, height and width of the alveolar processes. In the edentulous subject loss of width is not uniform but is most marked on the buccal aspects of the alveolar plates in the anterior and premolar areas; this results with ageing in a posterior displacement of the alveolar process thus shortening the alveolar ridge as a whole. At the same time the oral and vestibular alveolar plates are reduced in height and are folded inwards towards each other. The net result of these concommitant actions is a reduction in the height and width of the alveolar ridges. The changes are of course seen in their most extreme form in elderly edentulous subjects, but it is certain that they are manifest whether or not teeth are present.

At this stage it becomes relevant to describe a clinical condition immediately recognizable to the experienced clinician. It is seen in patients in their twenties especially where there is a complete dentition and the dental arch width is large in relation to the basal bone; the condition, although not confined to the lower jaw, is typically seen there in relation to the canine and premolar teeth. Here the bone covering the buccal aspects of the roots of these teeth is thin and inverted interdentally. In fact the bone at the crestal margin shows no immediate cancellous structure between the buccal alveolar plate and the lamina dura of the socket. At the time of post-pubertal growth and during the period of anabolic activity in the early twenties the bone height and gingival margin are held in close relationship to the amelo-cemental bone and gingiva are seen to recede and cemental exposure of the root of the tooth becomes evident. In the presence of good oral hygiene no gingivitis accompanies this change and the structural integrity of the marginal tissues is maintained. Exposure is most marked where a tooth or one of its roots is displaced into the cortical bone outside the general contour of the arch. Gingival recession is permitted by resorption of the thin layer of bone in the absence of gingivitis. The recession of the gingiva and crestal bone has been a physiological response to depletion of the blood supply, a change which may take place in days rather than weeks.

A special case of this event deserves mention when there has been a fenestration in the alveolar plate just apical to an intact thin crestal ridge of bone. On atrophy there is a dramatic gingival recession to expose considerable depth of cementum. This results in dehiscence, a condition sometimes known as Stillman's cleft.

It is important to stress that these atrophic changes in the oral gingivae and alveolar plates are unassociated with regression in the corresponding interdental tissues. The appearance is of a very sharp and extended interdental papilla without gingivitis or oedema; it also appears to become more inverted and indeed may well do. At this stage there is no failure of the endosteal circulation and the interdental space is filled by normal bone, ligament and col tissues.

These observed macroscopic changes have their microscopic counterparts. Work by Atkinson *et al.* (1968) led them to conclude that 'once the mandible has reached maturity the resorption which contributed to the remodelling of the jaw during growth continues and becomes more extensive with ageing. Such resorption, when situated at specific sites along the alveolar crest, not only leads to an uneven distribution of porosity within the bone but also results in changes of shape typical of the edentulous senile mandible. The osteoporotic process is not dependent on the presence or absence of teeth for its patterns of distribution were similar in both cases. Although tooth extraction undoubtedly affects the crest height, we suggest that the pattern of osteoporosis is the result of an inbuilt predisposition to resorption which was established during growth. Such changes in the bone appear to be a major cause of tooth loss in the adult rather than a result of it'. The pattern of bone loss to which Atkinson refers is that the last bone to be deposited is the first to be resorbed. Again at the histological level Rowe (1983) concludes a study of bone loss in the elderly by stating 'the pattern of resorption seems the result of an innate predisposition of bone to resorb at specific sites along the alveolar crest, which had been established during the period of growth. This resorption which contributes to remodelling during growth, becomes more extensive with increasing age and leads to the uneven distribution of bone density and changes in shape characteristic of the edentulous senile mandible. *The resorption may be the cause rather than the result of tooth loss*'.

So far we have considered the early atrophy of the crestal bone of the alveolar plates where the arch is crowded or where there may even be a genetic disposition to an underdeveloped alveolar process. But later the atrophic process centres, not on the alveolar plates, but especially on the interdental bone. The form of this bone had previously remained stable or in rarer circumstances even slightly hypertrophied, but in the thirties and forties interdental atrophy is liable to ensue. The first signs of this in macroscopic terms is a blunting of the interdental papilla which reduces in height and becomes more everted. Especially in the buccal molar areas it appears that the gingival margin inverts less into the interdental alveolar depressions and the appearance of the gingival margin becomes more linear antero-posteriorly. With atrophy of the interdental bone a space is very quickly opened up between teeth. This is the outcome of the interdental bone having only an endosteal blood supply; there is no periosteal supply to impose the preservation of a genetic bony form. The lamina dura of the socket can rightly be considered as a condensation of cancellous bone even although its histological appearance may show areas of whorled bone, compact bone, callus and fibrous tissue. The essential feature of this bone is that in atrophy, unlike the cortical plates and like a soft tissue, it is free to recede and to re-establish at a level at which it is capable of being supported by the depleted blood supply. In fact this does happen and the characteristic lesion of periodontal disease is established; an interdental, intrabony pocket has been created. Observations on dried anatomical specimens are few but very revealing. Tel Haim (1984) describes how with age the interdental bone becomes successively convex, straight, then concave. Later frank craters appear in the interdental bone and these occur with increasing frequency from the anterior to posterior regions. This frequency coincides with the greater width of the interdental bone in the molar area. With this change in form the surface of this bone presents a changed appearance; its surface becomes less regular and is perforated by many canals. Above all its porous surface has retracted below that of the crest of the alveolar plates and with the eversion of the latter a stepped condition comes to pertain between the two rather than the smoothly curving crestal extremity of the circumferential alveolar bone. But such an irregular bony form precludes the existence of an intact marginal ligament as far as the individual tooth is concerned.

Still considering macroscopic change, if for any reason the teeth are permitted to move more closely together, the length of the composite marginal ligament will be reduced and its dimension will more closely approximate that of the atrophying alveolar process. In purely mechanical terms a strained condition would have been relieved.

Various clinical conditions often permit the teeth to approximate:

(i) *Horizontal stepping.* This is illustrated in Fig. 6.1. The original slightly buccal position of the lower first premolar is accentuated when the tooth tilts further buccally and the distance between the canine and second premolar decreases. There may also be a slight lingual displacement of the second premolar. Although the case illustrated is not uncommon, the continuing imbrication of a lower incisor is frequent.

It should be stressed that these horizontal tooth movements must be permitted by the occlusal condition. They do not arise where a positive occlusion permits no movement. Loss of an opposing tooth, a local open bite situation or flat cusps are all conditions which would favour horizontal stepping. It is also necessary to point out that a lateral tooth displacement in an atrophying alveolar process is necessarily accompanied by increased root exposure on the side towards which movement takes place.

A Perspective on Periodontal Disease

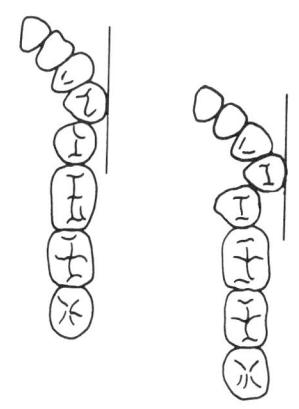

Fig. 6.1. Horizontal stepping. The original slightly buccal position of the lower first premolar is accentuated when the tooth tilts further buccally and the distance between the canine and the second premolar decreases. There may also be a slight lingual displacement of the second premolar.

(ii) *Vertical stepping.* Again the condition is best illustrated by reference to Fig. 6.2. The convex distal surface of the second premolar is accommodated into the concave mesial surface of the molar following hypereruption of this tooth. The shortening of the arch is also facilitated by the crown of the molar having a smaller circumference at its junction with the root than at its occlusal surface. Again the movement can only take place when the occlusion permits.

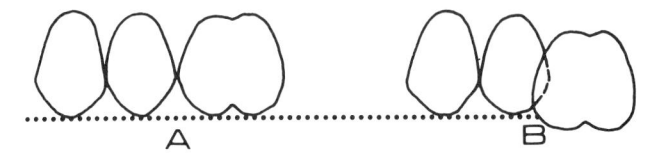

Fig. 6.2. Vertical stepping.
A The original condition.
B The situation following stepping of the molar.
The convex distal surface of the second premolar is accommodated into the concave mesial surface of the molar following the eruption of the tooth.

(iii) *Presence of an edentulous space.* The reduction in size of an edentulous space is noted in the absence of an occlusal stop. Space closure in this case is especially noted when a lower incisor tooth is extracted.

(iv) *Interstitial caries.* A sound tooth in a compressed arch is often seen to migrate into a large carious cavity on the interstitial surface of a contiguous tooth.

(v) *Attrition.* In primative peoples occlusal and interproximal attrition of the teeth is noted in considerable degree. The occlusal attrition frees the restrictions of cuspal interference and permits the reduction in mesio-distal tooth dimensions to result in a shortening of the arch and composite marginal ligament. This reduction is always dependent on the integrity of the marginal ligament and is greatly facilitated if the roots of the teeth are wholly accommodated within a core of cancellous bone. Where the cross sectional width of the alveolar ridge is small and all the roots indent into the cortical bone of the alveolar plate, tooth movement is restricted.

As a sequel to the shortening of the composite marginal ligament and the arch length, the volume of the cancellous bone between the roots of contiguous teeth is reduced. This would then permit a higher inter-radicular bony septum to be maintained at a level approximating to that of the alveolar plates; a physiological condition would be assured and a viable intact marginal ligament maintained on its interdental aspect.

Thus approximation of the teeth in the atrophying jaw most favourably permitted by abrasion is a natural compensatory mechanism preventing the onset of periodontal disease. Begg (1938) wrote: 'This continuous process of attrition must necessarily be considered along with the process of recession of the tooth investing structures in relation to the sequence of events which lead to pyorrhoea. It has been observed by the present writer that in the presence of active and marked occlusal and interproximal attrition, common to primitive man, pyorrhoea does not occur, while, in the absence of attrition pyorrhoea occurs. These studies would seem to amply demonstrate that in primitive man in whom attrition is generally found, there is a normal progressive obliteration and atrophy of the tooth, gingival periodontal fibres and alveolar bone, which when occurring in a proper sequence, diminished the possibility of pyorrhoea manifestations'.

It is postulated that for oral health an optimal relationship must exist between changes in the dentition and atrophic changes in the alveolar bone. However, naturally there is no possibility of adjusting the degree to which each class of change takes place. In contradistinction to many regulatory mechanisms, there is no feed-back process. There is a genetically inherited and environmentally influenced plan for change in the vascular bed and associated changes in bone atrophy and reduction of the marginal ligament. That such a mechanism is far from perfect is apparent from the prevelance of periodontal disease in modern man. Murphy (1964) put the case well when he wrote 'nature works to an anticipated degree of tooth attrition'.

At the histological level the diagram reproduced in Fig. 6.3 clearly shows how the volume of the interdental bony septum has been reduced giving a structure only somewhat reduced in height and one comparable with that of the alveolar plates. Generally speaking, and always with conically shaped, single rooted teeth, the form of the interdental bone is not quadrilateral but triangular in longitudinal section with the apex at the crestal margin. The consequence is that a small dimunition in blood supply to this structure is going to result in a considerable reduction in the crestal height of the septum.

A Perspective on Periodontal Disease

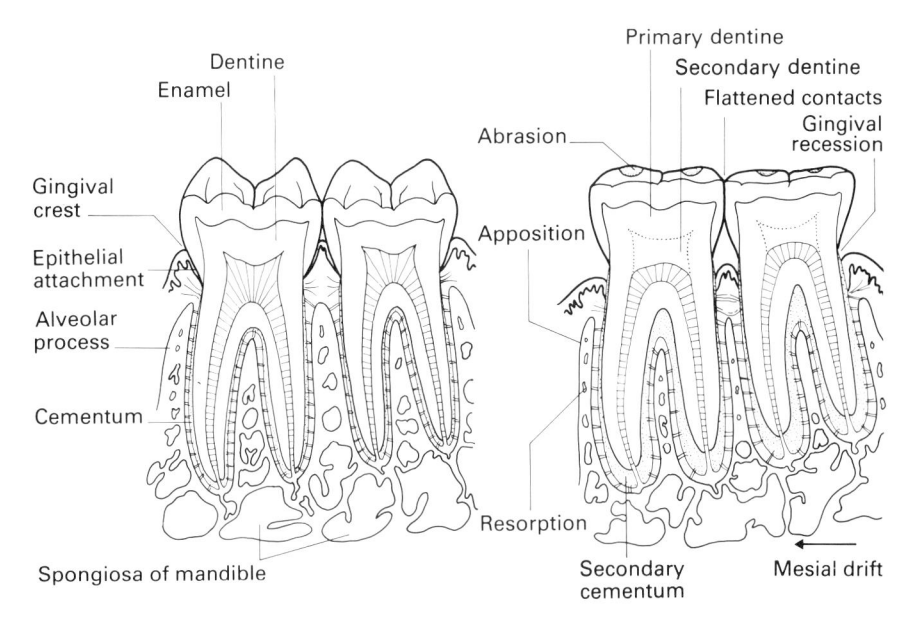

Fig. 6.3. Diagram of the changes in the tooth and their supporting tissues which occur in the presence of attrition. The presence of occlusal and interstitial attrition, cemental deposition and reduction in volume of interradicular bone should be noted.

It is now necessary to introduce a complication which is seen especially in the molar and even on occasion in the lower incisor area. In the molar areas buttressing of the crestal terminations of the alveolar plates may be considerable. In other words a substantial volume of cancellous bone lies between the compact plate of the alveolar process and the lamina dura of the socket. Whereas, say in the premolar area, the face of the compactum of the alveolar process is vertical and closely approximated to the lamina dura, in the molar area the terminal approach to the crest of the socket is definitely oblique and sometimes more closely approaches the horizontal. When atrophy of the alveolar plate occurs inward realignment of the plate as a result of resorption and remodelling does not take place in the molar area as it does elsewhere; this is especially noted where there has been some associated hypereruption of the tooth (see later). Examination of dried anatomical specimens clearly shows that the smooth periosteal bone terminates just short of the rim of the socket and the bony surface in this area is rough and perforated. The reason for the lack of recontouring of the alveolar plates is not only their original form but also the presence of muscle insertions immediately proximate to the crest of the socket. Reference to Fig. 6.4 shows the areas of insertion of the buccinator, superior constrictor and mylohyoid muscles relative to the margin of the molar sockets in the mandible. In the

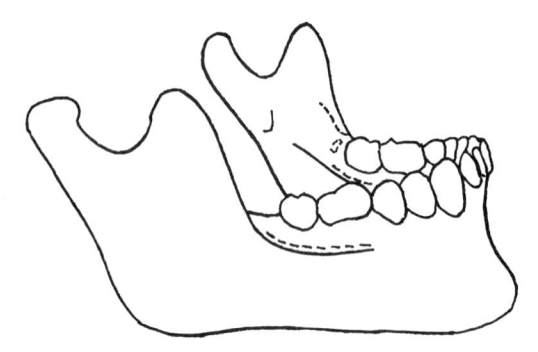

Fig. 6.4. Shows the proximity of muscle attachments of buccinator, mylo-hyoid, superior constrictor and temporalis muscles to the crestal bone of the molar alveoli in the mandible. The proximity of the heavily buttressed bone of the oblique ridges is also apparent.

maxilla the buccinator again has a proximate origin and one of the heads of the medial pterygoid originates from the distal aspect of the maxillary tuberosity (Fig. 6.5). Every dentist has noticed how in an old edentulous person with the most severe ridge atrophy the genial tubercles giving origin to the genioglossus muscle do not resorb and come to protrude as a bony elevation into the atrophic mucosa of the floor of the mouth. Areas of muscle attachment to bone are very resistant to remodelling; muscles cannot lengthen perceptibly to accommodate a change in bony form. Thus it arises that the alveolar plates in the molar areas are restrained from remodelling into closer apposition with the socket and a narrow ring of bone without periosteal blood supply comes to encircle the tooth. This ultimately may give rise to a compound periodontal intrabony pocket encircling the tooth rather than confined to its interproximal aspect.

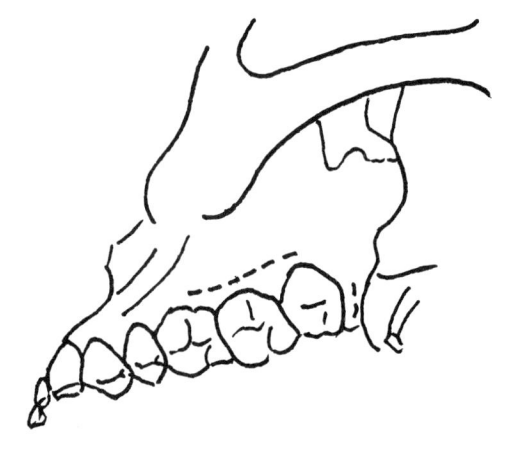

Fig. 6.5. Shows the proximity of muscle attachments of buccinator and small head of medial pterygoid muscle to the crestal bone of the molar alveoli in the maxilla. The proximity of the heavily buttressed root of the zygomatic process is also apparent.

If it appears that the role of atrophy has been more concerned with the crestal bone of the alveolar socket this is because it is much more readily observable than the overlying marginal ligament. However since this is a more terminal tissue in an end organ blood supply, ischaemic embarassment must be even greater than in the more distal bone. Newman (1982) reviews the position well: 'Tissue damage proceeds from the gingival connective tissue until the transeptal fibres are involved. The main body of the ligament shows little inflammatory change throughout the disease process (James and Counsel, 1927; Wade, 1965). The principal alteration is progressive destruction spreading apically from its coronal periphery. The alveolar bone seems to show more dramatic changes than the periodontal ligaments (James and Counsel, 1927). The ligament fibres initially lose their attachment to bone and then to cementum. If occlusal trauma be a complication, the ligament may be involved before the bone'.

Although the suggestion is sometimes made that the periodontal tissues 'retreat in good order' it should be appreciated that the tissue that more deeply replaces the atrophied transeptal fibres in the absence of abrasion has not its dense structural integrity and has begun to show zonal inflammatory infiltration. It cannot be expected that a highly organized tissue can be replaced by one of substantially increased area in the face of a compromised blood supply. Most importantly this granulation tissue, well developed as it may be, falls short of its predecessor in resisting inflammatory extension, imposed horizontal loading and hypereruption. The previous compartmentalization of gingival and periodontal zones is compromised. The structural integrity of the marginal ligament interdentally can only follow approximation of contiguous root surfaces permitted by interproximal tooth abrasion.

Causes of periodontal ischaemia

So much emphasis has been accorded to the depletion of the endosteal blood supply that it becomes necessary to summarize the different causal mechanisms which might well act conjointly. All of these have been shown to be associated with the incidence or increased progression of periodontal disease. It is not however proposed to deal with these conditions other than superficially. These conditions may be classified:

(i) *Continuous pressure imposed on terminal vasculature.* Continuing pressure resulting from tooth eruption into an overcrowded arch leads to pressure on the terminal vasculature, causes relative stasis and chronic oedematous marginal gingivitis. After a considerable time a strained condition acting on the arteriolar endothelium may contribute to a hyaline type of arteriosclerosis.

(ii) *Insufficient provision of blood to the peripheral circulation.* Cardiac failure is present when the diseased heart is unable to maintain a cardiac output adequate for the needs of the body. This arises when the heart is required to meet an increased mechanical load, when the performance of the cardiac muscle is impaired or when disease processes interfere with cardiac filling. When cardiac failure is sustained for a long time all organs suffer, among them the periodontium.

Another condition, considered physiological rather than pathological, which is associated with compromised peripheral circulation is pregnancy. Hormonal change has often been invoked to account for pregnancy gingivitis but the more likely cause is direction of the available circulation to the developing fetus.

A condition representing the antithesis of peripheral vascular failure was seen in a patient with considerable periodontal disease who developed a thyrotoxicosis; the increased cardiac performance resulted in an improved periodontal status.

(iii) *Obliterative ateriopathies.* This is a generic term used synonymously with arteriosclerosis to describe degenerative lesions in the walls of arteries which intrude into the lumen and cause a mechanical impedence to the circulation. When the lesion affects the elastic arteries it is known as atheroma and is associated with increased diastolic blood pressure and increased cholesterol blood level. In the muscular distributing arteries (maxillary, mandibular, lingual, palatal) similar lesions have been described and are calculated to embarass blood flow through the reduced lumen. At the level of the small arteries and arterioles arteriosclerosis characterized by the deposit of an eosinophilic, hyaline material within the vessel wall is seen. It is believed that this material derives from the circulating plasma and as in the case of atheroma a strained condition on the endothelium favours its permeation into the vessel wall and causes occlusion. This type of lesion is particularly associated with diabetes mellitus. A rarer type of atherosclerosis seen in larger periodontal vessels is more fibrotic and resembles the endartitis obliterans of vessels seen at the base of a gastric ulcer. There is abundant evidence in the dental literature of the association of these types of occlusive, degenerative arteriopathy and early periodontal disease. Much of the work on this aspect has been done in Eastern European countries where in the last four decades the aetiology of periodontal disease has been considered as arising entirely from them, whereas in Western countries it has been considered entirely inflammatory. The truth, as stated earlier, probably lies in the combination of the two processes within a more complex aetiology.

(iv) *Peripheral action of stressors on the terminal vascular bed.* Drug action, axon reflex and hormonal action are important stressors which act on the small arteries and arterioles of the gingivae and periodontium through contraction of the smooth muscle component of the media. Again two or all of these mechanisms may act in association or implement the ischaemic effect of the previous conditions. These conditions are:

(a) Action of nicotine in smokers
(b) Axon reflex following exposure to cold
(c) Protracted mental stress acting through the vasoconstrictors adrenaline and noradrenaline. (The hypothalamic–pituitary–adrenal cortical axis also acts by producing an increase in the level of the circulating glucocorticoids, which have a facilitatory effect on the catecholamines.)

Specific deficiency states. In addition to the above conditions which produce an ischaemia, some deficiency states act in the presence of an adequate circulatory status; their effect, however, is very similar and results from depleted delivery of specific chemicals necessary for metabolism to the tissues of the periodontium. All of these are metabolic requirements of fibroblasts and their near relations, osteoblasts. All are required in the complex synthesis of collagen. Too often in this greedy world we have seen evidence of starvation and depleted protein intake; the necessary amino acids are not available to form the polypeptide chains in the formation of collagen. Ascorbic acid, deficiency of which causes scurvy, and ferrous iron are also required in the concatenation of biological sequences needed for collagen formation; calcium is necessary for the modification of the ground substance characteristic of bone formation. Above all oxygen is required; the early intracellular stages of collagen formation can procede in the absence of oxygen but it becomes necessary for the still *intra*cellular synthesis. Oxygen is also critical to the action of both osteoblasts and osteoclasts. In conditions of anaemia periodontal involvement is frequent. But at other extremes in a patient treated with hyperbaric oxygen for disseminated sclerosis, resolution of a chronic oedematous marginal gingivitis was noted. Furthermore it is recalled that in the fifties a rather creative Canadian dentist Box, was treating periodontal disease with oxygen therapy.

(iii) Traumatism

It has become obvious that traumatism is not the rather simple physical issue it used to be considered. The mechanical concepts, although more complex than were formerly realized, remain more straightforward than the associated biological changes that precede and follow traumatism. It is certainly not now sufficient to dismiss the whole biological reaction by stating that up to a certain critical and variable level imposed load is stimulating, but above that load tissue destruction takes place.

Picton (1984) noted that after protracted loading a significant extrusion of a tooth continued in diminishing degree for several hours provided all occlusal contact was prevented during this period. Since the extrusion was accompanied by rhythmic pulsations due to heart beat and to breathing, it was concluded that the extrusion was caused by forces generated in the periodontal membrane resulting from biochemical changes rather than by alteration in the vascular status. This experimental finding accords well with the functional observation of Berry *et al.* (1984) who found that after a period of stress the teeth had moved so that the previously existing tooth position could not be re-established exactly; some teeth had been extruded more than others; they also found that following a period of relaxation and presumably the removal of protracted interocclusal loading, the occlusal status quo was re-established.

Picton considered that the lack of intrusive loads would have enabled progressive repolymerization of ground substance, with rebinding of water in the ligament. This would have resulted from more water entering the ground substance from the capillaries. Such an increase in periodontal fluid would have caused the pressure to rise and the tooth to be extruded proportionately. This would have continued until the restraining force of tension developed in the gingiva and in the apical and alveolar crest fibres to equal the force from the expanding ligament.

The above descriptions refer to the healthy periodontium, but a different situation pertains when the marginal ligament has been depleted by either inflammation or ischaemia. Considerably increased extrusion of the tooth is permitted and its mobility is clinically demonstrable.

It is apparent that this mechanism is a reaction intermediate in time between the evanescent extrusion of a tooth immediately following a single imposed thrust and tooth movement within the jaw bone accompanied by structural alveolar change which requires a time period of weeks or months. It should be regarded as a probable necessary precursor of this later established architectural change in relationships of tooth, periodontal membrane and alveolar bone. The long term favourable outcome is the re-establishment of all of these tissues in previously existing structural form but accommodating a changed tooth position.

In this mechanism and considering the more studied and less complicated situation pertaining in horizontal tooth movement, histological changes are first noted in the side of the periodontal membrane towards which horizontal movement is affected, as indicated by the appearance of osteoblasts and increased DNA production. On the contralateral aspects a strained condition is evident in the collagen fibre groups, but it is only later that osteoblasts appear active. On the compressed side osteoblasts remove the lamina dura of the socket provided a low order of force is operating. After a balanced tooth position has been attained osteoblastic activity supercedes and woven bone is laid down to reform the lamina dura in the newly established tooth position. Again on the side under tensile stress following primary osteoblastic endeavour considerably delayed osteoblastic activity generates within the cancellous bone. The structural status quo is re-established but with the tooth in a new equilibrated position.

It should be remembered that bone is a living tissue which grows in the young and repairs itself in the adult, but it can only do these things if it is supplied with oxygen and the other necessities for bone formation including glycogen, amino acids, vitamins, hormones and mineral ions. It is probable that bone tissue is specially sensitive to oxygen tension and that the osteoclastic potential of the osteocyte is favoured by a small decrease in oxygen tension whereas the opposite trend favours osteoblastic action. Another explanation invokes piezo-electric property of living bone. It is known that a distorted trabeculum develops a negative charge along the concave surface and a positive charge on the surface rendered convex. The negative charge is believed to be the stimulus for the appearance of osteoblasts and therefore bone deposition; whereas osteoclasis is stimulated on the side showing a positive charge. This observation accords well with the observation that whereas bone resorption is constantly seen, cemental resorbtion is rare. This arises since strain in the cementum is not conspicuous because of the resistance of the more rigid tooth substance to deformation and therefore change.

It is necessary to discriminate at this stage between two actions of the marginal ligament. The first is its ability to resist load and extrusion and these qualities are dependent on the quality of the collagen component. The higher the collagen component the greater its resistive potential and the stronger the ligament. But this is not the whole story for the capacity of the ligament to absorb load without permitting tooth movement is also dependent on the maturity of the constituent collagen fibrils and its association with cross linkages between fibrils. The organization of fibrils into fibres and fibres into ligament also significantly affects the strength of the tissue. All of these conditions are controlled by the ability of the fibroblasts to effect regeneration and repair of the ligament. In a condition tending towards ischaemia the cells can only accomplish this by reconstituting the ligament as a tissue in equilibrium with its blood supply at a lower level on the tapered root of the tooth. But this cell activity is necessarily preceded by three distinct processes:

(i) apoptosis
(ii) reactive hyperaemia
(iii) fibroblast stimulation.

(i) *Apoptosis.* Neither frank coagulative necrosis nor inflammation is present in the atrophying marginal ligament. However there is a constant loss of mature cells and replacement by the mitotic activity of their fellows. Recently the concept of apoptosis has been introduced to account for these observations. The degenerating cell condenses, apparently due to the loss of water, to form a pycnotic nuclear mass surrounded by a depleting cytoplasm and is known as an apoptic body; this body eventually disappears in a process known as 'cell defaecation'.

(ii) *Reactive hyperaemia.* It has already been emphasized that the regenerated, more economically sustained marginal ligament can only be reformed as a result of a temporarily increased metabolism. This demands a temporary, local hyperaemia. The existing vascular bed is opened up by an axon reflex and the creation of a new vascular bed stimulated by the action of chemical mediators such as histamine, various kinins and prostaglandins. The biochemistry of all the mediators proposed for establishing the hyperaemia, many with independent cascades of enzymes and interactions, is so complex that the workings of 'the soup' remains an enigma.

(iii) *Fibroblast stimulation.* The fibroblasts concerned in regeneration appear to originate in adjoining tissue and migrate into the field of repair. Two actions are proposed for the initiation of this activity. The first presumes the restraining action of a chalone which holds mitosis in check in the physiological condition. In regeneration the action of the chalone is inhibited locally. The alternative or additional method is by the release of a specific growth factor.

The nature of the forces that bring about tooth movements which in the past were known as mesial drift when horizontal, and continuous eruption or hyper-eruption when vertical, is still speculative. In the case of horizontal movements the cause is clearer as it can be prevented by severing the marginal ligament interdentally; it is reasonable to assume from this that the recently discovered contractile ability of the fibroblast provides the generative force.

The importance of the strained marginal ligament in resisting extrusion of the tooth has already been described, but the apical fibre system must also be accorded some place in resisting tooth movement and stabilizing tooth position and occlusion. The tooth cannot erupt without placing its apical fibres under tension, a condition calculated to resist movement. The importance of the contribution of this action is revealed in the local deposition of the cementum in the apical region to regenerate new tissue, a condition which is not seen to the same degree in other areas of the root other than in sites of function; the apical area being nearer to the source of the endosteal blood supply is more favourably placed than the marginal tissues of the tooth to respond to imposed strain in an ischaemic state. The conclusion is probably justified that the apical and marginal fibre systems are jointly concerned in the control of the degree of tooth movement and the preservation of a structural integrity in the face of atrophy.

The site of ischaemia and resulting tooth movement is very often localized and the outcome is that movement vertically and horizontally may well be, and very often is, restricted to one tooth. This means that in the absence of attrition the whole of the masticatory force comes to be imposed initially on this tooth when the jaws are occluded. Such is the genesis of traumatism or traumatic occlusion. Traumatic breakdown of the marginal ligament is inevitable and a vicious circle has been entered. Not only are the fibres more stressed and disrupted but damage to the small blood vessels in the marginal area where tooth movement is greatest, is likely; a further ischaemia of traumatic origin is added to that of atrophic origin and regeneration is sadly embarrassed.

The imposition of occlusal traumatism may be avoided when the periodontium of the tooth is not in an ischaemic condition and when its circulatory status favours anabolism. Such a condition is frequently seen clinically and has been studied experimentally when a filling in a tooth has been left in a high position. The extrusion of the tooth is opposed by a sustained intrusive force reflexly imposed by the opposing occlusion and the reaction is entirely different. Without change in tooth position the initial hypermobility is accommodated by a widening of the periodontal membrane especially marginally and hypertrophy of the marginal ligament ensues. It should be emphasized that the type of reaction that actually occurs depends on the vascular status of the periosteal tissues at the time. In youth and early adult life the reaction is likely to be stimulating and the marginal apparatus responds with hypertrophy; in middle adult life and old age the effect will more surely be catabolic.

Traumatic occlusion is unlikely to be a primary cause of marginal ligament breakdown as in the case of inflammation and atrophy, but it most certainly augments the primary action of these two and more quickly effects ligament dissolution and the inception of deeply progressive periodontal disease.

So far the genesis of traumatic occlusion has been envisaged in one particular case, that when it results from local tooth movement following ischaemia and atrophy. But it may arise in several other ways and again the reaction in the affected periodontium may be either hypertrophic or destructive:

(a) loss of teeth
(b) straightening of the mandibular core
(c) eruption into an overcrowded arch
(d) interocclusal intrusions.

(a) *Loss of teeth*. Every experienced clinician has seen that loss of a large number of teeth resulting in the loss of even more opposing occlusal contacts results in traumatic overloading of the periodontium. In such a situation the provision of partial dentures may make a significant contribution to treatment simply by reducing the load the periodontium is required to accept and retrieving the situation from a pathological one to a physiological one. Here the edentulous ridges and hard palate are required to accept a share of the imposed load.

(b) *Straightening of the mandibular core.* This anatomical change was first described by Murphy (1958). As a result the mandibular dental arch moves anteriorly in relation to the maxillary arch. If there has been considerable occlusal abrasion, posterior traumatic occlusion is not generated but where the cusps are marked this safeguard does not operate. It is, however, in the anterior segment that special results of this condition are most evident. Where the overbite is small and where there has been some incisal abrasion a normal overlapping incisor relationship comes to be replaced by an edge-to-edge bite and trauma is avoided.

When, however, the overbite is marked and the change in mandibular form extreme, damage in one of two possible directions is inevitable. If abrasion is marked and compensatory action for the development of periodontal disease evident, palatal loss of upper incisor tooth substance can be extreme; in the fifties and sixties this can result in the upper incisors being reduced to thin labial facings of enamel poorly supported by a thin layer of sclerosed dentine; eventually fracture occurs. The alternative when the tooth structure is preserved is the inception of marginal ligament breakdown of the maxillary anterior teeth with characteristic elongation and splaying greatest at the incisal edges. A third very rare alternative is the development of a temporomandibular arthrosis. Satisfactory treatment of this class of condition has been extraction of one lower incisor.

(c) *Eruption into an overcrowded arch.* This event generally takes place with the advent of the eruption of the third molar in the early twenties when the outcome is likely to be hypertrophy and some hypermobility. This is especially noticeable in the most posterior molar and the first premolar, as the latter is restricted in forward movements by the stability of the long rooted canine.

(d) *Interocclusal intrusions.* Two specific examples of this event are so commonly seen as to warrant description. First, after the inception of periodontal disease in the upper anterior teeth hypereruption results in the downward movement of the incisal edges. Associated with the breakdown of the transeptal fibres a forward tilting of these teeth takes place under the traumatic action of the lower incisors as they occlude. Especially where the overjet is marked the previous stable condition when the lower lip lay in repose over the labial surface of the upper incisors, may come to be changed with the interposition of the lower lip between the palatal surface of the upper incisors and the labial surface of the lower incisors. An additional, constantly acting, traumatic insult is thereby imposed which, happily, can be dramatically treated simply by grinding the incisal edges, and later the proximal contacts of upper and lower incisors. Not only is the previous lower lip position restored and the trauma averted, but the appearance is agreeably restored. In this therapy the lower lips again come to exert a backward pressure against the labial surface of the upper incisors and movement of these teeth to re-establish proximal contact is induced, and tightening of the loose teeth is spectacularly effected. This comes about through harnessing a natural orthodontic force and suggests a place for orthodontic appliance therapy to restore proximal tooth contacts after grinding in the posterior segments of the mouth.

In the second condition in this class a foreign body is habitually interposed between the dental arches and may act traumatically. The commonest is a pipe, but a pencil or pen may be the offending article in a stress idiosyncrasy.

All of the above descriptions apply to a situation which may be described as chronic traumatism, to distinguish them from another group of acute events of traumatic genesis, fortunately much rarer in incidence. In the most severe trauma a tooth may be completely evulsed. More commonly acute trauma may cause a subluxation when the tooth is displaced from its original position with some alveolar fracture and tearing of the marginal ligament. Various degrees of looseness of the tooth reflect the magnitude of the damage. In such an event whether recovery is likely or not depends on the repair potential again dependent on the blood supply. It must be borne in mind that gross damage to the marginal ligament and periodontal membrane not only decreases tooth support but opens the whole periodontal membrane to infection and the possibility of abscess formation.

Another example of acute traumatism arises with an oblique root fracture; this may arise from a traumatic accident or as a fatigue fracture in a crowned tooth where the post is supported by an inadequate root volume. The significance of such an event is that a communication between the exterior oral environment and the periodontal membrane may be created, and bacteria may invade the latter, bypassing the barrier action of the marginal ligament.

Abrasion as a compensatory mechanism

Although reference has been made to the role of abrasion as a compensating mechanism in the preservation of the structural integrity of the periodontal membrane, it would help to give an integrated description of its mode of action.

Abrasion may occur naturally or as a result of grinding as an operative dental procedure. In the former the abrasive material may be included in the food and in primitive populations because of the methods of food preparation there is significant abrasive contaminant resulting in enamel wear; an example of such an action is the incorporation of sand in the cooking of meat by Australian Aborigines. Even in modern society abrasive material in the form of small enamel particles may be autogenously developed in grinding; another less frequent source is the abrasive inclusions in tobacco used for chewing. Natural abrasion occurs slowly and is accompanied by a peripheral occlusion of the underlying dentine so that a patent outlet for dentinal fluid and caries is avoided as dentine is exposed. In the development of occlusal abrasion, the first stage is the formation of a circumscribed, highly polished, enamel facet without penetration of the enamel layer. However, eventually the dentine is exposed, first as a small area in the centre of a facet. This event releases enamel fragments from the edge of the lesion and this accelerates the rate of surface breakdown. Enlargement of the facet is followed by coalescence of several to give a large exposure of sclerosed dentine. Finally the whole occlusal surface comes to consist of exposed dentine with only a peripheral encircling wall of enamel. On the interstitial aspect the wear facet simply increases in diameter and again eventually involves the dentine.

Occlusal abrasion has two distinct advantages in preventing the progress of periodontal disease. First the cusps of the tooth are gradually reduced and eventually a flat occlusal surface results; this then permits horizontal movement of the teeth of opposing arches without cuspal interference and the development of traumatic occlusion. Wear of the incisal edges of the anterior teeth as the mandibular core lengthens can be considered a special case of the same principle. Additionally as the tooth erupts further its crown is shortened. Reduction in the length of the clinical crown reduces the torque acting in horizontal tooth loading and effectively preserves the vasculature and marginal ligament. Reduction in the height of the crown also preserves the height of the interocclusal clearance and does not require muscle lengthening.

Interstitial abrasion acts beneficially on the tissues of the periodontium by allowing contiguous teeth to approximate as the need arises for the marginal ligament to shorten. Tooth contact is preserved by the contractile effort of the fibroblasts of the transeptal fibres, while the volume of the interdental bony septum is reduced permitting its failing blood supply to support a crestal bone level proximating to that of the alveolar plates. A structural condition is thereby created for the integrity of the marginal ligament. When interstitial abrasion is absent as atrophy proceeds the integrity of the marginal ligament is lost and the granulation tissue which replaces it is less well adapted to prevent extension of a marginal gingivitis and to splint adjacent teeth and thereby distribute lateral load. This tissue is also less well equipped to effect closure of a gap between adjacent teeth. Since the teeth may now be prised apart in mastication, interdental packing of food fibres becomes an unpleasant consequence of eating meat and vegetables; the teeth are torqued in their sockets and the small vessels further stressed to compromise the blood flow. Again after the application of a matrix band when filling a compound cavity, space closure is not effected.

3 The Spread of Periodontitis Following Marginal Ligament Breakdown

The background condition against which the further advance of periodontal disease must be viewed is one of continuing ischaemia. As with growth, however, atrophy is not a continuous process but progresses by short sporadic incidents. This view accords well with the similar progress of periodontal disease. Therefore one can never say the disease has been cured or even permanently halted, as would logically be possible if inflammation were the sole cause. The progress of the disease may, however, always be retarded even when a mixed aetiology is granted. The view at this stage must be one of trying to reduce the destructive mechanisms and facilitating repair. The further progress of periodontal disease will be considered from the viewpoints of infection, tissue configuration and tooth mobility; these are the very same factors as an orthopaedic surgeon would consider when treating a bone fracture or ligament damage.

(i) *Infection.* Unless the structural integrity of the marginal ligament is preserved at the same qualitative and quantitative level it must be said that the barrier action to the extension of inflammation is depleted. In practical terms it is probable that this circumstance prevails. However, the repaired tissue does have a considerable but variable value as a barrier. One fact on the debit side is that the crestal bone covered by the defective fibrous tissue is structurally more vulnerable to the spread of inflammation on account of its porous structure.

Although not considered as important as formerly, pocket formation now deserves consideration. The bacterial plaque, the source of the toxins accredited with antigenic capacity lies in contact with the junctional epithelium lining the periodontal pocket. With the dissolution of the marginal ligament at its most coronal level and its replacement more apically along the root, the epithelium is free to migrate deeply and increase the depth of the pocket, with the reconstituted ligament acting as a barrier to its further downward growth. In this way the plaque extends rootward to maintain its antigenic influence at a more apical level and thus at least maintain its pathogenic effect. In practical terms, however, it always becomes more difficult to remove plaque in any oral hygiene regime as the pocket becomes deeper.

But a further mechanism is liable to act as ischaemia and pocket depth increase. The oxygen tension in the gingival transudate or exudate is bound to reduce; this arises because of the embarrassed circulatory competence and the high demand for oxygen by the fibroblasts active in tissue repair. This accounts for a changed bacterial flora of the plaque; there is a shift to more anaerobic organisms, both facultative and obligatory. Such organisms are generally considered more pathogenic and introduce the potential to invade the previously sterile tissue. It is these organisms that are responsible for the odious taste and odour characteristic of this progressive stage of the disease.

In summary it may be said that because of the decreased quality of the barrier action, the porous nature of the crestal bone, the deepening of the pocket and the shift to an anaerobic flora, the harmful potential of the plaque is in every way enhanced. Especially at this stage attention to oral hygiene becomes a much more important principle of treatment.

(ii) *Tissue configuration.* Approximation of abraded teeth must be the aim of treatment. The more gradually and earlier this can be achieved the better, as the preservation of the transeptal fibres is the essential component in the tooth movement. Where breakdown is advanced orthodontic movement should be contemplated to give a tissue configuration amenable to repair.

(iii) *Tooth mobility*. Although prior concern has been given to the marginal ligament, the principal fibres of the periodontal membrane have a significant role in stabilizing the tooth. Thus a long rooted tooth such as a canine often remains immobile while shorter rooted incisors and premolars succumb after becoming hypermobile.

Increased mobility always means increased rate of collagen destruction and the greater need for reparative anabolism. Thus treatment must always be directed towards reducing the load on a tooth by reducing traumatism. This is accomplished by grinding and splinting which should be regarded as replacing the depleted transeptal fibre action subgingivally by a rigid metal component supragingivally. However there is a degree of mobility, which once entered upon, defies all treatment other than extraction. Such a hypermobility infers damage to vessels and lymphatics with the extravasation of plasma into tissue spaces. When circulation is sluggish ideal conditions pertain for the incidence of a periodontal abscess.

The Extended Concept of the Marginal Cuff

The concept of an epithelial attachment whereby a physical bond was considered to exist between the reduced enamel epithelium and the junctional epithelium was rightly replaced by the idea of an epithelial cuff. However, the concept was still specially directed to the epithelium and the nature of its relationship to the tooth surface. The epithelial attachment was considered to be at least substantially derived from an adhesive bond between the junctional epithelium and the surface of the enamel, the chemical phase of the bond being secreted by the epithelial cells and being associated in some rather undefined way with the hemidesmosomes of the surface cells of the junctional epithelium. The writer's view would accord much more physical than chemical importance to the nature of the epithelial attachment. Simply, it is viewed as being substantially dependent on the action of a constraining force applying the epithelial cuff more tightly against the enamel surface of the teeth, or even in later years after hypereruption, against its cemental surface. This force is envisaged as being derived from the contractile nature of the component fibroblasts of the subepithelial corium acting through their close physical relationship with associated collagen fibres. Collagen fibres of three groups of the marginal ligaments are especially implicated in this action. The dento-gingival fibres attach the gingival tissue to the cementum; the free gingival fibres attach the gingival tissue to the crest of the bone and the superficial circular fibres course completely around the tooth in a continuous band. The action of the first two groups cuts through their exclusive insertion into the gingival epithelium of the marginal tissue. This action is facilitated by the well developed rete pegs in this epithelial structure and the consequent formation of deep corial extension into which the collagen fibres extend. There is no equivalent structure in the junctional epithelium, nor is there any concentration of fibre direction into this epithelial surface.

The contractile action of these fibres is, therefore, to apply the gingival cuff tightly against the tooth surface. The net outcome of a similar action of the circular fibres is identical, as this band seeks to establish a complete band of smaller circumference. It will also be appreciated that this anatomical concept is in physiological terms rather a dynamic one. The ground substance approximating to the collagen fibres of the corium shares in the structural unity applying the epithelial surface against the tooth. When this is in a gel phase the applying force is greater than it is in a sol condition, imposed force being one critical condition which specially affects the gel–sol distribution. Again the interface between ground substance and collagen fibres is an intermediate zone in which a constant biochemical flux between soluble and insoluble collagen exists; the more insoluble form present the greater the magnitude of the adapting force. As is well known, the effect of bacterial endotoxins and the extracellular products of some inflammatory cells is to reduce the fibre content of the marginal corium; here especially there is a marked reduction in the tightness with which the cuff is applied against the teeth, a fact which may be clinically demonstrated by freely lifting the cuff away from the teeth with a blunt probe or by applying a jet of warmed compressed air against it.

The writer would agree with MacPhee & Cowley (1981) where they state that 'Disruption of this anatomical arrangement of the connective tissues, and loss of continuity of buccal and lingual papillae through the embrasure, are the first major clinical signs of an established periodontitis'. The fibres most concerned in this dissolution are the superficial circular fibres, and since their blood supply is essentially endosteal in the interdental segment this is a very early indication that there is a trophic breakdown interdentally. Thus the apposition of the papilla to the tooth is seen to reduce before a like effect can be demonstrated in that part of the gingival margin related to the oral surface of the teeth.

The foregoing seeks to extend the concept of an epithelial cuff to a concept embracing the corium additionally, and even emphasizing the importance of the contribution made by the crestal alveolar bone to the idea that the whole marginal compartment is critically concerned in the healthy adaptation of the cuff.

However, the writer would seek to extend the concept of the cuff further, by applying it to the deeper tissues especially to the most marginal tissues of the periodontal membrane proper. Another way of saying the same thing is that the whole marginal apparatus should be implicated in this concept of a marginal cuff. When, in early periodontal disease, the integrity of the marginal ligament breaks down interdentally and when its structural unity is still preserved buccally and lingually, the fibre bond between the two alveolar plates which formerly acted interdentally is lost. It was the force generated by this component of the marginal ligament that moulded the base as well as the interdental papilla into close approximation with the teeth; this was accomplished as always by a remodelling process in the bone. Thus, in early periodontal disease the alveolar plates come to flatten out interdentally and the indentation of the bony plates in the interdental area as already noted is lost. In the interdental area the alveolar plates move away from the teeth and expose a depressed bony surface, triangular in shape interdentally which consists of cancellous bone, unprotected by an overlying marginal ligament. This bone is immediately exposed to advancing inflammation from the marginal tissues, as it is now unprotected by the barrier action of a dense marginal ligament and an underlying surface of indented cortical bone. This pathological sequence accounts for the extension of the interdental intra-bony pocket into the first stage of the compound intra-bony pocket as it extends especially onto the buccal surface of the molar teeth.

The compound intra-bony pocket is specially noted in the molar rather than the premolar regions for several reasons. In the molar area the alveolar plates are more horizontally inclined and are therefore much less amenable to a moulding force aimed at approximating these against the tooth surface. The heavy bone buttresses and proximate muscle insertions in the molar areas also generate forces which act against the toothward deflection of the alveolar plates. The condition in the premolar areas is opposite; the alveolar plates are vertical and may therefore be readily adapted to proximate towards the roots of the teeth with a minimum of remodelling activity. Moreover buttressing and muscle insertions are absent and no contrarily directed, modelling force is generated. Yet again, in the molar situation because of the substantially greater width of these teeth the interdental volume of the septal bone is large, making it more vulnerable to trophic deprivation; it therefore tends to break down when the equivalent premolar interdental bone is maintained.

The veracity of this viewpoint is given credence when the sequence of events following extraction of premolars and molars in the same segment is considered. In the early phases of healing, the underlying bone structure is readily appreciated on visual, tactile and radiographic inspection and shows little change. The alveolar plates remain disparately placed with sharp margins and the interdental bony margins are sharply defined and depressed below the level of the bone of the confining alveolar plates. The most noticeable change is a complete resolution of inflammation, following which the resulting edentulous alveolar ridge comes to be covered by a complete, if immature, epithelial surface. Gradually this epithelial surface matures into a stratified squamous epithelium of substantial thickness. At the same time, a process that we regard without question as alveolar resorption proceeds. In this context the alveolar plates bend over towards each other seeking to approximate but always failing to do so completely. Ridge height and ridge width are lost.

In fact, what has happened is that a volume of bone has been created that can be sustained by the prevailing endosteal circulation. Meantime, the area of the covering ridge mucosa is reduced and its supraperiosteal blood supply is enabled to sustain a more mature stratified squamous epithelium even with some keratinization. But the point to emphasize is that the residual ridge is not characterized by a substantially greater width in the molar area than the premolar area as previously existed before the teeth were extracted. Nor does any suggestion of a remnant of the interdental depression of the alveolar plates remain. Quite simply, the cortical plates of the edentulous alveolar ridge come to take the form of smooth surfaces. Some little additional width of the alveolar ridge does remain posteriorly due to the effects of buttressing and muscle insertions but these are confined posteriorly and are not marked. In the maxilla the tuberosity which was formerly well developed, gradually becomes a vestigial characteristic. What has happened in this process of ridge resorption extending over many months and even years is that a new modelling force has been generated, probably locally, not so strong as the previously existing force generated in the action of the marginal ligament interdentally. However, as judged by the smooth contour of the resultant alveolar plate, the force must be viewed as acting over the whole length of the ridge and not, as previously, in segmented interdental regions. The writer suggested thirty years ago that the moulding force resulted from the covering epithelial surface seeking to establish a reduced area; he would now add that this was affected by a reducing blood supply and the overall action is one previously described as an atrophy. This section might well be concluded and gain in meaning by quoting a very old piece of writing from a very famous book. Reneé Lereche's *'Surgery of Pain'* (1937) '. . . if the (edentulous) gums of these patients are carefully examined it will be seen, in fact, that their mucous membrane appears to be too restricted for the bulk of bone, however atrophied, that it has to cover. It is stretched over the bone as over a frame, and has lost is pliancy'.

Thus, the concept of a cuff action having reference not only to the junctional epithelium but the whole of the superficial marginal gingiva and additionally to the subjacent tissues of the marginal apparatus, is advanced.

References

ARNIM S.S. and HAGERMAN D.A. (1953) Connective tissue fibres of the marginal gingivae. *J. Amer. dent. Ass.* **47**, 271.

ATKINSON P.J. and WOODHEAD C. (1968) Changes in human mandibular structure with age. *Arch. oral Biol.* **13**, 1453.

BEGG P.R. (1938) Progress report on observations on attrition of the teeth in relation to pyorrhoea and tooth decay. *Dent. J. Aus.* **42**, 315.

BERRY D.C. and SINGH B.P. (1984) Effect of electromyographic feedback therapy on occlusal contacts. *J. pros. Dent.* **51**, 397.

JAMES W.W. and COUNSEL A. (1927) Histological investigation of so-called pyorrhoea alveolaris. *Brit. dent. J.* **48**, 1273.

LERECHE R. (1937) *The surgery of pain.* Ballière Tindall & Cox, London.

LOE H. (1983) Principles of aetiology and pathogenesis governing the treatment of periodontal disease. *Int. dent. J.* **33**, 119.

MACPHEE T. and COWLEY G. (1981) *Essentials of periodontology and periodontics.* 3rd Ed. Blackwell Scientific Publications, Oxford.

MURPHY T. (1958) Mandibular adjustments to functional tooth attrition. *Aus. dent. J.* **3**, 171.

MURPHY T. (1964) Reduction of the dental arch by approximal attrition. *Brit. dent. J.* **116**, 483.

NEWMAN H.L. (1982) Infection and the periodontal ligament. *In*: Berkovitz B.K.B., Moxham B.J. and Newman H.L. (eds) *The periodontal ligament in health and disease.* Pergamon Press, Oxford.

PICTON D.C.A. (1969) The effect of external forces on the periodontium. *In*: Melcher A.H. and Bowen W.H. (eds) *Biology of the periodontium.* Academic Press, London.

PICTON D.C.A. and MOSS J.P. (1984) Short term extrusion of isolated teeth of adult monkeys (*Macaca fascicularis*) *Arch. oral Biol.* **29**, 425.

ROWE D.J. (1983) Bone loss in the elderly. *J. pros. Dent.* **50**, 607.

SOCRANSKY S.S., HAFFAJEE A.D., GOODSON J.M. and LINDLE J. (1984) New concepts of destructive periodontal disease. *J. clin. Periodontol.* **11**, 21.

TAL HAIM (1984) The prevalence and distribution of intrabony defects in dry mandibles. *J. Periodontol.* **55**, 149.

WADE A.B. (1965) *Basic periodontology.* John Wright, Bristol.

7

TREATMENT PLANNING AND MOUTH PREPARATION

The success of a partial denture depends upon many factors of a purely technological nature, some which are carried out at the chairside and some in the laboratory. It is dependent also upon the knowledge of the practitioner and his technician, and upon the skill with which they each carry out their respective tasks. However, unless the mouth upon which they work presents conditions favourable for partial denture construction, there is little hope that their efforts will be successful. The problems that should receive attention before actual denture construction is commenced must therefore be considered. The ultimate success or failure of the denture may well depend upon the initial diagnosis and treatment planning.

Consideration must be given not only to the purely dental factors involved but also to the personal factors appertaining to the particular patient. These have already been discussed in Chapter 3.

When teeth have been lost or it is planned to remove them there are five alternatives:
1 complete upper and/or lower dentures
2 partial dentures
3 bridges
4 leaving the condition as it exists without replacing the missing teeth
5 any combination of 1, 2 and 3.

1 Complete upper and/or lower dentures

Total extraction of all teeth is usually necessitated by gross caries or periodontal disease, but may sometimes be advised in one jaw only owing to a grossly abnormal occlusal relationship of the teeth. In some cases a mere cursory examination will show that any other treatment is impossible; other cases will just as obviously require only one or two teeth to be removed or conserved and partial dentures supplied. Between these extremes are the doubtful cases where a decision has to be made between total extraction and complete dentures or selective extraction and partial dentures. In arriving at a decision the practitioner should bear in mind the personal factors, to which may be added the patient's preference for one or the other form of treatment. It is futile to advise a patient to embark upon a lengthy treatment ending in the fitting of partial dentures if he has firmly made up his mind that he wants all his teeth removed and complete upper and lower dentures.

When oral hygiene is poor and there is little reason to believe it will improve, it may be advisable to recommend total extractions. A combination of poor oral hygiene and a mucosa-borne denture may well result in the premature loss of the remaining teeth.

If the construction of partial dentures is proposed, it must, as far as possible, be assured that they will be worn. It is generally uneconomic from both the patient's and the practitioner's point of view to make partial dentures, whose expectancy of life is less than two years unless the dentures are recognized as a temporary line of treatment to accustom the patient to denture wearing before being supplied with full dentures.

Where the alternative to full dentures is a lengthy and expensive course of treatment the former may have to be preferred on economic grounds.

2 Partial dentures

There are two circumstances in which it may be decided to make partial dentures. In the first, a successful long-term prognosis is anticipated and in such cases the best partial dentures should be expected to give service for many years. To do so, however, they will require inspection and adjustment, including saddle rebasing, at regular intervals.

The second situation is when it is apparent that in the foreseeable future the patient will require complete dentures. It is most important that the transition from the natural dentition to the complete artificial dentition is as comfortable as possible for the patient. This is particularly so with the highly strung, nervous individual, and with the elderly. One of the most useful procedures is to provide such patients with partial dentures, even though the expectancy of service may only be for a short period. Such treatment is temporizing, and the day when complete dentures will be needed is merely being delayed. However, this period gives the patient experience in denture wearing and in adaptation to an artificial dentition.

Partial dentures constructed in such circumstances should be relatively simple in design and should permit the easy addition of further teeth, which may be immediate replacements of condemned natural teeth. It is likely by this means that the partial denture may ultimately be converted into a complete denture, 'immediate' in respect of the last two or three teeth added. This type of denture has been aptly called the 'additive' partial denture by De Van; it is particularly indicated in the lower jaw. It is often advisable to retain standing lower teeth, especially single standing canines, to delay or avert recourse to the complete lower denture. In this way lower denture stability and retention are more assured. Single standing canines can often be retained for long periods provided the incisal surface is adequately reduced and the denture components are constructed so as not to exert horizontal pressure on the teeth when the jaws are out of occlusion. It may also be possible to utilize such teeth to carry the stud or bar types of precision attachments which may enable a denture with a longer term prognosis to be supplied. Canines are favourable teeth for retention because they possess long and comparatively slender single roots, which may be free to move within the cancellous bone of the alveolus. Retention of the canines also requires a partial denture with three saddles of nearly equal size, a condition which favours stability.

One of the most difficult problems that the practitioner has to face is when to advise changing from these temporizing partial dentures to complete dentures. The patient's desire to retain the remaining natural teeth must not be allowed to influence a decision to extract if the practitioner has decided that further alveolar loss will seriously jeopardize the success of full dentures. The alveolar resorption that follows extraction is always greater where rapidly advancing periodontal disease is present. Therefore, the day of total extraction should not be delayed until there is so little bony support that the teeth are grossly loose, and there is little hope of securing a reasonable edentulous ridge.

3 Bridges

In many cases a fixed bridge is a superior restoration to a partial denture. In arriving at a decision as to which will be the better in any particular case the following *advantages* of fixed bridges should be remembered:
- They have minimal bulk, do not encroach upon the tongue space, and do not cover the gingivae to the extent a partial denture does. In consequence they 'feel natural'.
- Their aesthetic value can be high since little metal work need be visible.
- In many cases more efficient mastication is possible than with any removable type of restoration.
- A fixed bridge will give superior splinting and will prevent increasing tooth mobility by reinforcing the resistance of the single marginal ligament and to some extent by replacing the failing interstitial fibres of the composite marginal ligament.
- Some patients prefer a fixed restoration and abhor the idea of having to remove and insert a denture.

Fixed bridges have certain *disadvantages*, however, which may be listed as follows:
- They may often necessitate the removal of a considerable amount of healthy tooth tissue. However, modern methods of tooth preparation make this factor less serious than formerly.
- There is a limit to the number of teeth which can be replaced by a single fixed bridge. Stresses may be borne by the abutment teeth only; it is not so easy for

these stresses to be distributed over a large number of teeth as with partial dentures. Teeth with maximum healthy bony support are, therefore, essential for abutment purposes.

- Fixed bridges should only be constructed for patients whose standards of oral hygiene are high, if the possibility of proximal gingivitis is to be avoided. Removable appliances are more readily cleaned.
- Fixed bridge work is more time consuming at the chairside and generally more expensive.
- Repairs are difficult and additions impossible.

Additional factors in deciding between a fixed bridge and a partial denture must be the operator's own capabilities and preferences in these respective fields. Additionally, it is imperative that the original diagnosis and decision to construct a bridge or bridges is correct. Considerable time and expense are involved in this type of work and bridges can never halt a progressive failure of the blood supply and a deteriorating periodontal status. Full mouth rehabilitation by fixed appliances, following an incorrect diagnosis of the original condition, can result in painful cementum and periodontal abscess formation.

4   Leaving the condition as it exists without replacing the lost teeth

Every partial denture may be potentially harmful to oral health. When it is decided that the possible damage which may result from fitting a partial denture will be greater than the possible beneficial results, then it is better to leave the condition as it exists. The loss of a few teeth is often better left untreated by partial dentures.

The harm done by a partial denture will necessarily vary according to its type and design. For example, a mucosa-borne acrylic resin denture without clasps or rests, inserted in the lower jaw is likely to be far more detrimental than an adequately rested and clasped denture of hygienic design. The type of denture that it is possible to make will, therefore, be a big factor in deciding whether or not to leave the condition as it exists.

The concentration of force transmitted by a lower denture to the underlying tissues is always greater than an upper owing to the reduced area of supporting bone in the former. In the upper jaw vertical and lateral forces are partly resisted by palatal bone, and consequently less load has to be met by the teeth and ridges. This indicates that an upper denture should be less damaging to the edentulous ridge than a lower, a fact which is borne out in clinical practice.

The number and position of the missing teeth must be an important factor in deciding whether or not to fit dentures. Anterior teeth must usually be replaced for aesthetic reasons, but some posterior teeth can often be lost without being replaced by a denture. The longer the edentulous space in the posterior region the greater is the need for replacement.

Arch form, the nature of the occlusion, tooth size, jaw size and whether natural or artificial teeth oppose the spaces are additional factors which must be considered together with those already discussed. Lastly, the points discussed in previous chapters regarding the significance of oral hygiene must be considered seriously before deciding to make partial dentures.

Planning Surgical, Periodontal, Muscular and Restorative Treatment

When it is decided that partial dentures are to be made, other dental treatment is usually required. Normally, the prosthetic work is undertaken after all other forms of treatment have been completed, since dentures must be constructed to relatively stable conditions in respect of tooth shape and tissue form. Consequently it is essential that any surgical, periodontal, muscular or restorative treatment be undertaken with the denture requirements in mind. Partial dentures are more likely to be successful when other dental treatment has been correlated with the proposed denture design and construction.

The first types of treatment to be undertaken must be those concerned with surgical, periodontal and muscular requirements, since the mouth may take a protracted period of time to stabilize before partial dentures can be commenced. Allowing weeks even months to elapse following treatments in these classes permits time for tooth movement and reorganization of bone and soft tissues in positions harmonious with their blood supply. On the other hand, restorative treatment requires no such period and may be carried out immediately prior to commencing prosthetic work.

Surgical treatment

Extraction of teeth is often necessary prior to constructing partial dentures. When deciding whether or not to extract a tooth particular attention must be paid to its mobility. The degree of mobility indicating extraction is a matter of clinical judgement based on experience, but a tooth which is freely mobile between the alveolar plates has a poor prognosis and should be removed. Also the position of the tooth is important when arriving at a decision as to whether to extract or not.

The removal of a tooth from a crowded segment is often a wise procedure as it will effect arch decompression, following the same principle as interstitial grinding. A misplaced or stepped tooth often shows periodontal involvement, and its earlier rather than later extraction is advisable. This is especially so if the teeth in the segment are single rooted and lie within a well-developed alveolar process.

Grossly carious teeth must be extracted and careful assessment made of heavily filled teeth, particularly if it will be necessary to use them as abutments.

When partial dentures are required the best interests of both patient and practitioner may be served by the removal of certain healthy teeth. Single standing teeth and misplaced teeth come into this category.

Single standing teeth. Single standing teeth often present a problem; in some cases they are of the greatest value and in others there are strong indications for their extraction. Single standing posterior molars should be retained since they enable the saddle to be tooth-supported distally. A single standing tooth that interrupts what would otherwise be a long free-end saddle is often worth retaining. For example, if a lower second premolar is the only standing tooth posterior to the canine, part of the masticatory stress can be placed on it in the interests of ridge preservation. Also, the problem of retention and stability is eased since it is often difficult to utilize a lower canine successfully, whereas the premolar can be of considerable assistance. However, to prevent such a tooth from being subjected to stresses beyond the physiological limit it is often helpful if it is united to the canine by means of a fixed bridge. The abutment then, effectively, becomes two teeth instead of one. Also, the problem of a single tooth saddle on the denture is removed (Fig. 7.1).

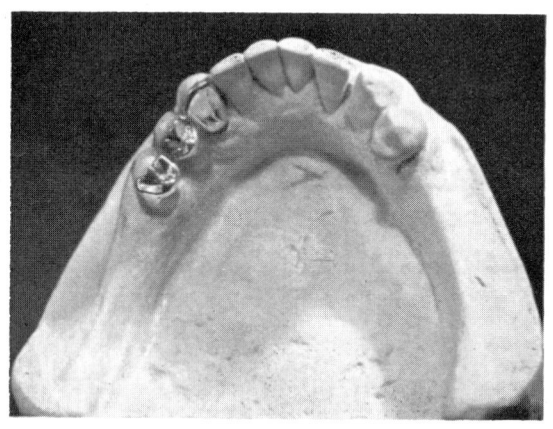

Fig. 7.1. The use of a fixed bridge to strengthen the single standing premolar.

As discussed earlier in this chapter, it may often be advisable to retain two lower canines only and construct a partial instead of a complete denture. Such a denture may be a temporizing form of treatment, but is often valuable in that the patient learns to control such a denture more readily than a complete denture and often such dentures last many years.

It is often advisable to extract a standing tooth that has a single tooth saddle on either side of it. This is particularly so if the other abutment teeth are healthy and the single tooth is tilted or has a very bulbous contour.

Misplaced teeth. Teeth that are grossly misplaced in the arch should be removed in the interests of both function and aesthetics. Anteriorly misplaced teeth that are unsightly may be extracted and replaced on the denture. Sometimes cases present where no space retainer has been inserted after the extraction of a central incisor, and closure, up to half the width of the tooth, has occurred. Overlapping the replacing tooth may give a reasonable appearance but often the most satisfactory result is achieved by extraction of one of the contiguous teeth.

Lower posterior teeth with gross lingual inclination may prevent the correct positioning of a bar and, therefore, warrant extraction. A posterior tooth or teeth which have over-erupted into a space created by the extraction of their opponents may interfere with occlusion. When this displacement is more than slight and cannot be corrected by grinding, extraction is often necessary (Figs 7.2 and 7.3).

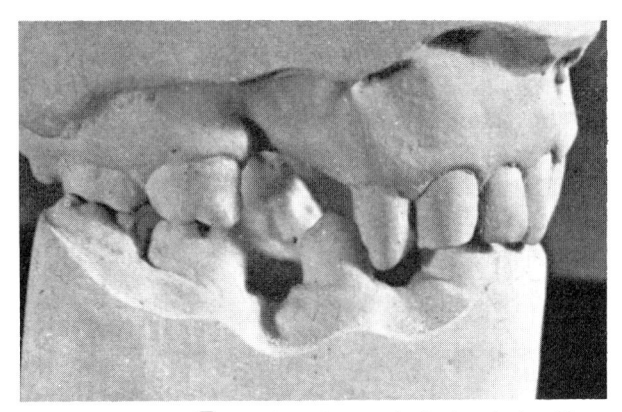

Fig. 7.2. Continued eruption of $\overline{5|}$ and $\underline{4|}$ producing a locked occlusion. Fortunately in this case the overbite is large, and it is doubtful if a marked protrusive movement would be used in mastication.

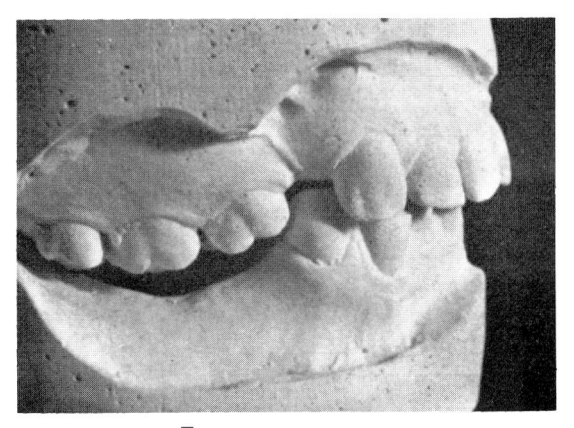

Fig. 7.3. Continued eruption of $\overline{4|}$ and $\underline{876|}$. As well as producing extra stress on the premolar, little space is available for a lower dental saddle.

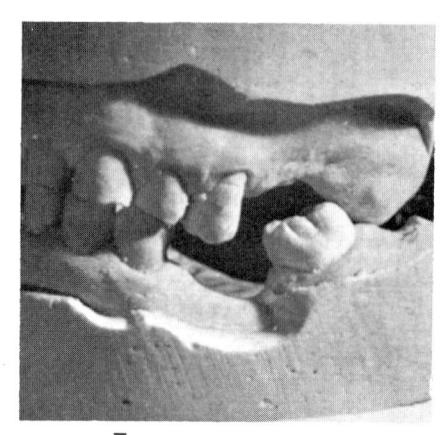

Fig. 7.4. Continued eruption of $\overline{7|}$ obviating the possibility of inserting an upper saddle above it. The bulbous tuberosity is often accompanied by a marked downward extension of the maxillary antrum thus contra-indicating alveolectomy.

Sometimes a lower molar is found impinging upon the tuberosity, rendering an upper denture impossible unless the vertical dimension is increased. If this is not indicated the offending tooth should be extracted or surgical reduction of the tuberosity undertaken. The choice will depend upon the value of the lower tooth for support and retention (Fig. 7.4).

Although extractions are the commonest and simplest surgical procedures carried out prior to partial denture construction, other surgical measures must sometimes be undertaken when circumstances dictate. For example, the removal of buried roots and unerupted teeth the presence of which has been revealed by radiographic examination is a necessary preliminary. Ridge shape may also be modified by the reduction of undercut areas, massive tuberosities, and prominent anterior ridges. Graty, Tomlin, and Fox have described a surgical procedure for the resection of a superficial and prominent mylohyoid ridge covered by atrophic soft tissues. Such a condition may cause pain and ulceration if a free-end saddle is placed over it. Soft tissue attachments that might interfere with the positioning of a bar clasp or denture saddle may require resection, but this operation is best carried out after the denture has been completed. In rare cases a torus mandibularis may require removal to allow positioning of a lingual connector.

Periodontal treatment

If the exclusive inflammatory concept of periodontal disease is accepted it would be logical and reasonable to expect that cure of the disease should be anticipated from measures directed at a resolution of the inflammatory process. Thus a combination of adequate oral hygiene, soft tissue and/or bone surgery, and drug therapy should not only ameliorate the symptoms of the disease, but should prevent its further progress. Treatment of traumatism by any means does not refer to the inflammatory aetiology and would therefore be unacceptable as a rational therapy for the inflammation. But the clinical experience of many dentists and the statistical results of recent epidemiological surveys have cast serious doubts on the efficacy of these treatment methods in completely curing periodontal disease. Also attempts to ascribe all blame for the shortcomings of the approach on the patient's failure to respond adequately to oral hygiene instruction and motivation have been unimpressive.

Immediately the exclusive inflammatory hypothesis is abandoned in favour of one also implicating atrophy and traumatism a changed situation exists. The concession that atrophy has a major aetiological role implies that, unless compensated, some progress of the disease is inevitable. However pessimism should not be uncompromised as the targets of treatment have now been widened to include means of retaining or even re-establishing a structural integrity of the marginal apparatus of the periodontium. Optimism, rather, is substantiated and at least considerable amelioration of the disease is anticipated; this may accept a reduction in hope but promises an increase in expectation.

The therapeutic treatment of periodontal disease

It is not considered that a book on partial dentures is the appropriate place to consider a rational programme of preventive treatment of periodontal disease, nor even to describe in detail accepted therapeutic techniques which have made unquestioned contribution in ameliorating disease progress. Rather it is considered desirable to describe in detail those techniques especially appropriate to obtaining the best periodontal status prior to constructing partial dentures. Further it must be appreciated that since the aims of the clinical procedures advised are to facilitate repair and even regeneration of tissues, time must be allowed for these healing reactions before results or further progress can be assessed. Oral hygiene, scaling, decompression of the arch, occlusal adjustment, drug therapy, surgery, splinting and the provision of temporary partial dentures are the approaches requiring description and emphasis in the individual case.

1 *Oral hygiene.* The sound basis of good oral hygiene must always be regular tooth brushing. As the gingiva becomes more atrophic the need for the use of a softer toothbrush must be emphasized, but compensation demands that more time should be given to the pursuit. Time spent on cleaning can well be raised to three minutes at each session and whereas twice a day was very adequate in the twenties it should be supplemented by a third session in the middle of the day in middle adult life. Its aim should always be twofold; the removal of dental plaque is obviously pertinent, but equally so is the encouragement of a deep axon reflex aimed at producing a longer acting local hyperaemia.

With atrophy and the creation of an actual rather than a potential interdental space, regular interdental irrigation is highly recommended. It is always a sound investment in middle adult life to purchase, and regularly use, one of the irrigation machines on the market today; not only do they remove accumulated exudate from the depth of the interdental pocket but viable pathogenic bacteria which may be present in the more anoxic conditions. After all this is only complying with the oldest principle of surgery, too often neglected today; where there is pus let it out. The equipment must dispense a pulsating jet of water through a tip designed to give easy access to all interdental spaces. Tepid to warm water should be used and an oxygen liberating or chemotherapeutic drug such as chlorhexidene added.

A satisfactory standard of oral hygiene is related to the ability of the patient to control the formation of dental plaque in his mouth. Although this is commonly achieved using mechanical methods these are not completely efficient and efforts have been made to develop a chemical agent for plaque control.

At present the most effective chemical anti-plaque agent is chlorhexidine which is widely used as a topical antiseptic with both bacteriostatic and bacteriocidal properties. In controlling plaque formation it is thought to act either by direct antibacterial action, or by suppressing the oral flora to a level at which colonization does not occur. It is also possible that a reversible interaction may occur with tooth enamel, the chemical being adsorbed on to tooth surfaces and slowly released, so preventing bacterial colonization.

For plaque control chlorhexidine may be used as a mouthrinse, topical application, or a dentifrice. Side effects are rare, but include a bitter taste, and staining of the teeth and restorations. The latter may be linked to dietary factors, but is not permanent, being removed by conventional toothbrushing.

2   *Scaling.* The writers would still advocate that regular scaling confers some benefit in the treatment of periodontal disease, but would insist that it could only help. The concept of a calcified mass of either supra- or sub-gingival calculus containing any significant source of viable organisms is to be doubted. The deleterious action of calculus is much more likely to stem from a mechanical action than an increase in its infected potential. Once again the method is dependent on the age old adage, where there is pus let it out. The flow of transudate or exudate through the gingival cuff or pocket must be slowed by the presence of calculus, not only because it presents an impedance but because its rough surface makes onward flow sluggish. Pressure of the overlying gingiva against such a surface in mastication might well add to the traumatization of the delicate and even inflamed or ulcerated epithelial surface lining the pocket. Also the rather pleasant feeling resulting in the mouth after thorough scaling is appreciated by the patient and may well be motivating to further personal care.

Whereas the writers would accept the conclusion that equally good results are to be obtained by hand as with ultrasonic technique their distinct preference is for

Treatment Planning and Mouth Preparation 139

for the latter method, as it is less time consuming and often more acceptable to the patient. But there can be no denying that the ultrasonic machines utilize a considerable amount of energy and dissipate this as heat against soft and hard tissue surfaces. The technique demands copious water irrigation to cool the area and this imposes problems in removing the water. Whereas the introduction of high volume aspirators has done much to facilitate the removal of large volumes of water, the writers feel there is still a real need to improve the design of attachments used to remove the water from the area of operation. But there is another very real disadvantage which applies more especially to ultrasonic scaling and that is hypersensitivity. The pain generated by the heat in ultrasonic scaling can actually contra-indicate the method in favour of hand instrumentation. But another approach is to attempt to treat the hypersensitivity before scaling is attempted. Durkacz (1976) introduced the use of a soluble, relatively stable, hydrocortisone sodium phosphate as a desensitizing agent which must be accorded merit. Likewise the longer term use of a strontium containing toothpaste may help, and recourse is made to both of these methods. However previous decompression of the arch, especially by an interstitial grinding method to be described, is the most hopeful approach to overcome hypersensitivity. This would appear to substantiate anoxia as the cause.

Very recently the use of an abrasive technique has been advocated. It is understood that this is more effective against the soft plaque than the calcified deposits.

3 Arch decompression techniques. This concerns a technique introduced by one of the writers in the latter half of the fifties and used by him in a huge number of cases ever since. Its aim is to reduce the length of the dental arch and this can be effected either by extraction or by the removal of small amounts of tissue interdentally, a technique known as interstitial grinding.

Extraction of teeth can only be expected to reduce the arch length when it is possible for the teeth to move. Generally some degree of shortening of the arch can be expected after extraction but this is variable. Tooth movement in one arch is always resisted by a positive occlusion between the teeth. Where the occlusion is held by a cusp to sulcus relationship movement is restricted and should never be counted upon. Likewise the presence of high cusps in the presence of such an occlusal pattern would be expected to prevent horizontal tooth movement in the arch following extraction. When, however a cusp to cusp relationship exists, a condition favouring tooth movement pertains. Again if the cusps are inconspicuous either as a result of natural form or attrition tooth movement giving a reduction in arch length is to be expected. One situation where the extraction of a single tooth as a decompressive method is especially rewarding is the removal of a single lower incisor. This is always accompanied by a favourable tooth movement, a regular arch resulting from a backward movement of the remaining three incisors, the periodontal health of which often improves dramatically. If one of the teeth is considerably displaced this tooth should be sacrificed. Again (and it often amounts to the same thing) a loose tooth should be preferred to sounder teeth when a decision is made regarding the selection of a tooth for extraction. Although the more noticeable effect following such an extraction is on the health of the remaining lower incisors, advantage also accrues to the upper incisors. This may take the form of reduced palatal attrition where these teeth are firm or cessation of incisal edge proclination when their periodontal status is not good. A good general principle when considering extraction to accomplish arch decompression is to remove the most displaced tooth as it is the one whose movement is most likely to be restricted by the outer or inner cortical alveolar plate; teeth will always move more favourably through cancellous bone. A narrow alveolar process is also to be regarded with less favour. One final point to be made when considering extraction is that a point is reached in the mobility of a tooth when resolution just cannot be hoped for. When this stage is reached with any tooth, it should be extracted without delay. Some favourable shortening of the arch may be accomplished or the space may afterwards be used by a partial denture to accept a share of the occlusally applied load. Most of all the improved comfort of the patient when eating is likely to be appreciated. By and large, the use of extraction to decompress is resorted to later rather than sooner, but in the forties the writer has always liked to see a posterior break in the arch, provided sufficient teeth remain in a healthy condition to accept the masticatory load.

Interstitial grinding is the alternative method of effecting arch decompression. In this case the advantage is that the release of pressure upon the vasculature is spread throughout the arch and is not concentrated locally as when extraction is carried out. Three methods may be used for interstitial grinding:

(i)   by an abrasive strip
(ii) by ultrasonics
(iii) by an abrasive disc.

(i) *The abrasive strip method.* A fine steel strip on which sapphire dust is bonded is required. It should have a thickness of about one-eighth of a millimetre so that it can be inserted with some pressure between the majority of healthy teeth. If tooth contact is specially tight, a wooden wedge should be pushed between the teeth concerned and allowed to remain in place for a few minutes.

In order to grind interstitially these strips are cut into one-inch lengths and one end is rounded. The square end is firmly locked in the curved jaws of a Spencer Wells forceps (Fig. 7.5). The strip is inserted between the teeth at the end nearer the forceps and is drawn through the interspace towards the lips or cheeks keeping it as nearly straight as possible to minimize the chances of breakage. Should this occur a new grip is made on the extruding end of the strip which is finally drawn completely through the contact. The procedure is repeated some six times, then another series of draws is made with the cutting surface

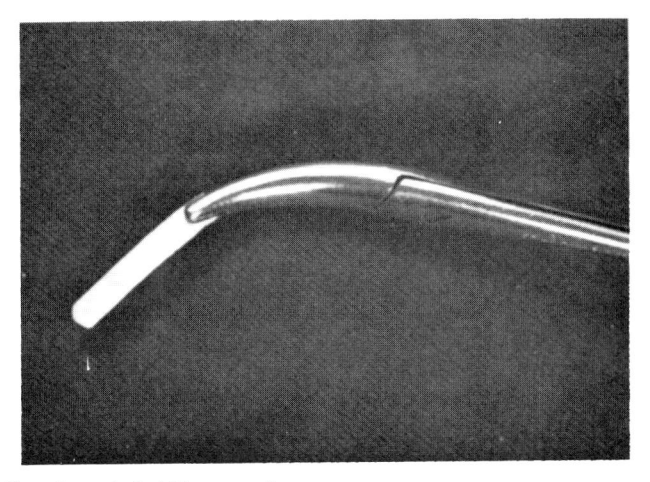

Fig. 7.5. Abrasive strip held in artery forceps.

acting on the opposite contact. It is advisable to use two artery forceps with strips mounted so that their cutting surfaces face in opposite directions.

During this operation pain should be avoided and the patient's tissues subjected to minimal trauma. Since the operation is carried out over the whole mouth at one visit local anaesthesia is inappropriate. Nor is any anaesthesia necessary where the contact points are near to the occlusal surface or incisal edge, as in the lower incisal and premolar areas. Here, precise placement of the strip can avoid contact with the interdental papilla. However, where the contact point is more gingivally placed, as in upper anterior and molar areas, or where tooth inclination is marked, it is advised to apply a surface anaesthetic as deep placement of the strip in unavoidable. Pain from pricking the tongue can be avoided by rounding the free end of the strip.

Damage to the corner of the lips and the interdental papillae is avoided by careful attention to technique. The tongue and corners of the mouth should be held back by the operator's fingers, both for protection and to give a clear view of the area being cut. Cutting is carried out by holding the forceps with the third and fore fingers while the thumb is used as a levering contact against the tooth mesial to the concerned area. In this way a short controlled movement is ensured. Control is liable to be lost when excessive force is employed to withdraw the strip especially when the thumb is inadvisedly removed from its pivotal position to generate more power. It is always better to do a preliminary separation of the teeth rather than to use force. Following the use of these strips it may be thought necessary to use further strips of finer grade to ensure that as smooth a surface as possible is left on the enamel.

(ii) *The ultrasonic method.* Ultrasonic instruments, although generally accepted for scaling, can also be used for cutting tooth structures in orthodontics where interstitial enamel stripping has been advocated to provide the space required to effect minor tooth movement. It has been estimated that interproximal spaces of one-quarter to half a millimetre may be created in this way.

The Cavitron orthodontic tips P20D and P20M may be used for interstitial grinding, but they are bulkier than the abrasive strips and the manufacturers recommend the preliminary use of rubber, wood or brass separators. However the use of abrasive strips may be more convenient. The tips wear in use and their expensive replacement is a disadvantage of the method, which is, however, comfortable to the patient.

A side-to-side movement of the curved tip is used with light pressure against the surface to be cut. A high energy setting is used. Cavipaste is applied to the tip and tooth surface and is mixed to a slurry by an instrument water flow of three to four drops per second. From time to time the field is flushed with water to inspect the surfaces and ensure that the tooth contour is being maintained.

Surfaces prepared in this way have a dull appearance due to minute uniform pits created by the impact of the abrasive particles. The manufacturers recommend finishing with fine cuttle-fish strips.

(iii) *The abrasive disc method.* This method which removes tooth structure easily and quickly, uses a single sided steel separating disc of 2.2 centimetres diameter. In the anterior and premolar regions a conventional straight handpiece with water spray is used at a speed of about 5,000 r.p.m. No tongue or cheek guard is used on the handpiece, but the operator manipulates the lip, keeping it out of the operative field (Fig. 7.6). In this way good vision is obtained. The writer no longer uses the method in the molar area because of the risk to tissue and lack of good access and visibility. In all areas it is advisable for an assistant to manipulate a saliva ejector with a tongue shield which provides better access for the operator, and protection for the patient. The patient is asked to keep still and to avoid swallowing during the short duration of the cut. This method requires especial care when operating because of the danger from the sharp edge of the disc.

The biggest issue in applying the interstitial grinding technique is in judging at what stage to start and to what degree of removal to work. Ideally one presumes an uncrowded condition in the formed dental arch, when the aim of the arch reduction is to compensate for the atrophic process. Then interstitial grinding may well be deferred until the thirties and then only mild but widespread reduction undertaken. The more gradual the change is effected the better and the more truly preventive the procedure becomes. However, so very often the patient arrives in the twenties with an overcrowded arch. In this event interstitial grinding may well be necessary in the twenties and the additional use of early extraction especially of misplaced teeth or partially or unerupted third molars,

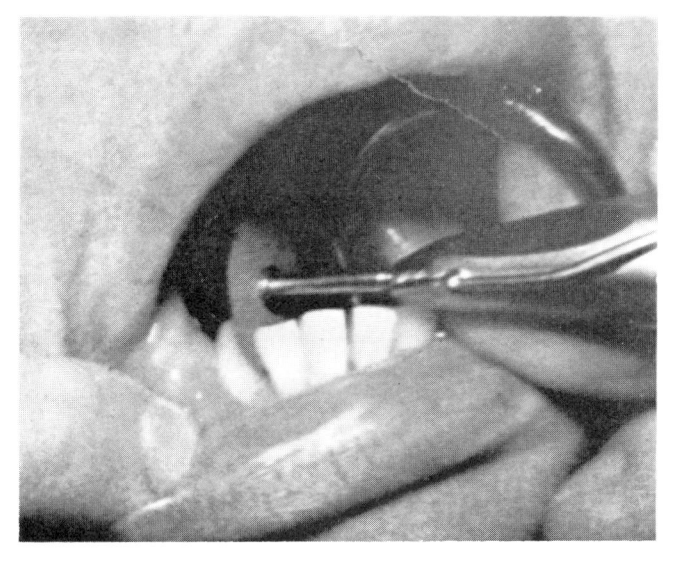

Fig. 7.6. Diamond disc used for interstitial grinding.

seriously considered. At this stage very tight contacts between individual teeth may be noted; these should always be eased by grinding. But there is one considerable disadvantage to the method. Removal of enamel tissue cannot be effected without weakening its structure and making it more vulnerable to comminution under imposed stress especially that acting in an overcrowded arch. From the viewpoint of caries prevention, ideally one would wish to defer interstitial grinding as we know the dentinal tubules are sealed by intratubular deposit of calcific tissue with the passage of the years especially at their terminal ends. This action is one calculated to seal the most superficial dentine and curtail the availability of tissue fluid necessary for the carious process. But we cannot defer indefinitely in the face of evidence of periodontal breakdown. After all caries can be treated successfully by filling and may be viewed as a preferable lesion to periodontal disease. In part this dilemma can be overcome by being selective in the site chosen for grinding. Teeth with a thick covering of enamel and a high contact point are best selected in the first instance; this would especially indicate work on the lower incisor area in the younger patient. Conversely where the contact point is situated near to the gingival margin in an area where the enamel is thin, grinding should be deferred; such a situation usually exists in the upper molar area. Quite often, however, in the periodontal disease-prone jaw the amount of interstitial caries and filling present mitigate against caution and indicates rather heavy interstitial grinding. The need for disciplined attention to recall examination should be emphasized to the patient in view of the increased risk of dental caries. In cases of established periodontal disease seen for

144 Chapter 7

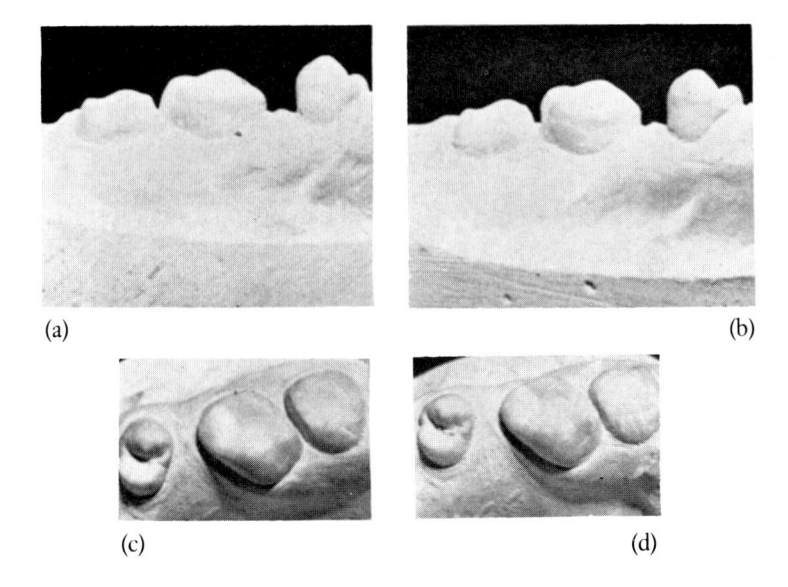

(a) (b)

(c) (d)

Fig. 7.7. Models showing (a) the original condition, (b and c) after grinding interstitially with a needle diamond and occlusal grinding, and (d) the closure that has resulted.

the first time rather later than one would have wished, extraction and interstitial grinding should be much more radical. The use of a very fine needle diamond in the conventional turbine handpiece has application in the molar area in such situations, but the cut areas should be carefully assessed for caries at frequent intervals. The result of such an intervention associated with freeing of occlusal contacts is shown in Fig. 7.7. Lastly it would be wise to caution against the use of the disc technique where tight application of the tooth is associated with irregularity. Here with a disc it is very easy to misalign the disc and to cut a groove into the enamel at the cutting edge. Feeling one's way with a strip is safer if slower. Interstitial grinding is always carried out in association with occlusal grinding at the same operative session.

(iv) *Occlusal adjustment.* Whereas interstitial grinding is a relatively new procedure, occlusal grinding has been advocated for many years. Its development was an extension of occlusal concepts formulated in the first instance to maintain the retention of full dentures during function. However, the technique now described is based on the biological requirements of the supporting tissues of the teeth, and aims at obtaining even tooth contact, with cusp reduction in the tooth position.

Treatment Planning and Mouth Preparation

Occlusal grinding may also be required to establish improved occlusal contacts as a treatment of muscular symptoms and to eliminate premature contacts causing non-coincidence of tooth and muscular positions. Although this may well have a significance in periodontal disease it is much more important as a therapy in the treatment of temporo-mandibular arthrosis, and for this reason will not be considered in the present description.

Occlusal grinding is carried out all round the mouth and may be done either as a preventive or therapeutic measure. A straight handpiece is used together with a barrel-shaped fine grained diamond instrument and water cooling.

When the periodontal status is reasonable and the aim is prevention, the amount of grinding is small but is graded according to the cuspal inclination; where the cusps are prominent more grinding is done. The patient is instructed to open and close several times into the tooth position on to thin blue articulating paper which has previously been warmed over a flame. The marks are ground away from the summits and slopes of the cusps; the fissures are left untouched. In this way, over a long period of time the cusps are reduced and a flat occlusal surface obtained. Grinding of the anterior teeth is carried out from the palatal aspect of the upper teeth; this reduces the chance of exposing the dentine of the lower incisor edges which may become stained.

After this stage the patient is again asked to tap the teeth together in the tooth position. He will often comment upon the changed feeling and is able to appreciate which teeth contact first. The sudden creation of a new occlusal pattern changes the sensory engram significantly and patients are immediately aware not only of a changed occlusion but of any irregularities therein. They are asked to indicate any tooth which seems to meet first or feel hard. Most patients readily indicate such hypercontacts. The few who find some difficulty are asked to take their time, concentrate and then make a series of light taps followed by a series of heavy taps. There may be some hesitation and concern and the patient may then indicate some tooth as a possibility only. This tooth is immediately ground and an improved tactile sensation gives the patient confidence in their ability to make the required judgement. Hypercontacts, as indicated by the patient, are reduced one at a time, always reducing the cusp height. The condition is satisfactory when the patient says that the contact is even.

The final stage of grinding the occlusion is necessary in a small minority of cases only, and concerns the incisal edges of the anterior teeth. When the path of mandibular closure into the tooth position is via an initial contact in the incisor region and then a slide distally into maximum intercuspidation, it is necessary to obtain even contact between the opposing incisor teeth when they first occlude. Aesthetic consideration will determine whether grinding on the upper or lower teeth is appropriate.

When treatment of existing periodontal disease is being undertaken grinding is more radical. First all the teeth are assessed individually for hypermobility. The teeth are moved laterally when the patient maintains an open mouth. Any particularly loose teeth are noted as this is likely to indicate that the tooth is in premature contact. The patient is then asked to tap the teeth together heavily in the tooth position while the forefinger is placed over each of the crowns successively. Displacement of any tooth is felt as a tactile sensation; the development of this clinical skill requires much practice and the operator will become more discerning in assessing hypercontacts which move the teeth. Thereafter the teeth are visually observed during tapping together with the lips and cheeks retracted, and it may be seen if one or more teeth is making a primary contact which causes its displacement; this in turn permits the remaining teeth to occlude apparently evenly in the tooth position. The patient does not experience any heavy contact or other sensation when these hypermobile teeth occlude. These teeth are ground first until they are stable under occlusal load as judged by tactile and visual evidence.

Thereafter occlusal grinding is carried out as described for prevention but the amount of tooth substance removed can be greater because occlusion of the dentinal tubules in relation to the enamel has usually occurred before periodontal disease is evident. The amount removed should be proportional to the degree of atrophy and to the extent of the periodontal destruction, and must compensate for the continued and accelerated eruption of the teeth which has taken place. Grinding into the dentine may be inevitable but it may have to be restricted because of pain.

It is also necessary to balance the occlusal glide from the ligamentous position of the mandible to the tooth position. The patient must practise closing into the ligamentous position and then gliding forward to the tooth position. This should be a smooth uninterrupted glide. If it is not, it is necessary to discover and reduce the offending contacts. In established disease hypermobilities rather than hypercontacts are the commoner, when the operator rather than the patient must diagnose their presence and location; the most posterior molars are the common site. This reduction is important because in mastication when a tough or hard bolus is being comminuted jaw closure takes place with the condyle head braced into its most retruded position, where it is most capable of resisting the heaviest loads the masticatory muscles can generate. On penetration through the bolus the first tooth contact is in the ligamentous position; it is desirable that this load be well distributed and not concentrated on the most posterior occluding teeth. Its importance lies in the magnitude of the applied load rather than in the frequency of its use. It is now nearly thirty years ago since on electromyographic and attritional evidence one of the writers described this as the 'power stroke' in mastication.

By examining the degree of attrition on the incisal edges of the upper anterior teeth it is generally possible to discover whether or not the patient is engaging in bruxism. The condition is very common, and is generally most actively practised in the lighter sleep before waking. Because of its continuous nature and the fact that the muscular force used is considerable it is highly desirable to share the load on a segmental basis. Certainly distribution of contact over the three anterior teeth in the lateral glides is highly desirable. When analysing this movement it is necessary to appreciate that the extent of the glide is usually extreme. The patient is asked to try several directions of glide to an extreme mandibular position while the operator watches for coincidence of attritional facets between upper and lower teeth. The constituent bruxismal pathway can always be demonstrated and it is a simple matter to induce the patient to perpetuate the particular movement while grinding is carried out to the incisal edges to involve more than one opposing pair of teeth.

A final tactile and visual assessment should ensure that hypermobile teeth have not been brought into hypercontact when the occlusal vertical dimension has been reduced.

Lastly a particular case needs to be described which may complicate advanced periodontal disease. When the disease process involves the upper anterior teeth migration of these teeth takes place initially due to premature contacts as upper and lower teeth continue to erupt. Diastemata make their appearance with the space being greater at the incisal edges than at the gingival margin. Hypermobility can always be demonstrated in these teeth and their movement on closure easily verified. It is of course always necessary to eliminate this movement by grinding. But additionally it is sometimes found that with elongation of those upper anteriors the lower lip has in the resting state become interposed behind the incisal edges of the fronts. Here it is essential to reduce the clinical crown length greatly by grinding the incisal edges. The engagement of the lip behind the incisal edges must be freed. In such cases the appearance is greatly improved by the grinding, a fact appreciated by most patients. Where radical interstitial and occlusal grinding of the lower anteriors accompanies this measure, rather spectacular improvement can often be achieved.

Let it be reiterated that interstitial and occlusal grinding cannot cure periodontal disease; the atrophic process will continue inevitably. However, the process will contribute in greatly extending the useful life of the periodontally diseased dentition. By grinding it is necessary to arrange for the teeth to move together in the absence of traumatism; it is also worth reiterating that when a tooth has become substantially diseased it is a mistake to persevere in its retention.

(v) *Drug therapy.* A consideration of the use of drugs in the treatment of periodontal disease centres on the use of antibiotics. There can be little doubt that antibiotics can, and do, have some part to play in the control of the rate of advance of periodontal disease. This is especially so in ameliorating the symptoms of gingivitis and an early periodontal abscess. But periodontal disease advances in spite of the use of antibiotics, as has been noted in those cases where a patient is taking regular doses of antibiotics for life; this is one of the telling observations emphasizing that the present exclusively inflammatory paradigm on the disease is insufficient and that atrophy and traumatism have an essential role in the aetiology.

No one can doubt that the removal of a locus of inflammation can only contribute to an improved health status. The resistive capacity of the body is conserved and the sense of well being and confidence deriving from a 'clean' mouth is natural, even if it is misleading. But the sporadic use of antibiotics has a part to play in that it prevents destruction of tissue, even though, as in the case of gingivitis, that destruction is relatively superficial; it also by eliminating inflammation makes some contribution to the circulatory economy. Where there is an acute or subacute gingival inflammation systemic antibiotics are critical to treatment. The use of antibiotics must be commended in certain cases of early periodontal disease associated with gingivitis. Here patients are usually middle aged with the majority of the teeth present, firm and with tight contacts. The gingival mucosa is taut and thin and the margins are red, very oedematous and glazed. There is considerable false pocketing, bleeding and often some more acute exacerbation. Such cases are slow in their response to grinding.

However a two week course of phenoxymethyl penicillin V 250 mg four hourly can be used with great benefit. This suggests that the elimination of the inflammatory process by chemotherapy also eliminates an ischaemic element which is secondary to the inflammatory process. This is always of less significance than the ischaemia due to intrinsic change in the vasculature, since if grinding has not been carried out, the inflammation quickly returns upon withdrawal of the drugs. When grinding has been done, and implemented by antibiotics, results are more apparent and more permanent.

The writer recalls the case of one patient in this class whose gingival condition was very intractable to treatment. The patient contracted a serious appendicitis and peritonitis which necessitated the use of large doses of antibiotic. When the patient returned for dental treatment the gingival and periodontal status had improved remarkably. This experience has stimulated the writer to use increased antibiotic doses in intractable cases in the class described.

Generally speaking wide-spectrum antibiotics are to be recommended, as the infections are generally mixed. Phenoxymethyl penicillin V in one of its proprietary forms has always been the first choice and is generally successfully used in normal dosage. In cases of sensitivity tetracycline and erythromycin are useful alternatives. One drug, however, needs to be considered for use in difficult cases and especially where penicillin-resistant staphylococci are suspected of involvement. Fusidic acid and its salts are narrow-spectrum antibiotics specially effective against staphylococci, a bacterium often found in osteomyelitis. It has the added advantage of concentrating in bone. The drug in 500 mg doses is given eight hourly in cases where liver function is sound.

In addition, the writer would call attention to the use of one other drug he found by accident to have some use. Nicotinic acid is sometimes used in the treatment of peripheral vascular disease and hyperlipidaemia; it is one of the water soluble B group of vitamins. One of its side effects is 'flushing' and it is the selective hyperaemia it induces in the head and neck which is harnessed to improving the periodontal blood supply. Its use is limited to healthy patients and to restricted and selected periods of use. It is only used as a booster to local circulatory performance immediately following the use of interstitial and occlusal grinding. As a digression it has also been noted that the use of this drug helps in cases of particularly hypersensitive dentine. It has been reassuring to learn that nicotinic acid is also used by some ear, nose and throat specialists.

(vi) *Surgery*. Rationally and logically Fish introduced the operation of gingivectomy following upon his advancing the inflammatory concept of periodontal disease. It has since been used in the restricted form as papillectomy and its use has sometimes been segmental. It has been advocated by all periodontal specialists for over forty years but after the sixties it suffered a decline in popularity and its use now is very restricted. Its decline from favour has not stimulated any reappraisal of concepts on aetiology as should have been the case; it is simply seldom used today on account of its lack of success and patients often found it was followed by a protracted period of pain. Stimulated doubtless by lack of success, the vogue of soft tissue surgery was replaced by enthusiasm for more radical bone surgery of the alveolar process. The reasons for justifying this are interesting. Initially the method was undertaken to facilitate exposure of root surfaces to permit their scaling and planing in meticulous manner. At a later stage a modification of this type of surgery was advocated to permit a remodelling of the alveolar process; the aim was to reduce the height of the alveolar plates to eliminate the interdental bony pocket. The concept of remodelling was never rationalized, although what reference it could possibly have to inflammation still remains obscure. Today conservative and radical surgery are not widely practised.

Frenectomy, however, is a single example where surgery has been helpful. Gingivae and periodontal healing cannot take place in the presence of movement of the peripheral soft tissues through constant muscle action.

(vii) *Splinting*. This approach in the treatment of periodontal disease is both rational and effective. The destruction of the interdental component of the marginal ligament isolates the tooth mechanically from its fellows in the arch. This means that it must totally accept load which was previously shared segmentally. It also means that the tooth is freer to erupt selectively in the arch and lead to a damaging hypercontact. Splinting is quite simply the supragingival replacement of the destroyed interdental marginal ligament, and certainly extends the life of periodontally diseased teeth.

The principle may be applied through fixed bridgework or partial dentures or increasingly nowadays in the combination of the two. However again the method cannot be relied upon to give assured results, as experienced clinicians have all encountered loosening of the teeth or even periodontal abscess formation in a segment in which fixed bridgework has been undertaken.

But bridgework is a superior method to partial denture construction in attaining effective splinting. However it is still such an expensive form of treatment as to put it in the luxury class. It therefore has little application where the prognosis is at all doubtful. Two suggestions should be added where bridgework is selected; take impressions only after the teeth freed from occlusion have been given opportunity to move together (even if this involves the consideration of orthodontic force) and do not jeopardize the reconstruction by failing to extract teeth with a poor prognosis.

(viii) *Partial denture prosthetics.* Partial dentures should be used in two ways to contribute to the treatment of periodontal disease. The first is the use of temporary, short term, simple acrylic dentures, and the second, hopefully more permanent appliances which are always cast.

The first type of denture is used to distribute occlusal load. This is especially important when the teeth are few in number and the edentulous spaces long. At least some of the occlusal load is taken through the overlying denture saddles but nearly all of it may be directed on to the hard palate and saddles by the simple expedient of increasing the vertical dimension of occlusion. This not only reduces trauma but facilitates tooth movement within the alveolar bone, hopefully into a position to allow repair of the marginal ligament. In its most extreme form this type of denture may take the form of an upper bite plate disengaging all the teeth and having the lower anteriors only occluding on a platform of acrylic resin.

The second type of denture is a more permanent appliance. It is always cast and embodies the principle of splinting, albeit this being relatively inferior to that achieved by fixed reconstruction. It does not involve increasing the vertical dimension and is constructed to an even occlusion in the tooth position. Its design often includes the principle of stress breaking. Its construction is not undertaken until the best possible periodontal result has been obtained following all indicated treatment approaches including the use of a temporary partial denture.

Treatment of muscular or joint symptoms

This phase of treatment is required only when symptoms of the temporomandibular syndrome are apparent; this is a relatively small number of cases. Pain especially in the region of the temporomandibular joint is a constant symptom but more remote pain related to the masticating muscles may be present. Paraesthesias are generally referred to the skin and usually involve thermal sensations; these may precede and outlast the pain but are not a constant complaint. Limitation of joint movement is always present and may be associated with clicking of the joint. More rarely ear symptoms such as tinnitus, deafness and vertigo may be the primary complaint.

The diagnosis of temporomandibular syndrome is based on the patient's description of the symptoms enumerated and the demonstration of signs by the following approaches:

- *Visual signs.* Face often thin with comparatively well developed active muscles.
  Limitation of movement; maximally open jaw cannot contain width of three fingers.
- *Palpation.* Extraorally for smoothness of joint action and pain over insertions of muscles.
- *Auscultation.* Intraorally for painful areas in specific muscles.
  This is referred to the teeth and temporomandibular joints. The method may be direct or by Watt's method using a stereostethoscope.
- *Radiography.* Several techniques of radiographing the temporomandibular joint have been described; the writers generally use that of Grewcock. Evidence of a posterior and superior displacement of the condylar head on occlusion would confirm a tentative diagnosis but would not be pathognomonic.
- *Electromyography.* The availability of this instrument is the limitation of the best single method of demonstrating muscle spasm.
- *Otoscopic examination.* This is undertaken to exclude ear pathology in the presence of symptoms referrable to the auditory apparatus.
- *Occlusal analysis.* The method is less useful in diagnosis than is usually believed, as it is only applicable when no muscle spasm exists.

However treatment (if not diagnosis) may be facilitated by occlusal analysis which is carried out using stone casts mounted on a fully adjustable articulator. In many cases it will not be necessary to place casts on an articulator since it will be possible to make an assessment directly in the mouth; many operators prefer to do this routinely. Very often it is found that little or no additional knowledge is gained from studying the casts on the articulator; although vision is better from the lingual aspect there is no assurance that the movement patterns used by the patient in function are reproduced on the articulator.

When it is decided to mount study casts on an articulator the following procedure is undertaken. Casts in artificial stone are poured from accurate impressions. Great care must be taken to avoid air blows on the occlusal surfaces of the impressions since these will cause small pimples on the casts which will give artificial errors in the occlusion. It is necessary to have these casts duplicated so that, after those mounted on the articulator have been scraped to modify occlusion, comparison can be made with the original casts. An articulator of the Dentatus pattern should be used since it is possible with this instrument to provide both anterior and posterior movement from the muscular position; in addition, the upper cast can be mounted in natural relation to the Frankfort plane horizontal. In order that the upper cast may be mounted in the correct condyle–maxillary relationship on the articulator a face bow recording must be made as described in Chapter 16.

The lower cast must be mounted with the aid of records obtained from the patient in the muscular position but just short of cuspal contact. However, the muscular symptoms (the permanent treatment of which by grinding or an appliance is the ultimate object of the occlusal analysis) usually prevent such a recording being obtained, due to muscle spasm. Hence, the first objective is to eliminate the muscle spasm so that a relaxed recording in the muscular position can be obtained. Often there will be a discrepancy between the tooth and muscular positions which has caused the muscular spasm and symptoms. The provision of an acrylic resin overlay splint with a flat occlusal surface will eliminate premature tooth contacts which may be deviating the mandible and so causing spasm. Such an appliance is easily constructed and its occlusal surface easily modified, and it usually alleviates the symptoms in a relatively short time.

Additional measures to eliminate the spasm such as short wave therapy, infra-red radiation, and light massage are designed to increase the volume of blood flowing through the muscles and thereby remove the offending metabolites. The use of muscle-relaxant drugs, for example Diazepam, may be effective in relieving the symptoms, but the patient should be warned of possible side effects. When the relief of pain indicates that the spasm has been relieved a recording may be attempted. The whole essence of this procedure is an unhurried approach to a suitably conditioned patient.

The patient may be prepared by the use of tranquillizing drugs, and by resting a short time before the clinical session. However, the success of the record depends on the approach of the operator and his ability to induce in the patient a state of complete relaxation. This, in essence, is a light hypnotic state and the operator would be well advised to acquaint himself with the techniques of those expert in this field of therapy.

The first essential is to make a quiet, simple statement to the patient of what is required and the necessity for relaxing the arms, then the shoulders, and finally the jaws, emphasized. Constant repetition of phrases such as 'just relax your shoulders', 'let the cheeks feel soft', 'just concentrate on relaxing your jaw', will be helpful, as also may a regular light tapping on the side of the chin.

The position of the patient in the chair is with the body inclined only slightly backwards and with the head and body in the same straight line. When relaxed entirely the patient is asked to open and close the mouth, when it is evident by the slow easy nature of the movement if the desired muscle pattern is being reproduced. When this movement is being repeated the record is taken in soft wax. After thorough softening, a strip of aluminium filled wax is placed over the premolars on each side and the patient is asked to close slowly into the wax. The metal filling in this type of wax increases its heat capacity and maintains a well-softened state long enough for the recording to be made. The patient is instructed to stop closing at a point before there is cuspal contact. The opposing arches should, however, approach as closely together as possible without actual contact, as there is often some degree of translation of the mandible in its movement from the rest position to the muscular position.

After chilling with cold water, the hardened wax strips are removed carefully from the mouth and examined to ascertain that at no place has there been complete cuspal penetration. The wax projecting over the buccal aspects of the teeth is now trimmed away with a sharp knife so that, when the wax records are replaced, a clear view may be obtained of the movement of the cusps into their markings in the wax; in a satisfactory and acceptable record this movement should be direct. If it is not, the wax should be resoftened on its upper surface and the process repeated. Two small records confined to the first molar and premolar areas are preferred to the common horse-shoe wax record as fewer extraneous muscle patterns involving either protrusion or retrusion are initiated. Protrusive movement is the usual complication and is often due to stimulation of the nerve endings in the periodontal membranes of the anterior teeth.

The lower cast can now be mounted on the articulator by means of these two wafers. The other information that will be required from the patient is a record of the mandible in a protrusive position so that the individual condyle paths can be recorded on the articulator. For this record a horse-shoe shaped wax wafer can be used. Care must be taken to ensure that the mandible takes up a position at least 6 mm in advance of the muscular position and in a purely sagittal plane unaccompanied by any marked lateral deviation. The record so obtained is placed upon the casts on the articulator and the condyle path angulations set in the usual manner.

When working with casts on an articulator the operator must be aware of the limitations of this instrument. Where the occlusion is being studied in the static tooth position it is reasonable to assume that an accurate reproduction of the mouth conditions is being seen. However, when horizontal mandibular movements are made on the articulator, only an approximation to functional movements can be expected.

When the casts are mounted, the occlusion of the patient is examined in all its phases. Thereafter, adjustments can be made by scraping the occlusal and incisal surfaces of the stone casts, such procedures being repeated later in the mouth, by grinding, if thought desirable. However, before describing the methods to be followed in analysing the occlusion and the steps to be taken, it is necessary to consider the situations which may present. Not all the situations will be those in which the patient has muscular symptoms, but may be cases in which occlusal premature contacts are suspected and some occlusal grinding may be helpful as a preventive measure.

First, there may be the case that, on clinical examination, shows no evidence of mandibular deviation or premature contacts in function. An occlusion analysis on the articulator may be carried out as a check but if this confirms the clinical opinion no form of occlusal equilibration will be required.

Second, there is the case that shows non-coincidence of the muscular and tooth positions. Often, such a case will show muscular symptoms and occlusal grinding will be necessary to make the two positions coincident and hence eliminate the painful muscle spasm.

Third, there is the case that requires grinding of the occlusion in order that adequate distribution of load in function may be achieved. These cases may or may not be periodontal problems but in either event occlusal grinding is carried out as described earlier in this chapter. It may be helpful to have casts on an articulator so that an assessment can be made of the amount of grinding that will be necessary to achieve widespread contact in the tooth position.

The fourth group of cases are those in which a decision has to be made regarding the possible necessity of increasing the vertical dimensions as well as restoring an acceptable horizontal position of the mandible. This form of treatment should never be undertaken unless it is assessed that the case is one of overclosed occlusion. By this is meant a condition in which the free-way space appears to be grossly in excess of what would appear to be normal for the particular patient.

The causes of this condition are usually deranged tooth eruption or loss of a varying number of posterior teeth, but cases may present where excessive attrition has resulted in such a condition. The results of overclosure may be aesthetic disfigurement through shortening of the lower third of the face, dysfunction of the temporomandibular joints or muscular spasm. Any of the above symptoms caused by overclosure may be treated by the provision of partial dentures carrying onlays to restore the occlusion.

Before any such treatment is carried out it is necessary to differentiate between an overclosed occlusion and a condition in which a deep anterior overbite is normal; an Angles Class II Division 2 occlusion. If, after clinical examination, any doubt exists as to whether an increase of vertical dimension is desirable, it is advisable to make a simple acrylic resin onlay appliance and let the patient wear this for a few days. Should the patient report that the appliance is quite intolerable and produces painful symptoms, then no attempt should be made to increase the vertical dimension permanently. As a further aid to differential diagnosis temporomandibular joint radiographs may show retrusion of the condyle in cases of overclosure and normal condylar relationship in all those cases where the vertical dimension has not diminished.

It may be helpful, therefore, when modifications to the vertical dimension are under consideration to obtain radiographs of the joints. A simple technique for this purpose has been described by Grewcock.

The patient is seated comfortably in the dental chair and the head adjusted to the Camper plane position. An imaginary line drawn from the upper border of the external auditory meatus to just below the anterior nasal spine (in practice it will be found much easier to work to the ala of the nose) gives the Camper plane, and the head is regulated until this line is horizontal (Fig. 7.8).

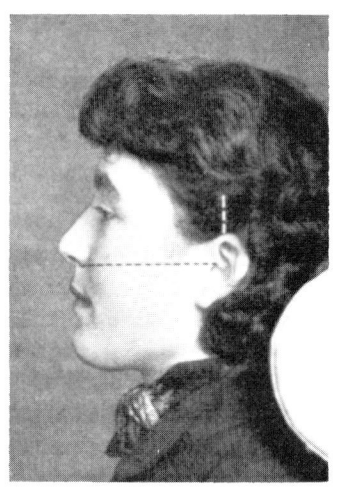

Fig. 7.8. Shows the head in the Camper plane position. The horizontal line is drawn from the upper border of the external auditory meatus to the ala of the nose.

The importance of maintaining immobility during and between the two exposures of each joint is emphasized to the patient. The cone of the tube is not removed, but is applied directly to a point 2.5 cm above the upper border of the pinna, on a line immediately above the external auditory meatus..When directed straight at the opposite condyle head, this gives an approximate downward deflection of between 20 and 25° and a forward inclination of 15–20° towards the face (Fig. 7.9). Figure 7.10 shows the path of the rays at this angulation.

A cassette, with intensifying screens, suitably lettered in lead to differentiate each position, is applied centrally over the joint and maintained in position during exposure by the patient's own hand pressure. To obviate recharging during exposures, four cassettes measuring 9 by 12 cm (or smaller) are used, so that all four exposures can be made within a minimal period. Exposure time is a matter for experiment with the individual apparatus. A Smit Golden Grid may be used to obtain greater definition and contrast by eliminating the scattered rays, in which case the exposure time must be increased by about 50 per cent. Opening movement of the mandible is normally accompanied by upward movement of the maxilla and although gross alteration in head position is unlikely during the brief

156   *Chapter 7*

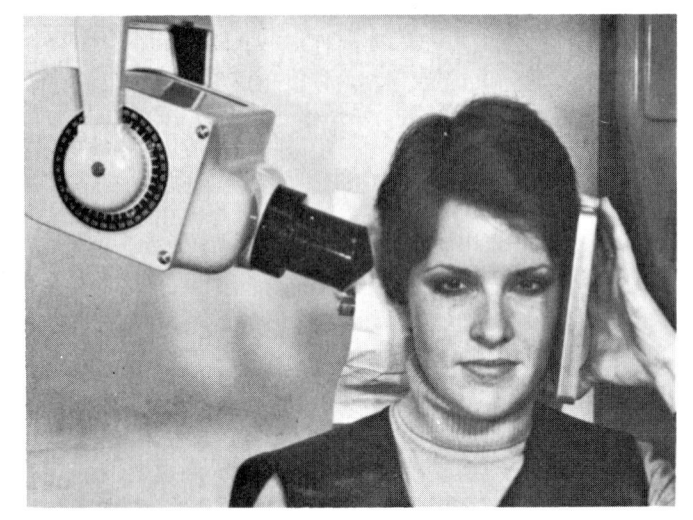

Fig. 7.9. Position of the X-ray tube and cassette.

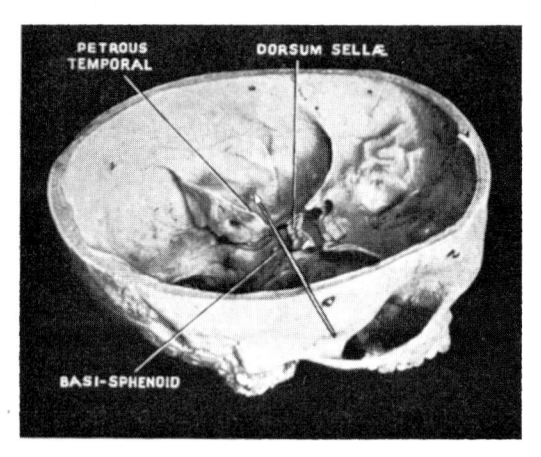

Fig. 7.10. The arrow shows the direct path of the rays, avoiding the petrous part of the temporal bone, the basi-sphenoid and the dorsum sellae.

hinge movement, immobility must be observed between and during exposure. For this reason it is convenient to radiograph the rest position first, the teeth being lightly closed on a wax wafer which has been taken beforehand. Following this exposure, the patient's head and the X-ray tube are maintained in the same positional relationship, the wax withdrawn and the mandible gently guided into occlusion. A second cassette, charged and suitably marked with lead indicator letters, is positioned and the exposure made. The process is then repeated for the

Treatment Planning and Mouth Preparation

opposite side (Fig. 7.11). If so desired a third, open position can be taken, in which case a prop should be inserted between the teeth in order to correlate each condyle in a predetermined opened position. It is of utmost importance that all exposures of any joint are taken with the patient and the tube in exactly the same position. Berry and Chick have pointed out the marked differences in apparent condyle head position which may appear due to even small variations in tube angulation.

The temporomandibular joint radiograph should not be regarded as the sole diagnostic approach; clinical assessments may be more revealing. When the two sources of information do not give corroborative results the evidence of the radiograph should be disregarded. However, condylar displacement which is obvious on the radiographs, especially in an upward and backward direction from the position of rest to that of maximal intercuspidation, is suggestive of a discrepancy between the muscular and tooth positions of the mandible.

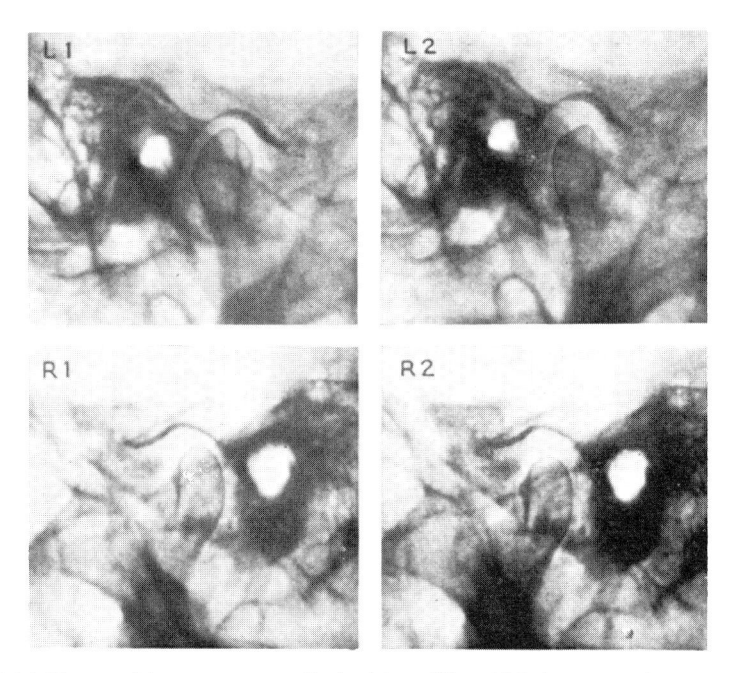

Fig. 7.11. X-rays of the temporomandibular joints. R1 and L1 show posterior displacement of the head of the condyle in a case of closed bite. R2 and L2 show normal joint spaces in the rest position.

When the condition is associated with overclosure it is often possible to obtain coincidence of the two positions by increasing the vertical dimension using partial dentures carrying onlays. When, however, the free-way space is considered normal no increase in vertical dimension should be attempted. In this situation occlusal grinding may be used to re-establish a coincidence of muscular and tooth positions; this is true regardless of the extent of anterior overbite present. If onlays are used misguidedly and the free way space is obliterated discomfort will ensue due to continued muscular contraction and collection of metabolites. Resulting pain may be so severe as to necessitate the patient's removing the denture; this could only be considered as a fortunate happening. If the patient persists in wearing the denture the standing teeth may be depressed into the bone which supports them until a free way space is re-established; this process takes place at varying rates in different individuals.

The following occlusal analysis procedures can be carried out on the casts mounted on the articulator as preliminary diagnostic assessments prior to occlusal grinding in the mouth. Alternatively they may be carried out directly in the mouth if the operator prefers. The clinical procedures for mouth grinding have been described previously (p. 144).

Coinciding muscular and tooth positions

The mounted casts are brought together with thin blue articulating paper between them, the articulator being locked to prevent any lateral or protrusive movement. Only sufficient closure to make the first contact should be carried out, as soon as this is felt the casts should be separated. The common premature contacts that may be found have been described by Cross:

(a) Buccal slope of palatal upper cusp in contact with lingual slope of buccal lower cusp (Fig. 7.12a).

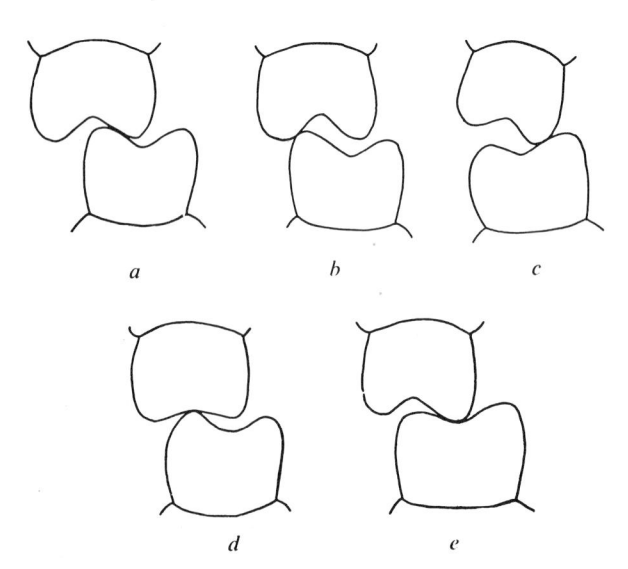

Fig. 7.12. The five premature contacts described by Cross.

Treatment Planning and Mouth Preparation 159

(b) Lingual slope of buccal upper cusp in contact with buccal slope of buccal lower cusp (Fig. 7.12b).
(c) Palatal slope of palatal upper cusp in contact with buccal slope of lingual cusp (Fig. 7.12c).

These are corrected by scraping both contact surfaces until contact is no longer premature, as shown by the blue articulating paper.

(d) Upper fossa, lower buccal cusp (Fig. 7.12d).
(e) Lower fossa, upper palatal cusp (Fig. 7.12e).

In all these types of premature contact the cusp should be scraped or ground. In this way the cusps are reduced and a flat occlusal surface is obtained which permits horizontal movements without the possibility of cuspal hypercontacts. During the scraping of cusps or other contact surfaces notes should be made, step by step, of the areas so treated, so that this can be repeated by grinding the actual teeth in the mouth at a later stage (Fig. 7.13).

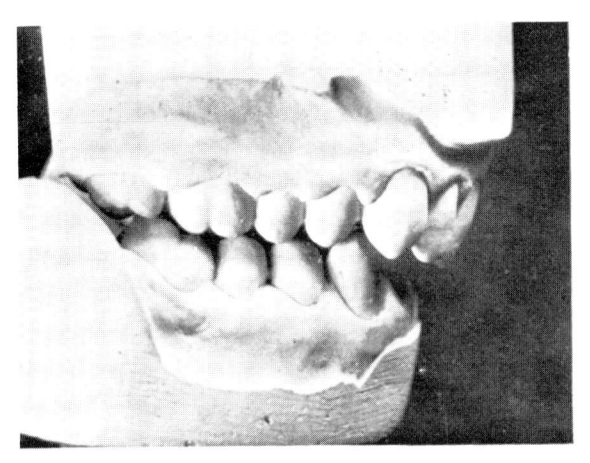

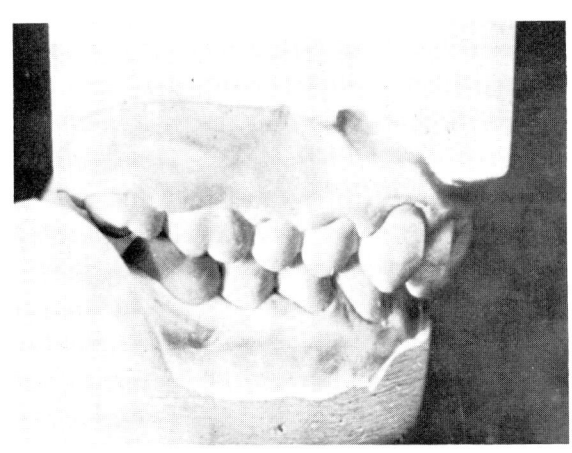

Fig. 7.13. Non-coincidence of the tooth and muscular positions (above); corrected by occlusal grinding so that the two positions coincide (below).

Whereas protrusive, lateral and retrusive mandibular movements may be provisionally studied on the anatomical articulator it is always necessary to make any decisions on occlusal adjustment with reference to the mouth. Here it is possible to define actual jaw movements used by the patient both in terms of direction and extent; the definition of occlusal and incisal facets on the teeth makes a more precise matter and may also indicate the degree to which bruxism is practised. The methods used have already been described when considering occlusal adjustment in periodontal disease.

It will be appreciated that the value of occlusal analysis using casts mounted on an articulator is less than was formerly believed. In practise its principle use is in locating small prematurities on firmly retained teeth which deflect the mandible from its habitual path of closure, often these can be detected in the mouth but sometimes occlusal analysis facilitates their discovery and precise localization.

Restorative treatment

Restoration of natural teeth may well be necessary before partial dentures are constructed. Carious teeth may require restoration for their preservation over a protracted time. In general terms conventional restorative techniques should be expected to give a prognosis commensurate with the anticipated life of the partial dentures. If the denture is planned as a more temporary one, accepting some doubt in the prognosis of a restored tooth is justified. However, as is usually the case when cast appliances are fabricated the prognosis must be expected in terms of years. Two particular conditions come into the doubtful category and deserve special consideration. The first involves deep caries related to the gingival margin; here the base of the preparation must be absolutely caries free and should at no point be proximate to the marginal ligament of the tooth. In the event of deep extension gingivally and the continuing presence of decalcified dentine as deeper cutting is effected, it is always wise to extract. Reference should also be made to the carious activity elsewhere in the mouth; where this is widespread and where carious advance is fast extraction rather than restoration should be favoured. When carious involvement is so deep as to expose the pulp of the tooth, root filling should be considered. Certainly pulp capping procedures with or without pulp debridement confined to the pulp chamber should not be countenanced unless the patient and dentist are prepared to defer denture construction for several months, when an assessment may be made as to the successful outcome of the procedure. The preferable method is generally root filling. Modern endontic therapy should assure a predictably successful result with an excellent long term prognosis, provided two conditions are met. The first is that the periapical tissues are sterile and this can only be assured if no pulpitis preceded the root treatment. When this condition is judged to pertain, confidence in the root filling is justified and denture construction should proceed forthwith. However where infection of the pulp has been in evidence it is essential to allow a proving period before commencing denture work. Apicectomy may well yet be considered but its application should be restricted to a young mouth. It will be recalled that in a more atrophic condition the periapical fibres of the periodontium played a considerable part in restraining hypereruption of the teeth; reliance upon a tooth requiring apicectomy in the presence of periodontal disease would be a decided gamble. However the retention of an apicectomized tooth which had proved its functional use over a period of several years would be favourably regarded and would indicate neither extraction nor deferment. The second condition stipulated for a good endontic prognosis prior to denture construction would concern the form of the root canals especially in the periapical region. When there is confidence that the pulp can be completely extirpated and the canal completely and permanently filled without the possibility of a dead space where tissue fluid would stagnate and provide a substrate for bacteria, there is no reason not to proceed with the final treatment. However when the root canal is tortuous especially in the apical area it is doubtful if such confidence is justified and a wait and see approach would be sensible. The infection of such a static pool of tissue fluid could occur after a protracted period, especially where poor oral hygiene was associated with some periodontal disease. The innoculation of subgingival bacteria into the stagnant tissue fluid would occur via the lymphatics in a tooth subject to jiggling. The position with regard to prognosis where endontic treatment is contemplated is a matter for sound clinical judgement; it should be based on what the individual operator has observed over years of practise.

Restoration of some, or rarely all, of the standing teeth may be necessary or desirable, to produce a tooth form better able to accommodate the components of a partial denture. Greatly overhanging tooth inclines may require reduction. For example a very tilted lower molar may incline towards an edentulous space so much as to create an undesirably large space between the saddle and the proximal surface of the tooth. Again a lingually inclined lower molar may embarrass the favourable placement of some lingually placed denture component. Thus a lingual bar or even the inferior edge of a lingual plate may have to be placed so far lingually near the floor of the mouth as to be unacceptable to the patient on the grounds of its encroaching on tongue space. Or the commonly seen straight lingual contour of a lower premolar or molar in a lingually inclined tooth may necessitate the placement of a clasp arm or indirect retainer at the occlusal level of the tooth where it could well provide an obtrusive and unacceptable impedence to tongue movement. The contour of surfaces of teeth planned for the reception of retentive clasp arms may also require modification to enable the placement of the tip of the clasp arm in an area of sufficient undercut; a more bulbous convexity may well need to be created. On the other hand the contour may have to be moulded to reduce the undercut so that the clasp arm can be placed about the middle of the vestibular or oral tooth surface out of occlusion from an opposing cusp and in a position likely to be well tolerated. The occlusal surfaces and palatal inclines of the upper anterior teeth may well need to be modified to allow the placement of occlusal rests, clasp arms, indirect retainers or onlays without providing a hypercontact in functional occlusal positions.

These modifications of tooth form may be accomplished by crowning, filling or grinding and it is pertinent to consider the merits of, and indications of each.

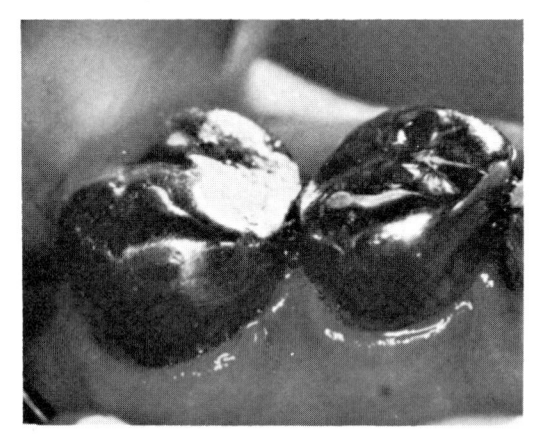

Fig. 7.14. Abutment and contiguous tooth crowned to improve contour and to give protection against caries.

The use of the full coverage cast gold crown has proved one of the most successful approaches of restorative dentistry; it is especially applicable in restoring grossly carious teeth assuring they can contribute indefinitely in load bearing; weak enamel walls associated with conventional amalgam fillings are hardly justified if cast partial dentures are to be provided. Their strength too eliminates the hazards of fracture where well supported enamel has been lost interstitially. But the use of the full coverage cast gold crown has especial advantage since in construction all the non-fitting surfaces of the crown may be modified to accept the approximation of a partial denture component in its ideal location; thus attending to the special demands catalogued above. Additionally the use of contiguous cast gold crowns allows the possibility of splinting; this may be extensive on a segmental basis and provides good therapy in periodontal disease. Such a splinting of two premolar teeth may provide an enhanced abutment couple (Fig. 7.14). In the molar teeth and the second lower premolar aesthetics is not compromised by the yellow gold coloration. However in the remaining premolars patients now usually request the use of aesthetic buccal facings on these teeth and happily for the last two decades this requirement has been adequately met by the use of porcelain bonded facings. However such facings are not suitable for the placement of clasp arms and other means must be devised for retention. This may be accomplished by clasp arms used on other tooth surfaces where deep rest seats stabilize the tooth. However the cast gold crown permits the use of a whole range of precision denture attachments, the use of which will be considered more appropriately later.

The conventional filling methods of restorative dentistry still have wide application in cases where partial dentures are planned. Caries may still be well treated in this way and additionally small changes in tooth form may be facilitated for example by placing an amalgam filling to form a rest seat preparation on the cingulum of an upper anterior tooth or a concavity on the buccal pit of a lower molar to receive a retentive clasp terminal. Whereas specially developed composites are now proving of value in restoring carious teeth it remains to be finally settled whether their use is to be recommended in association with different denture components; however initial observations are encouraging. But where such fillings are already *in situ* their acceptance is not conditioned by the associated use of a partial denture. It is only necessary to confirm that existing fillings are sound. However if it is decided that existing fillings would require recontouring to create room for a proposed denture component it would need to be ascertained that the reduced filling would still have adequate strength to assure it was not distorted or fractured thus permitting a recurrence of caries.

When a metallic portion of a denture has to come in contact with a metal filling it is preferable that the alloys should be of similar composition. The production of pulpitis in an amalgam filled tooth clasped with gold, although not common, is an example of the phenomenon that metals having different solution potentials are liable to induce galvanic action when they are in contact in the mouth. The fact that symptoms are not always evident may be due to the formation of a non-conductive layer on the surface of one of the metals, or by the poor conductivity of the electrolyte, in this case saliva or fluids taken by mouth. In addition to producing pulpitis this phenomenon can cause the familiar metallic taste when different metals come in contact. Corrosion of the metal parts involved in this process is an added complication.

Galvanic action may be prevented by using gold crowns or onlays for those restorations that will contact a gold based denture. However nowadays most partial denture bases are cast in cobalt chromium alloy and it is necessary to accept the fact that restorations must be made in a dissimilar alloy; in such cases gold may be preferable on the side of galvanic action and strength. It is not suggested that amalgam fillings are inappropriate; sound amalgam fillings are acceptable unless more than transient symptoms occur. The very low incidence of galvanic reaction with the cobalt chromium alloys is doubtless due to a fine ever present oxide film on the surface of the metal. Reaction from an immediately placed filling is likely to be transient and caused by the presence of free mercury.

But modification of tooth form may most often be accomplished without recourse to crowning or filling; generally grinding without restoration is acceptable. The criterion that must be met is that dentine with patent tubules should not be left exposed. Thus grinding should not be carried out until the third decade when some sclerosis of the superficial dentine may be expected. But it must be borne in mind that there is a considerable personal variation in the degree to which this takes place. Where considerable natural attrition of the occlusal surfaces has taken place it is safe to assume that superficial sealing of the underlying dentinal tubules has taken place. In general terms the older the tooth the more confidently can it be ground. However enamel thickness is also variable to a considerable degree. Rampant caries in the second decade is often associated with a deficient enamel thickness and such a history would alert the dentist to preferring restoration to grinding. Not all tooth surfaces are covered by a substantial thickness of enamel; fortunately the marginal ridges that are most often preferred sites for grinding are areas of deep enamel covering. Interstitial grinding of the teeth should be approached with more caution. Especially in the region of the gingival margin the covering enamel layer is thin and calcification of the dentinal tubules is not prevalent. This is just another area where clinical judgement stemming from the observation of large numbers of cases over many years is indispensible. However, the rare incidence of caries in sites which have been ground can easily be treated by conventional methods and should be revealed at routine recall examination; this is just another reason among many for commending routine dental examination following the provision of partial dentures.

Occlusal Rest Seat Preparation

Where the denture is to receive support from the teeth, these may require some preparation. Such support is provided by occlusal rests and the general principles involved in their use are discussed in Chapter 9.

A decision as to the teeth involved is dependent upon the design of the denture as a whole. Before this can be decided, study models and surveying will have to be considered. Certainly, the preparation of teeth for occlusal rests must be done before the final impressions are taken, but such preparation should follow any occlusal grinding.

Rest seat preparation may be undertaken for any or all of the following reasons:
1 To provide space between the occlusal surface of the upper and lower teeth to allow a rest of adequate thickness and strength to be used.
2 To provide more suitably inclined bearing surfaces for occlusal rests than those existing on the natural teeth.

3   To provide a shape of surface giving a desirable amount of bracing.

In general, preparation for the first reason is necessary in connection with the posterior teeth and for the second with the anterior teeth.

Preparation in posterior teeth

When contact between upper and lower teeth is close there may be no space available for the occlusal rest without interference with the occlusion. In other cases, if a space exists, the rest has to be made so thin and weak that it cannot withstand the load placed upon it and breaks. Hence, in such conditions, the teeth must be prepared for the reception of the rests. In addition most posterior teeth, even if adequate space exists, can have their surfaces improved for the satisfactory fitting of rests.

If caries is present in the teeth, fillings should be fitted and the rest seat preparations carried out in the alloy.

The most important principle to follow when preparing a rest seat is to ensure that its floor is at right angles to the long axis of the tooth. Preparations that slope towards the cervical margin must be avoided since they will induce a wedging action on the tooth. Such action may not be resisted adequately if the tooth is, for example, a single standing premolar. Rest seat floors at right angles to the long axis ensure transmission of vertical loading in the correct direction. Tilted teeth present a problem in this respect, but the correct application of vertical load in such cases can better be accomplished by variation in the rests themselves rather than in the preparation of their seats. These principles are discussed in Chapter 10.

All rest seat preparations in posterior teeth should have rounded proximal margins. If this margin remains angular then a similar angle is produced in the rest, which tends to induce strains at this point so that fracture may occur. In addition, a sharp proximal angle results in a reduction of metal at the point where strength is required and fracture is likely from this cause (Fig. 7.15).

The actual size of the preparation will vary with the bulk of metal necessary in the rest itself. This again varies according to the material of which it is made and the load that it has to resist. Rests made of chrome cobalt may be somewhat thinner than those made of gold. Powerful musculature and habits of clenching or grinding the teeth, evidenced by faceting or attrition, indicate that heavier and stronger rests should be used. If the partial denture is opposed by a complete denture in the other jaw then the load on the rests is not so great and accordingly they can be reduced in size. Natural tooth opposition indicates that greater strength must be provided.

The width of the seat should be such that it is broadest at the point of attachment of the rest to the saddle. At this area it should ideally cover two-thirds of the marginal ridge area. Towards the centre of the occlusal surface the width may be reduced, but it should never become tapered to a point. Wherever possible it should extend over the central axis of the tooth.

The floor and walls of the preparation should normally be saucer-shaped rather than form a box-shaped cavity. Much greater torque is produced when the rest preparation is of a box form, whereas the saucer-shaped seat allows very slight lateral movement of the rest over the tooth (Fig. 7.16). Box-shaped preparations may be advisable when little bracing action is obtained from the clasping and when it is estimated that the tooth can safely withstand a large lateral load. Box-shaped preparations should normally only be prepared in well-supported molar teeth and then only when no other bracing method is possible.

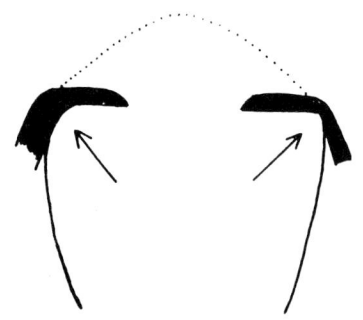

Fig. 7.15. The strengthening effect of rounding the edge of the rest seat (left) compared with angular preparation (right).

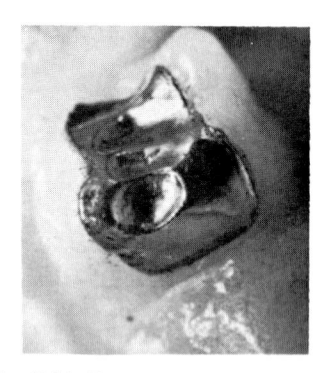

Fig. 7.16. Saucer shaped rest seat prepared in a gold inlay.

Normally, it is not necessary to penetrate enamel to prepare a rest seat that conforms to the general principle outlined above. However, should penetration of the enamel be unavoidable in a young patient it is essential to provide a restoration for the tooth. In older patients, when it is reasonably certain that sclerosed dentine deposition has taken place, exposure of dentine is not necessarily so serious.

Rest seats prepared in posterior teeth will usually be located either mesially or distally, but occasionally, particularly on lower first premolars, it may be better if they are prepared lingually. The lingual cusp of a lower first premolar is usually ill defined, and if it is ground off, a flat surface at right angles to the long axis of the tooth is produced on which an occlusal rest can be placed. Often, it can be built up to improve occlusal contacts but in any event there is usually adequate space between the upper and lower teeth in this area of the mouth (Fig. 7.17).

The initial preparation should be carried out with barrel-shaped, tapered, or round diamond abrasives. When the main preparation has been completed with the diamonds the surfaces should be further smoothed with carborundum stones and polished by rubber discs, brushes, and polishing paste.

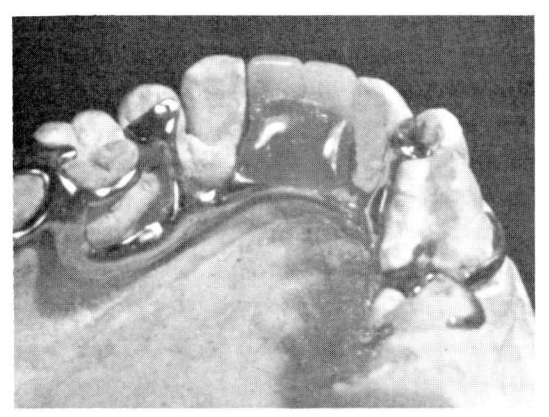

Fig. 7.17. Occlusal rests placed on the lingual aspect of the occlusal surfaces of the lower premolars.

Preparation in anterior teeth

The normal shape of an anterior tooth does not allow it to provide correct support for a denture. A rest placed upon the unprepared cingulum of an anterior tooth has its fitting surface at an angle much greater than 90° to the long axis of the tooth. Consequently an inclined plane effect can operate and one component of force will tend to displace the tooth labially. In the lower jaw this may be resisted by the overbite but in the upper jaw the force is unopposed. It is also obvious that the steeper the slope of the cingulum the less effective is the rest in providing support for the denture. Anterior teeth may be required to provide support, not only for anterior saddles, but, particularly in the lower jaw, for the connectors joining two posterior saddles.

The preparation of anterior teeth for the correct placement of rests can be carried out on the cingulum or on the incisal edge.

Cingulum preparations. A preparation on the cingulum of the tooth must provide a fitting surface for the rest which is at right angles to the long axis of the tooth. If the cingulum is pronounced it may be possible to do this by grinding the enamel to produce such a surface (Fig. 7.18). If this is done care must be taken not to penetrate the enamel owing to the risk of caries developing under the rest. In any event this method of preparation should never be used in the younger age group, or in any patient who appears to be more than normally prone to caries.

In the majority of cases preparation on the cingulum by grinding alone will not produce a sufficiently large bearing surface for the rest, without the removal of more tooth structure than is warranted. The angulation of the cingulum surface is often nearly vertical and hence grinding alone cannot produce an adequate area for support. In this respect lower anteriors are usually unsuitable for this type of preparation and hence it is more common practice to use the incisal edge preparation in the lower jaw, the cingulum preparation being confined to the upper. In the upper jaw canines are usually more favourable than centrals.

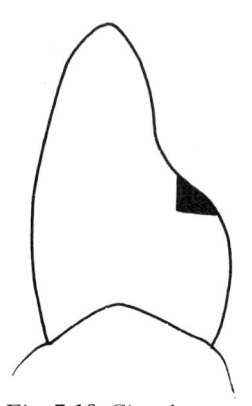

Fig. 7.18. Cingulum preparation on anterior tooth.

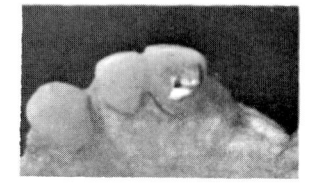

Fig. 7.19. Mesial inlay in a central, shaped to receive an occlusal rest.

There is no doubt that the best preparation is made by cutting an inlay cavity in the tooth and shaping a fitting surface to receive the rest in the inlay. Such inlays will vary in shape and outline form according to the type of rest that is to be fitted. Figure 7.19 shows a simple mesial inlay to receive an occlusal rest which will be attached to the anterior saddle. When the abutment teeth are laterals it will be wise to prepare the canines to receive the support of the anterior saddle. In this situation both canines should be prepared for three-quarter crowns, their cingulum surfaces being flattened to receive occlusal rests carried on continuous clasps (Fig. 7.20).

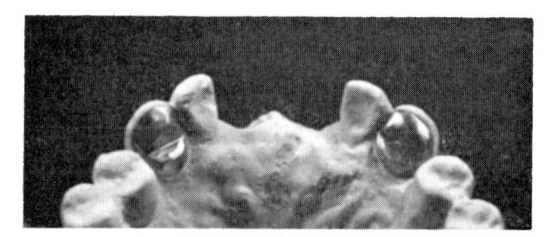

Fig. 7.20. Three quarter crowns on upper canines modified to receive occlusal rests.

One aesthetic advantage of preparing an occlusal rest seat on the cingulum aspect of the tooth is that there is no display of metal. It is also possible to apply the load to the tooth near to the long axis and low down on the crown, both advantageous from the stress point of view. The disadvantage of these inlay preparations is the time involved and the fact that it is often necessary to remove

Treatment Planning and Mouth Preparation 169

sound tooth structure. If the enamel is ground and no inlay is fitted then there is the potential danger of caries and also the fact that the exposed dentine may be hypersensitive.

Incisal edge preparation. This type of preparation is used more commonly in the lower jaw owing to lack of space on the lingual aspect of most lower anterior teeth. The type of preparation shown in Fig. 7.21 has been advocated by Kelly. The advantage of this preparation is that it gives a definite location for the rest and

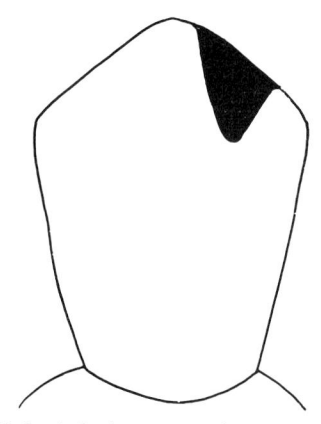

Fig. 7.21. Incisal edge preparation suggested by Kelly.

places it near to the long axis of the tooth. From an aesthetic point of view however, it is possibly more noticeable, owing to its outline form, than the preparation shown in Fig. 7.22. This is particularly suitable for use on a canine abutment tooth in the lower jaw. It should extend a little more than half-way across the incisal edge but care must be taken to ensure that the remaining

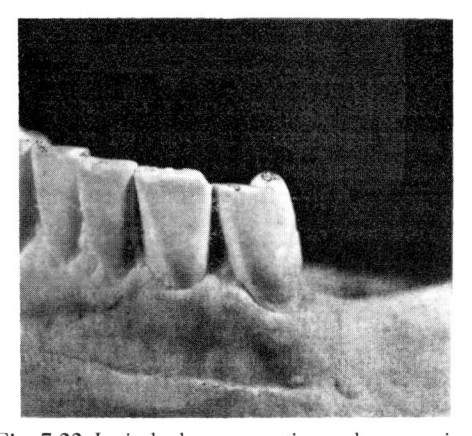

Fig. 7.22. Incisal edge preparation on lower canine.

segment of the incisal edge is adequately strong to resist backward movement. Preparation for an incisal embrasure hook is normally a simple matter of making a small recess in the enamel with a wheel stone.

The only other form of incisal edge preparation is the simple but somewhat drastic method of grinding down entire incisal enamel. This will result in adequate denture support with the load axially directed, but aesthetically is not always acceptable.

Preparation of opposing teeth. If it is not possible to prepare a rest seat of sufficient depth to accommodate a rest of the necessary thickness it will be necessary to grind away some enamel from the opposing tooth or teeth. Such a procedure usually involves the grinding of cusps only and is simple and not normally hazardous from the caries aspect.

Modifications of Occlusal and Incisal Surfaces

When one jaw, usually the upper, is completely edentulous and the other is to be supplied with a partial denture, it is important that an even, well-balanced occlusal contact is obtained in the tooth position. This is necessary to assist the stability and retention of the complete denture and to ensure that, as far as possible, stress is favourably divided between the partial denture, natural teeth and mucosal tissues of the opposing jaw.

In many cases these objectives will be easier to achieve if some modifications are first made to the occlusal plane, as presented by the remaining natural teeth. Usually this can be achieved by grinding the occlusal surfaces and incisal edges of these teeth. Any cusps of teeth that are likely to cause difficulty in obtaining good occlusal contacts should be ground flatter. Teeth that have over-erupted to a considerable extent may require extraction, but deviations from the occlusal plane to this extent should have been noted at the examination and treatment planning stage.

In particular, grinding of the incisal edges of lower incisors and canines will be most helpful in establishing a good protrusive occlusal contact when making a full upper denture when a number of lower teeth are still standing.

Adjustment to the tooth contour is indicated when attrition or abrasion has produced sharp angles between the occlusal and other surfaces of the teeth. Grinding to produce a bevel will remove the sharp edge from the notice of the patient's tongue and also make the insertion of the denture easier.

In certain cases of deep anterior overbite the incisal edges of the lower teeth will make contact with the palatal mucosa or the gingival margin of the upper teeth. Such a condition is an embarrassment to the fitting of an upper denture and may be treated by reducing the incisal edges of the lower teeth, even by as

Treatment Planning and Mouth Preparation

much as 2 or 3 mm. When the denture is constructed an incisal table must be provided behind the upper teeth to which the lowers can occlude.

Conditioning of the mucosa

This mouth preparation may be carried out in two different situations. When a new partial denture is to be provided for a patient who has been wearing such a denture for a considerable period of time, a chronic inflammatory condition of the underlying mucosa may be present. It is undesirable to take impressions when the mouth is in such a condition.

If the patient can be persuaded to discontinue wearing the denture for several days, the inflammation will subside, but such a request is unrealistic when missing anterior teeth are replaced by the partial denture. In such circumstances use should be made of one of the so-called 'conditioning materials'. A definition of a conditioning material has been given as 'a soft material which is applied temporarily to the fitting surface of a denture for the purposes of allowing a more equal distribution of load, thus permitting the mucosal tissues to return to their normal position' (Wilson *et al.*).

The fitting surface of the old denture should be covered with such a material and the patient allowed to wear the denture for two or three days. At the end of this time some degree of improvement in the condition of the mucosa is usually evident. Any areas of the fitting surface where the conditioning material is very thin, or absent, should be relieved by grinding and a fresh layer of material applied to the entire fitting surface.

This procedure may require repeating once or twice, but usually at the end of a week or ten days a marked improvement will have occurred and new impressions taken.

The second and more important situation when a mucosal conditioning technique is indicated is the preparation of an alveolar ridge and its covering mucosa for the reception of a new partial lower denture. The technique has special application in more elderly patients and in the case of free-end saddles which must be load bearing. In this situation if a denture were constructed without tissue conditioning pain would often be experienced in the covered mucosa. However when the tissue is subjected to a lesser load which may be gradually increased this situation is often overcome. Reduction of the load applied to the saddle of a temporary conditioning plate is effected in two ways; first the saddle area is covered by a soft conditioning lining and the acrylic resin occlusal table is first formed just out of occlusion with opposing teeth. After a short time an adjustment of the occlusal table is made to engage the occlusion but on a reduced table by the addition of self curing acrylic resin. This process may be repeated with increases in both the size of the occlusal table and mucosal compression. The principle is to establish a local hyperaemia without entering the traumatic range. The increased circulation terminates the local anoxia and the pain nerve endings accordingly show an increased threshold. But the aim goes much further than that, since the alveolar ridge is subjected to loading graded in magnitude but directionally exactly the same as that to which it will be subjected on completion of the new partial denture. During the conditioning period which may be extended into months change in alveolar form and structure is gradually induced under favourable vascular conditions and some thickening of the submucosa may be stimulated.

References

BERRY D.C. and CHICK A.O. (1956) Temporo-mandibular joint: interpretation of radiographs. *Dent. Pract.* **7**, 18.

CROSS W.G. (1952) Selective grinding as a means of prevention and treatment of periodontal disease. *Dent. Pract.* **2**, 300.

DURKACZ K.P. (1976) Hypersensitive dentine and cementum—treatment with hydrocortisone. *The Probe*, **17**, 276.

GRATY T.C., TOMLIN H.R. and FOX E.C. (1964) The mylo-hyoid ridge problem. *Brit. dent. J.* **116**, 203.

GREWCOCK R.J.G. (1951) A short survey of the principles involved in the establishment of balanced occlusion. *Dent. Pract.* **1**, 234.

GREWCOCK R.J.G. (1953) A simple technique for temporo-mandibular joint radiography. *Brit. dent. J.* **94**, 152.

LAMMIE G.A. (1966) *Dental orthodontics*. Alden, Oxford.

WILSON H.J., TOMLIN H.R. and OSBORNE J. (1966) Tissue conditioners and functional impression materials. *Brit. dent. J.* **121**, 91.

8
CAST SURVEYING

A removable partial denture which has been constructed correctly must be capable of being inserted into and removed from the mouth along a predetermined path without difficulty. Once in position it should have sufficient retention to prevent displacement during normal functions, particularly at right angles to the occlusal plane. In order to produce this situation it is necessary to survey casts obtained at different clinical stages, usually following recording of the preliminary impressions (the preliminary survey) and after recording master impressions (the final survey).

The necessity for two surveys is due to the fact that in order to provide a suitable path of insertion and removal together with sufficient retention, modifications may be required to the contour of the natural teeth either by grinding, the addition of an adhesive restoration, or even the construction of inlays and crowns. Surveying a preliminary cast will allow the need for such modifications to be identified and the necessary tooth preparation undertaken prior to taking the master impressions.

When these preparations have been completed in accordance with the information provided by both the preliminary survey and the clinical examination, the master impressions can be taken. A second survey is then carried out on the master casts to indicate the precise position of denture components and the angulation of the path of insertion and removal, so enabling the technician to prepare his master cast prior to producing either a refractory cast or a duplicate upon which the denture will be processed.

Principles of Surveying

All partially edentulous mouths contain undercut areas related both to the natural teeth and to the associated soft tissues. Those related to the teeth result from the natural bulbous shape of the crown, which is most marked in molar teeth and least in incisors. In addition, undercuts may result from the inclination of the long axes of the teeth, with teeth adjacent to saddle areas often subject to tilting, so creating or emphasizing the degree of undercut present. Soft tissue undercuts, which is a slight misnomer, are probably due to the pattern of bone resorption in the edentulous saddle areas.

All removable partial dentures contain both rigid components such as the base and the connector, and flexible components such as clasp arms. If a denture base is constructed so that it engages interproximal undercuts in a bounded saddle situation for instance (Fig. 8.1) there is a greater dimension between the gingival areas of the teeth than between the approximal areas of greatest convexity. Such a denture could not be inserted into the mouth as the rigid base would be of too great a dimension to pass between the areas of maximum convexity of the abutment teeth. If the proximal undercuts are masked out however, the denture can be inserted along the path of the solid lines. This will mean of course that the denture will not fit in the undercut areas, and in this respect it is important to ensure that the base is finished occlusal to the maximum convexity of the tooth, in order that it will fit snugly and prevent food packing between the denture and the teeth.

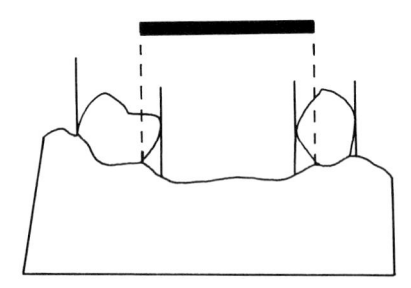

Fig. 8.1. The denture base as represented by the black bar, the length of which is equal to the distance between the proximal gingival areas of the abutment teeth. Such a base could not be inserted as it could not pass between the areas of maximum convexity of the abutment teeth.

Not all undercuts are masked out however, as some can be utilized for retention. This often depends upon the use of clasps, the flexible tips of which can be moved over the greatest convexity of the tooth until the tip rests in the undercut area. It is important to realize that clasps do not grip the teeth, and that their retentive properties depend upon their engaging an undercut. Their efficiency is dependent upon a displacing force during function being insufficient to pull the retentive portion of the clasp arm back over the maximum convexity of the tooth.

The purpose of surveying in partial denture design is therefore to locate undercuts that may prevent insertion of the denture along its selected path, and also undercuts that may be utilized for retention.

Fundamentally therefore the objective in surveying is to record the greatest convexity of the natural teeth relative both to the horizontal plane and a desired plane of angulation. In addition it allows the clinician to study the degree of parallelism between two teeth or groups of teeth, and to locate and evaluate tooth or mucosal undercuts in respect of their possible utilization. From the survey a decision can also be made on the location and preparation of guide planes which will direct insertion and removal of the denture along a predetermined path.

The majority of natural tooth crowns are bulbous in shape, but the area of maximum convexity may occur anywhere between the occlusal or incisal surface and the gingival margin. If a vertical plane is brought into contact with a convex surface, contact will occur only at the point of maximum convexity. If the convex surface is rotated, still in contact with the plane, an imaginary line will be traced at the greatest circumference. If a carbon rod is substituted for the vertical plane and a tooth for the convex surface, then a line will be produced which will indicate the maximum convexity of the tooth. This is known as the survey line (Fig. 8.2). The area of tooth above this line is the non-undercut area and below is the undercut area.

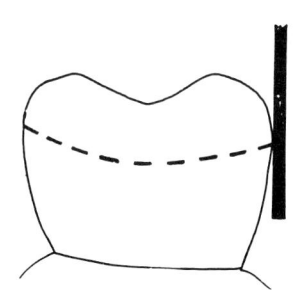

Fig. 8.2. The survey line dividing the tooth into undercut and non-undercut areas.

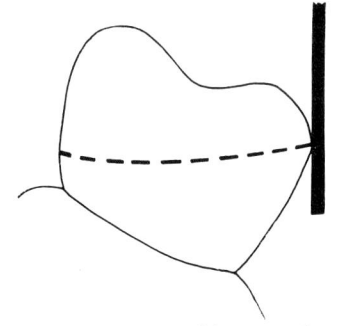

Fig. 8.3. Alteration of the survey line produced by tilting the tooth.

The position of a survey line and the loction and extent of the undercut areas are determined therefore by positioning the tooth in a vertical axis while a vertical carbon marker is passed around it. If the tooth should be tilted out of this axis and the carbon marker passed round again, the line shown in Fig. 8.3 will result. It will be noted that although the same tooth has been surveyed the level of the survey line, indicating the level of the maximum convexity, is now quite different. Consequently, the location and extent of the undercut and non-undercut areas have also changed considerably. This illustrates that the information obtainable from surveying can be varied by the angle at which the tooth is inclined to the carbon marker.

The principle of surveying has so far been considered in relation to a single tooth. In practice many of the teeth on the cast will have to be surveyed and they will not all be in the same vertical axis. Figure 8.4 shows how the location of the undercut areas can be varied by tilting the cast anteriorly and posteriorly. Comparable effects are also produced by lateral tilting of the cast.

When the preliminary cast is surveyed prior to mouth preparation it is necessary to decide on the most appropriate tilt. This is dependent upon two factors, the path of insertion and removal, and the path of displacement of the denture. Although ease of insertion and removal of the denture is important, its final success is dependent upon whether or not the patient will wear it. This is often directly related to its retention and stability during function.

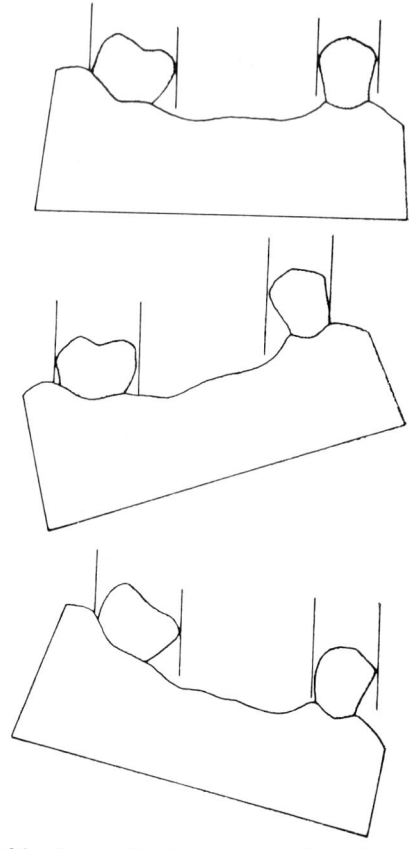

Fig. 8.4. Alteration of the degree of undercut by anterior and posterior tilting of the model.

Both upper and lower partial dentures tend to be displaced by the masticatory process whilst, in addition, upper dentures must also resist the force of gravity. Displacement of dentures during mastication tends to be in a *direction at right angles to the occlusal plane*. Lateral forces are also developed during mastication but, if the denture is correctly designed and constructed and there is freedom from cuspal interference, these forces should not cause displacement. Consequently, in deciding upon the tilt to be given to the cast, prior consideration must be given to the displacing forces acting at right angles to the occlusal plane.

In this respect it is essential that all casts are surveyed firstly with the occlusal plane at right angles to the carbon rod, in order that the degree of undercut

Cast Surveying

relative to the path of displacement can be identified. It is important to appreciate that if in such a survey no undercut areas are revealed, the denture cannot be made mechanically retentive against vertical displacement simply by altering the angle of tilt. Any apparent undercuts identified in this manner are only undercuts relative to the angle of tilt chosen.

It has been pointed out that one of the limitations of surveying is that it does not ensure that the path of removal of the denture will always be restricted to the single direction parallel to the surveying rod. If a denture can be removed in only one direction its retention will be greater than if it can be removed in more than one path. For example, if the cast has been surveyed with the occlusal plane at right angles to the surveying rod it may be found that removal is possible through a rotational pathway, in addition to that parallel to the surveying rod. Such displacement may be controlled by giving a small degree of anterior or posterior tilt to the cast without lessening the resistance to a displacing force at right angles to the occlusal plane. Conversely, increased resistance to displacement at right angles to the occlusal plane may be provided in free-end saddle dentures by an anterior tilt. This will allow the distal undercuts on the abutment teeth to be engaged by the denture and so increase resistance to vertical displacement; however, no resistance to rotating displacement about an axis located in or near the occlusal rests is provided in this way.

It is recommended therefore that all casts are first analysed and surveyed with a zero degree tilt, that is with the occlusal plane at right angles to the surveying rod. The resultant survey lines will indicate what undercut areas are available to provide retention against vertical displacement. Bearing in mind that this form of displacement is likely to be the most common, the majority of dentures will be well retained if the lines resulting from a horizontal survey indicate adequate

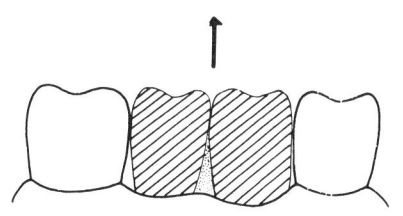

Fig. 8.5. Parallel abutments; the saddle can only be removed in a vertical direction.

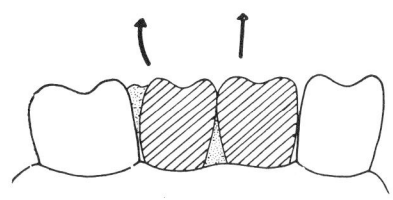

Fig. 8.6. Saddle can be removed by rotation as well as in a vertical direction.

undercuts for clasp engagement. However, when many teeth are found to be widely divergent or when there are gross differences in abutment tooth angulation to the occlusal plane, additional surveying may be required. In the case shown in Fig. 8.5, where the adjacent abutment teeth have parallel or practically parallel surfaces, removal of the saddle can be only in a vertical direction. In the case in Fig. 8.6, however, displacement of the saddle can also occur in a rotational manner, the distal part rising even though the mesial part is retained. In such a case an anterior tilt given to the cast will enable the operator to determine whether any undercut exists on the molar tooth which will help to resist this possible rotational displacement.

It is recommended in such cases that additional surveying is carried out with both anterior and posterior tilts. This will produce three survey lines on the teeth (Fig. 8.7). For the sake of clarity different coloured marking rods should be used for different tilts. The undercut area indicated by the anterior tilt survey line shows the area available for the positioning of a clasp arm that will resist displacement of the denture in a backwards direction. Conversely, the undercut present with a posterior tilt will show the area available for resistance to forwards displacement. If the clasp arm can be placed in part of the undercut area that is common to all three survey lines (the shaded area in Fig. 8.7) then that particular clasp will resist displacement of the denture in all directions. When this is not possible it must be accepted that no resistance to possible displacement in certain directions can be provided by clasping that particular tooth unless some modification of its contour is undertaken.

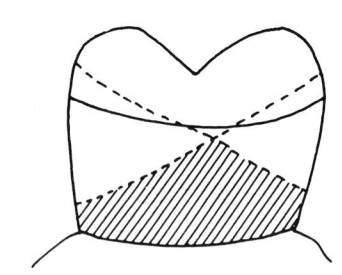

Fig. 8.7. Three survey lines on one tooth.

In this respect it has been suggested that the tilt given to the cast and hence the angulation of the path of insertion, should be determined by paralleling the carbon marker to the long axis of the weakest tooth to be clasped. By this means the weakest tooth would be stressed minimally during insertion and removal of the denture.

Resulting from the information derived from the various surveys, a decision should be possible regarding the tilt at which the final survey should be done to achieve the best results, not only in terms of retention but also with regard to the path of insertion.

The Cast Surveyor

All surveyors work upon the same basic principles which essentially allow a vertically movable arm to be brought into contact with the cast at any desired tilt (Fig. 8.8). The instrument usually has a heavy base which can often be rotated to allow easy access to the cast. On the base is positioned a table which can be tilted to any angle by virtue of a universal ball and socket joint on its base. Once tilted it can be locked in position. It is on this adjustable table that the cast is positioned and secured, usually by spring loaded or screw locking pins. Attached to the base of the instrument is a rigid vertical arm, which carries a horizontal arm able to pivot freely by means of two movable joints. This in turn supports another vertical arm which is adjustable in a vertical direction and which may be fixed at any required height by a locking screw. At the lower end of this arm is a chuck to which can be attached the various instruments used in surveying, cast modification and clasp positioning.

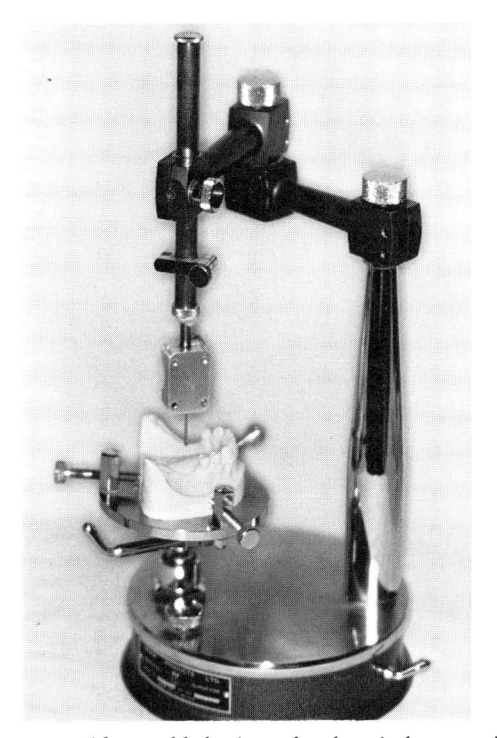

Fig. 8.8. A cast surveyor with movable horizontal and vertical arms and adjustable table.

The instruments which may be used with the surveyor are the analysing rod, the carbon marker, the undercut gauges and the wax trimmers (Fig. 8.9).

The *analysing rod* is a thin cylindrical metal rod which allows a preliminary

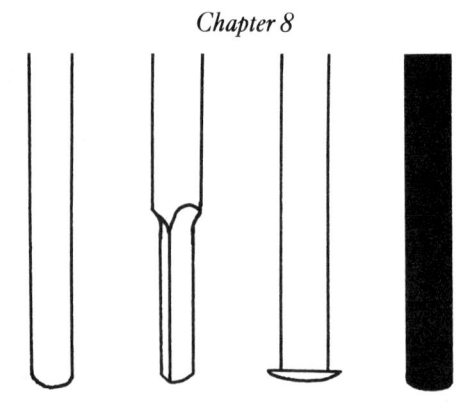

Fig. 8.9. The surveyor instruments. The analysing rod, wax trimmer, undercut gauge, and carbon marker.

surveying assessment without actually marking the cast. It is commonly used diagnostically to select the tilt at which the cast is to be surveyed. The *carbon marker* is used to trace the survey lines on the cast and so demarcate accurately the undercut area from the non-undercut area at the desired degree of tilt. It is normally attached in the long axis of the movable vertical arm, where its contact with the cast is assured irrespective of height. The *undercut gauges* are three in number and will measure the horizontal depth of the undercut present so allowing the operator to determine the correct position of the clasp arm according to the physical properties of the material to be used. The *wax trimmer* is used to trim wax which may have been placed in undercut areas in order to obliterate these for constructional purposes. It is usually (but not always) placed in the long axis of the movable vertical arm so ensuring accurate masking out of the undercut relative to the paths of insertion and removal.

Technique of Surveying

It has already been indicated that during function, any tendency for displacement of the partial denture will normally be at right angles to the occlusal plane, and that for clasp arms to be effective they must engage undercuts which are present relative to that path of displacement. All casts should therefore be surveyed initially with the occlusal plane horizontal, that is with zero degree tilt. As a result of the preliminary investigation it may be possible to decide that one survey at zero tilt will be all that is required, or that further surveys at different angulations of tilt may be necessary.

The cast in dental stone is mounted and secured on the adjustable table. The table should be positioned until the occlusal plane is horizontal. At this stage it is advisable to make a preliminary survey using the analysing rod fixed in the movable vertical arm. In this manner, by placing the rod against the various

Cast Surveying

abutment teeth, an assessment can be made of the degree of undercut present on different teeth, the angulation of these teeth, and the presence of undercuts in the area of the residual ridge. In free-end saddle cases it may be possible to decide whether the distal undercuts present on the abutment teeth are sufficient to indicate that an anterior tilt would be beneficial, and would allow the denture to be designed to engage these undercuts and so give increased resistance to vertical displacement (Figs 8.10 and 8.11). In addition it will also allow the denture to have a more ideal relationship to the gingivae.

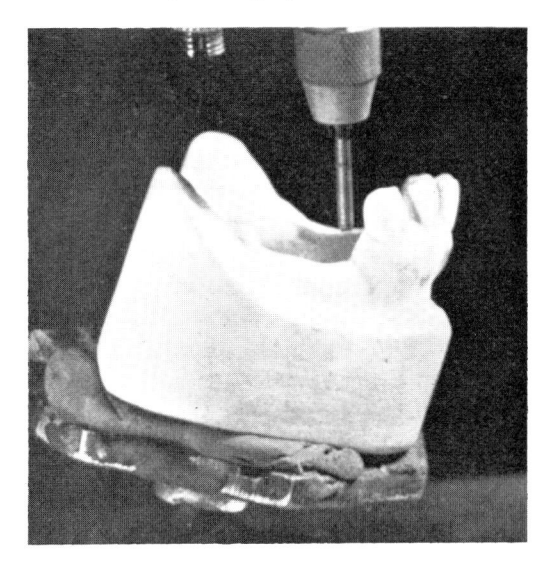

Fig. 8.10. A free-end saddle case tilted to allow an angled path of insertion to engage the distal undercuts.

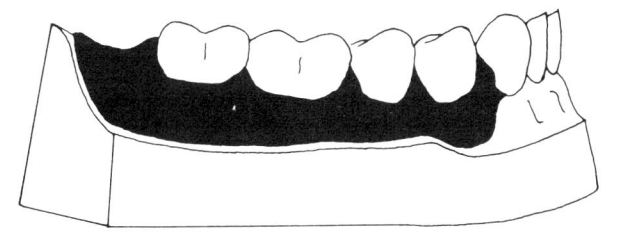

Fig. 8.11. Engagement of undercut to give retention.

Once the analysing rod has been used the table should be locked in position and the carbon marker placed in the chuck on the vertical arm. Lines are then traced around all teeth which may have to be clasped or have undercuts which require elimination. The marker should also indicate the extent of any soft tissue undercuts that must be eliminated prior to denture construction. This should be done with only light pressure to avoid abrading the cast.

Minor undercuts on the residual ridge areas need not be eliminated, as due to the nature of the soft tissues a denture can easily enter these areas and improve retention. Gross undercuts around upper tuberosities must be masked out, as also must undercut areas into which a gingivally approaching clasp arm might otherwise be placed. Lingual undercuts that will prevent placing of a lingual bar should also be eliminated.

If the path of insertion and removal and the path of displacement are similar, as will be so with the majority of cases, then only one survey will be required and the details of design can then be considered. Where these paths differ however, the cast must be surveyed again at a different angle of tilt and a second series of lines is traced round the same teeth. To avoid confusion between the two sets of survey lines different coloured leads should be used for the different angles of tilt.

The selection of a path of insertion/removal which is different from the path of displacement is influenced by the presence of abnormally tilted teeth and soft tissue undercuts which we might wish to engage for reasons of both aesthetics and retention. This is commonly seen where upper anterior teeth have been lost and there is a deep labial undercut interfering with insertion. If retention and aesthetics are to be satisfied by the rigid base engaging the undercut, then during survey the cast must be tilted to eliminate that undercut. If this is not done then the undercut will require to be masked out with possible adverse effects on retention and aesthetics. It must be appreciated however that besides eliminating some undercuts, tilting of the cast must create and emphasize others relative to the path of insertion. Tilting therefore should only be attempted after due consideration has been given to the effect on the positioning of the component of the partial denture particularly in relation to the creation of new undercut areas.

It has been suggested that in certain cases three surveys can be carried out using anterior and posterior tilts, but no mention has been made of surveying with lateral tilts. In only one condition is it likely that a lateral tilt survey could be of value and that is when the horizontal survey indicates marked lateral undercut areas on the tuberosities. Tilting the model laterally will mean using a lateral path of insertion for the denture in an effort to engage the undercut mucosal area to assist retention. Whilst insertion of the denture from one side will increase the retention of the denture against vertical displacement *on that side* it will usually only serve to decrease the retention against similar forces on the other side. Consequently when considering a lateral path of insertion for this purpose, careful consideration must be given to the position of the lateral tilt survey lines on the opposite side. If, as usually occurs, they are sited low on the teeth or ridge areas, then retention on that side will not be obtained, if a lateral path of insertion is used.

Cast Surveying 183

When the final tilt has been decided upon the cast table should be locked in that position and the final surveying carried out. Naturally, if the final tilt decided upon is one that has been used previously, for example the horizontal position, then a further tracing of survey lines is not necessary.

When the surveying has been completed consideration can be given to the details of the design. Prior to this stage the clinician will usually have decided upon the general principles of the design; for example, whether a lingual bar or a lingual plate is to be used, or whether an upper denture is to be of plate or skeleton design. Details regarding clasp design and position, however, cannot be decided until surveying has been carried out. It is after the completion of this surveying, which is done on the study cast, that decisions can be made regarding the necessity of any tooth preparation involving modifying tooth contours to produce better undercuts or reducing excessive proximal undercuts that have been shown to be an embarrassment to the path of insertion. The necessity for rest seat preparation will have been assessed previously by a study of occlusal contacts. The undercut gauges are not used until the master cast is being surveyed to decide upon the exact positioning of the component parts of the denture.

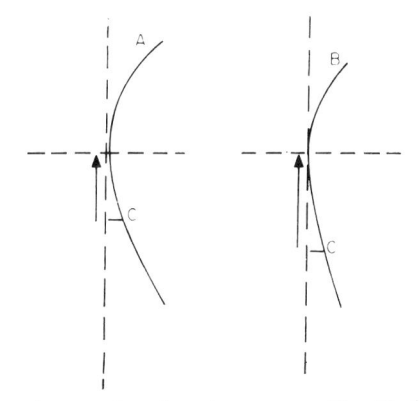

Fig. 8.12. Varying degree of tooth undercut controlling ideal position of clasp tip.

When a clasp is to be placed on a tooth one of the most difficult problems is to decide how far below the survey line the resilient portion of a retention clasp arm shall be placed. This is partly dependent upon the shape of the individual tooth being clasped (Fig. 8.12). In this case it is obvious that, although these two teeth have the same tilt and the same height of contour, tooth A is much more bulbous than B. Consequently, at an equal distance below the survey line on each tooth the degree of undercut is much greater on A than on B. Therefore, a clasp arm would have to engage tooth B much farther below the survey line than on tooth A, to engage an equal distance of undercut. Line C, which is the same length on both teeth, is much nearer the survey line in A than in B.

It is clear, therefore, that distance *below* the survey line is not the only guiding factor in positioning a clasp arm. The *horizontal* undercut, the length of line C, is a significant measurement that the operator requires to know. It is to measure these distances that the undercut gauges are designed. Figure 8.13 shows enlarged sections of the ends of the gauges which are designed to measure three dimensions of horizontal undercut; a quarter, a half, and three-quarters of a millimetre, these measurements being from the side of the shank to the rim of the head.

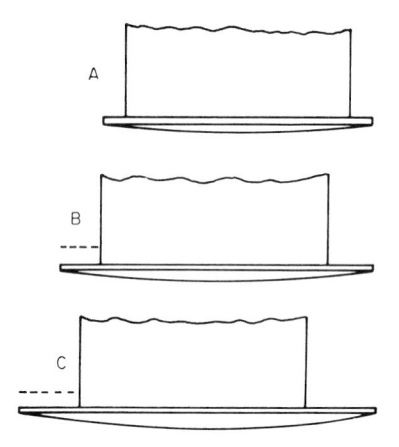

Fig. 8.13. Three sizes of undercut gauge.

The manner in which the head of the undercut gauge is positioned on the tooth is shown in Fig. 8.14. As a general principle the extent to which a clasp arm enters the undercut will be dependent upon the degree of retention which it is desired to obtain, and also upon the physical properties of the clasp material. Where multiple clasp arms are employed, they will not require to engage the same degree of undercut as might be necessary where a denture is dependent for its retention on only two clasp arms.

In relation to this the resilience of the clasp arms must be considered. Obviously, the greater the engagement of the undercut the more resilient must be the clasp arm. If this is not so then difficulty will be experienced in fitting the denture initially and the clasp arm may never engage correctly. At a later stage fatigue fracture of the clasp arm may occur, which will be a welcome relief for the tooth which will have been stressed excessively each time the denture was inserted or removed.

Cast Surveying

The degree of resilience will depend upon the shaping of the clasp arm and upon the alloy used. Wrought yellow gold wire makes the most resilient clasp arm and cast cobalt chromium alloy the least resilient. Variations in section, taper, and length, however, can produce great variations in resilience.

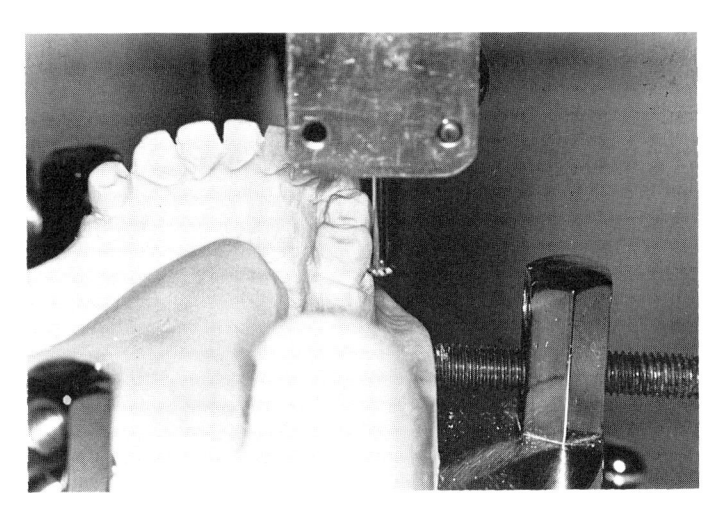

Fig. 8.14. The method of using the undercut gauge.

The last of the surveyor tools, the wax-trimmer, is used during the preparation of the master cast for duplication. Although it is always necessary to duplicate the master cast where a metal framework has to be used, it should be standard practice to duplicate every cast on which a partial denture is constructed. This has several advantages. Firstly possible damage to the master cast is minimized since the work is done on the duplicate, secondly, the completed denture can be fitted to the master cast, thus saving valuable chairside time that might be wasted in making adjustments to the contact points or peripheries; thirdly, check can be made of occlusion and any high spots adjusted prior to fitting; fourthly, it is easier to eliminate undercuts in wax than in cement, which is necessary if the working model is to be used for the final processing. There is no doubt that a higher technical standard is achieved if all partial denture construction is done on duplicate casts. With modern duplicating materials complete accuracy of reproduction should be guaranteed.

Prior to duplication, therefore, all unwanted undercuts should be obliterated by filling them with hard wax. In this way all structures can be paralleled with the path of insertion. To achieve this the wax trimmer is fixed to the vertical arm of the surveyor, an excess of wax is placed in the undercuts and the cast is placed on the cast table at the same tilt at which it was finally surveyed. Wax is now trimmed away until parallelism is secured (Fig. 8.15). The undercuts in which the clasp arm will engage are left free of wax. Before duplication it is helpful to build up a strip of wax to the lower border of the clasp arm (Fig. 8.16). This locates the position of the arm on the duplicate cast, on which no survey line will be marked. In the case of gingivally approaching arms the wax may be built up to a sloping ledge.

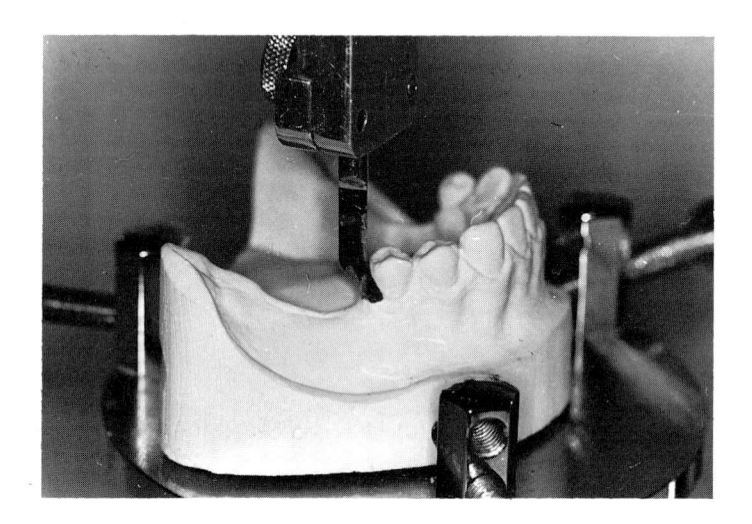

Fig. 8.15. Wax trimmer in use.

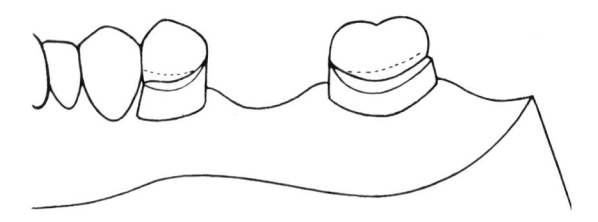

Fig. 8.16. Wax step locating position of clasp arm.

Particular attention should be paid to the waxing out of undercut soft tissue areas as well as those around the teeth. Also duplication will be aided if all other undercuts on the cast outside the denture-bearing area are eliminated.

It has been suggested that the elimination of undercuts in order to produce parallelism to the path of insertion is not in the best interests of gingival health. It

Cast Surveying

has been found that when saddles can be brought into close approximation to the standing teeth, the reaction of the underlying gingivae is good. If, because of mesial or distal undercuts, the saddle cannot be brought into this close relationship with the gingival margin of the tooth then chronic hypertrophic gingivitis and pocket formation are likely to occur. However, if the saddle is cleared well away from the gingiva, forming a large sluiceway, the gingival reaction is better.

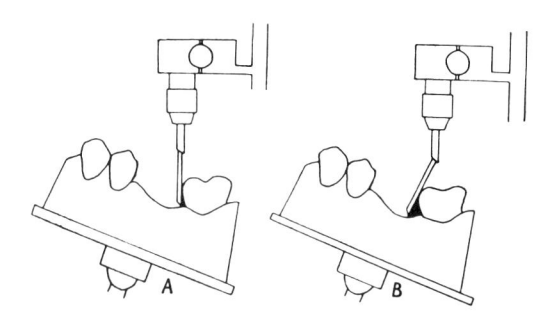

Fig. 8.17. A The use of the vertical cutting edge in the surveyor to wax out the undercut. B The use of the 25° tool to create a sluiceway.

Where the design of the saddle is intended to provide a large sluiceway a wax trimmer at 25° is useful (Fig. 8.17). This will result in a denture which fits accurately at and above the survey line but which possesses a bucco-lingual channel at the gingival margin large enough to prevent food packing between the denture and the abutment tooth. Such a tool can clearly be used only when long saddles are present.

References

ATKINSON H.F. (1953) Partial denture problems. *Aust. J. Dent.* **57**, 187.
ATKINSON H.F. (1955) Partial denture problems—surveyors and surveying. *Aust. J. Dent.* **59**, 28.
COHEN M. (1948) Principles of partial denture prosthesis with special reference to the use of the surveyor. *Journal of the Dental Association of South Africa*, **3**, 450.
CRADDOCK F.W. and BOTTOMLEY G.A. (1954) Second thoughts on clasp surveying. *Brit. dent. J.* **96**, 134.
CRADDOCK F.W. (1955) Clasp surveying and mysticism. *Aust. J. Dent.* **59**, 205.
DUNN B.W. (1961) Treatment planning for removable partial dentures. *J. pros. Dent.* **11**, 247.
DYER M.R.Y. (1973) Basic principles of partial denture designing. *Dent. Update*, **1**, 941.
LAVERE A.M. and FREDA A.L. (1977) A simplified procedure for survey and design of diagnostic casts. *J. pros. Dent.* **37**, 680.
The Ney Surveyor Book. The J.M. Ney Company, Connecticut.

PERRY C. and APPLEGATE S.G. (1948) Cast survey in partial denture prosthesis. *J. Mich. dent. Soc.* **30**, 151.

RUDD K.D., MORROW R.M. and EISMANN H.F. (1981) *Dental Laboratory Procedures. Removable Partial Dentures. Vol. 3.* C.V. Mosby Co. St Louis, London, Toronto.

SCHWARZ W.D. and BARSBY M.J. (1984) Tooth procedures prior to partial denture construction. Part II. *Dent. Update*, **11**, 167.

SHAFFER F.W. (1970) A method of analysing and surveying for removable partial dentures. *D. Digest*, **76**, 388.

9

MATERIALS USED IN PARTIAL DENTURE CONSTRUCTION

Throughout this text reference is made to the various materials that are used in partial denture construction. In view of the extensive literature in this area it is inappropriate to consider them in detail, but it is useful to compare their properties with reference to their use as components of partial dentures.

Such materials may be divided into metallic and non-metallic groups. The metallic materials are (*a*) yellow gold alloys; (*b*) cobalt chromium alloys and (*c*) stainless steel. The non-metallic group are (*a*) polymers or plastics and (*b*) porcelain.

Metallic

Metallic materials can be used for practically all the components of a partial denture. As saddle connectors in the form of plates and bars they are much stronger than plastic materials. Accordingly they can be constructed in thinner section with minimal tissue coverage, which makes them less obtrusive to the wearer. For all types of clasps, occlusal rests, onlays, and embrasure hooks, the use of metal is essential.

Alloys for any of these components may be employed in either the wrought or cast condition. Whilst cobalt chromium and gold alloys can be used in both forms, stainless steel is employed in the wrought condition, although currently a castable stainless steel alloy is undergoing investigation. Although cobalt chromium alloys often contain some nickel, alloys have also been used in which the total cobalt content is replaced by nickel. These have greater ductility but also a much lower proportional limit and it is questionable how useful they are in partial denture construction. In addition the operator should always be aware of possible tissue sensitivity to nickel containing alloys. It should also be mentioned that certain alloys contain a small proportion of beryllium and may create health hazards for the technician who finishes the denture, because of the toxicity of this element.

It is useful to consider the various properties of these alloys and to discuss the relative merits of each. In this respect it is essential that the clinician should have a knowledge of the physical and mechanical properties of the different alloys that may be used, so that he may prescribe the type of alloy most likely to meet the demands of the patient's present and possible future oral condition. Table 9.1 lists some typical properties of metallic denture base materials.

Table 9.1. Typical properties of metallic denture bases

	Yellow gold alloy softened	Yellow gold alloy hardened	Cobalt chromium alloy as cast	Stainless steel wrought
Density (g/ml)	15		8.3	7.9
Proportional limit (N/mm^2)	390	720	650	1440
Modulus of elasticity (N/mm^2)	—	96×10^3	207×10^3	200×10^3
Ultimate tensile strength (N/mm^2)	530	800	760	1800
Elongation (per cent)	36	9	4	8
Vickers hardness number	170	260	370	440

Density

The density of a denture base material, that is its mass per unit volume is important, particularly in the maxilla. It is this factor, together with the modulus of elasticity, that will in part determine the weight of the appliances which, in the upper, will act against the retention of the denture. In this respect it is reasonable to assume that the lightest possible denture is preferable.

The density of cobalt chromium alloys and stainless steel makes them superior in this respect to gold alloys. The greater the value of the modulus of elasticity the more rigid is the material and consequently its ability to resist distortion is greater. Hence high modulus materials can be employed in thinner sections, which reduces the volume, and therefore the weight, of the appliance. The modulus of elasticity of cobalt chromium alloys is approximately double that of gold alloys.

Hardness

The term hardness may be defined as resistance to permanent deformation in the form of indentation or scratching, which must be as high as possible in a metallic denture base. If such a material is liable to become scratched or abraded in use, a rough surface will be produced which will be difficult to keep clean and this will favour the formation of dental plaque and calculus.

Indentation hardness figures show that cold worked stainless steel or cobalt chromium alloys are superior to gold alloys. In addition it is found in practice that the former materials, particularly cobalt chromium alloys, maintain their high polish better than gold alloys. Hardness also increases the resistance to abrasion of the material, resulting in reduction in wear and a longer economic life.

The surface hardness of cast cobalt chromium alloy does however lead to difficulties in polishing and is certainly more time-consuming than the polishing of gold alloys. It is recommended that electrolytic polishing should be applied to all cobalt chromium alloys, particularly to their tissue fitting surfaces. In this way a lustre can be imparted without any significant affect upon the accuracy of fit. It is desirable that this surface of the alloy shall be as highly polished as is compatible with good fit as a protection against the deposition of dental plaque and calculus.

Tensile strength

Although figures for ultimate tensile strength are always quoted by manufacturer, their value is not very significant, as a metal will have undergone permanent deformation before its ultimate tensile strength or fracture point is reached. Fractures do occur in partial dentures particularly in relation to clasp arms. This may be due to metal fatigue however and there is not necessarily any correlation between fracture incidence and ultimate tensile strength. The tensile strength of cobalt chromium alloys is similar to cast yellow gold. In practice however, it is found that the incidence of clasp fracture with cobalt chromium alloy dentures is higher than in the case of yellow gold.

It has been shown that with cobalt chromium alloys, defects in the structure of the casting account for many of the fractures of clasp arms. It is also possible that an important cause of fracture of clasp arms that show no obvious structural defects is the fact that their inherent strength at the point of attachment to the denture base is often insufficient, due to the large grain size which is normally produced in this area. Clasp arms of a uniformly round cross section have been shown to have uniformly equiaxed grains and hence should withstand fatigue stresses better.

Proportional limit

In practice the proportional limit of a material may be taken as that stress beyond which deformation is permanent and not elastic. It is a property which is difficult to determine experimentally but proof stress, which is a property requirement quoted in standard specifications, can be measured and has a similar numerical value. Proportional limit is significant as far as the denture base is concerned, since it relates to its liability to permanent deformation by accident or in cleaning. It is, however, more important with regard to the clasps. Deformation of these in use and during removal and insertion of the denture must always be elastic. If a clasp arm is permanently deformed and displaced away from the tooth it is rendered ineffective in both its bracing and retentive properties. Similarly displacement in the other direction places undue stress on the tooth. Proportional limit must be considered together with the modulus of elasticity.

Modulus of elasticity

The modulus of elasticity is the description of the rigidity of a material. If the value is high then the material will be more rigid and require more force to bend it than would a material with a lower modulus. The modulus of cobalt chromium alloys is approximately twice that of gold—about 207×10^3 N/mm^2 against 96×10^3 N/mm^2. Therefore, a clasp of the same cross-sectional area is more rigid in cobalt chromium alloy than in gold alloy. This is clearly a disadvantage as additional force will be required when inserting and removing the partial denture, although retention during normal function may be enhanced. Since the proportional limit of cobalt chromium alloy is lower than that of cast yellow gold the possibility of permanently deforming a cobalt chromium clasp that has been too deeply engaged into an undercut cannot be overlooked. Clearly the high value for the modulus of elasticity of cobalt chromium alloy, coupled with its lower proportional limit compared to gold alloy, means that retentive clasp arms can be constructed in thinner section and will engage less depth of undercut.

Elongation

Elongation is a measure of the permanent extension which an alloy will undergo before breakage occurs, and is an indication of its ductility. If a clasp arm has to be adjusted a high value of elongation is desirable to minimize the risk of breakage. Also, if the alloy is accidentally stressed beyond its proportional limit a high elongation value will be some insurance against fracture. The alloy with the highest value of elongation consistent with satisfactory values of other properties, particularly proportional limit, should be chosen.

Corrosion resistance

Although this property of an alloy cannot be tabulated in figures, from the dental point of view it is of great importance. By corrosion is meant the attacking of the surface of a metal or alloy by some medium with which it is in contact, such as the oral fluids. The effect may vary from a surface stain or tarnish to complete disintegration of the material.

An important requirement of a denture base material is its ability to resist any degree of corrosion under all conditions of usage. Since the oral fluids are not constant in respect of acidity or alkalinity, mouth conditions provide a severe test.

Although gold alloys are particularly resistant to corrosion these are not commonly used nowadays, but the 'stainless' groups of base metals withstand the effects of the oral fluids equally well. Care must be taken however when using certain denture cleansers particularly those containing chlorine compounds.

Corrosion is essentially an electrolytic phenomenon and requires the presence of two dissimilar metallic alloys within an electrolytic medium. A single homogeneous solid solution is least likely to be affected by corrosion although its resistance will depend upon the nature and proportions of its component metals and it is known that at least 46 per cent by weight of gold must be present to provide adequate protection for the less noble metals.

Certain base metals such as aluminium and chromium form an oxide coating in air which protects them from corrosion. Such metals are said to be passive. It is this property of chromium which protects both the stainless steels and cobalt chromium alloys from corrosion in the mouth. From practical clinical experience the resistance to tarnish of the chrome alloys is found to be the best of all the metallic denture base materials. Stainless steel is very satisfactory as also is any yellow gold alloy of 18 carat or above. Low carat yellow golds leave much to be desired in this respect.

Heat treatment

It is necessary that all yellow gold alloys should be heat treated before being finished for insertion into the mouth in order to ensure that their properties are developed to the desired degree. In Table 9.1 it will be noted that two values are given for most of these properties in respect of yellow gold alloys and that there is a considerable difference between them. These examples indicate that it is essential to apply a *hardening heat treatment* to all yellow gold alloys so that their optimum properties are developed. Failure to do so may be responsible for clasp distortion or fracture. However, it has been shown that the more heat treatment a casting receives, the greater are the chances of distortion. Hence, it may be desirable to harden the gold casting without previous annealing.

Cobalt chromium alloys do not respond to precipitation forms of heat treatment and it is not possible to soften and harden them alternately as may be done with gold alloys. It is generally believed that better physical properties result from slow cooling of the material from the casting temperature, and that hardness and fatigue resistance are somewhat improved by ageing at 850°C for five hours.

Choice of alloy

In subsequent chapters preferences for any particular type of alloy in relation to its desired function are indicated. In general however, cobalt chromium alloys are to be preferred for rigid components such as lingual bars, palatal plate connectors and bracing and reciprocating elements of clasp arms. This is in addition to the fact that these alloys have a low specific gravity together with a high degree of corrosion resistance.

In some instances, different alloys should be used on one denture. A rigid reciprocating arm in cobalt chromium alloy on one surface of an abutment tooth can be combined with a resilient, wrought yellow gold retentive arm on the opposite surface. For palatal plates stainless steel has the advantages of lightness and lower cost when compared to gold alloys. Using a slow rate hydraulic forming process, stainless steel plates of minimal thickness with a good reproduction of fine detail can be produced easily and accurately.

Non-Metallic

Denture base

Of the non-metallic denture base materials the one used most widely is acrylic resin. When used for partial dentures however it has several disadvantages. Of those, the most important is its low strength compared to metallic bases and consequently its propensity to fracture. In addition it has a low abrasion resistance, absorbs moisture and may lack sufficient rigidity for satisfactory use as a connector. Where stress applied to the denture is likely to be severe, due to abnormal occlusal relationships or particularly strong masticating forces, a metallic base should be used.

The use of acrylic resin as the base material will also restrict the design of the denture. Usually this means maximum coverage of the mucosa in order to secure adequate strength with more delicate components such as bars or narrow plates being unsuitable for construction in acrylic resin. In some cases with a maxillary denture it is possible to position the border away from the gingival margins so reducing mucosal coverage without a significant loss of strength. An example of such an appliance would be a denture constructed to the principles suggested by Every.

When it is decided to use acrylic resin to form the denture base several factors must be considered. Firstly it should be adequately supported by the teeth in order to prevent excessive load falling upon the mucosa and particularly upon the gingival margins. When a plate has to be extended to the maximum size for reasons of strength it accordingly comes into contact with most of the standing teeth. Consequently, if it is not tooth supported it will impinge upon the gingivae causing traumatic damage to the gingival margins, particularly in the lower jaw. The denture must also fit accurately against the standing teeth occlusal to the maximum convexity (survey line) of the tooth. It has been suggested also that the denture should be relieved from contact with the gingival tissues by placing a layer of wax or foil over these regions prior to duplication of the cast. Current opinion however is that gingival enlargement will occur under all types of relief areas which will lead to false pocketing. This occurs to a much lesser extent where no relief is provided, and in situations therefore where the gingivae are covered, the denture should be adapted as closely as possible. It is however prudent to obliterate the gingival crevice as close adaptation in this region would result in a denture with a sharp edge which would be potentially damaging to the tissues.

Finally, every effort must be made to secure the maximum strength in the material itself. To this end, slow *initial* curing at low temperatures to eliminate gaseous porosity should be followed by a *final* curing at 100°C to ensure polymerization being as complete as possible. In addition, all possible precautions should be taken to minimize internal strain, whilst factors such as correct relief of hard tissue areas, good occlusion and denture shape will all contribute to the resistance to fracture of the appliance.

Owing to water absorption and the relative ease with which they are abraded, acrylic resin dentures are more difficult to keep clean and free from deposits and stains than metal bases. On this account they are less hygienic.

The main advantage of acrylic resin over metal lies in its aesthetic properties. If for instance a labial flange is provided on a partial denture it can be varied in colour, contour or surface texture to blend with the adjoining gingival and alveolar mucosa. It must be remembered however that when it is attached mechanically to an underlying metallic base, its colour may be affected by shadow of the metal, dependent upon the translucency and thickness of the resin.

Currently the majority of polymeric denture base materials are radiolucent. This creates problems of location if part of the denture base is inhaled or ingested as it will evade radiographic detection. Although some radiopaque denture base materials are available commercially, their physical and aesthetic properties are not always acceptable. There remains a need to develop a radiopaque denture base polymer therefore which will combine the physical and aesthetic properties with the ease of processing existing at present in the radiolucent materials.

Tooth Materials

The materials used for denture tooth manufacture are acrylic resin or porcelain although in special situations metallic inserts may also be used. The choice of material is governed by the clinical situation encountered, and also by the personal preferences of the operator and patient. Each material has its own advantages and disadvantages.

Acrylic resin teeth

These teeth are the ones most commonly used in denture construction. Being of a similar material to the matrix acrylic of the denture they form a chemical bond with it and are therefore easily attached. In the case of metal based dentures they can be reduced in thickness to allow an adequate intervening amount of matrix acrylic, ensuring a firm metal/acrylic mechanical union. In the same manner their contour may be modified easily and their polish rapidly restored after grinding. Their impact strength is greater than that of porcelain teeth and they do not require metal reinforcement except perhaps in the anterior region if there is a minimal horizontal overlap. The specific gravity of acrylic is low and the total weight of the appliance will be reduced. Furthermore during function they are less noisy than porcelain teeth, and therefore often more acceptable to the patient. However with a lower abrasion resistance than porcelain, they often lose their contour relatively rapidly with corresponding loss of occlusal contact. This may occur both with function and also by cleaning with abrasive pastes or powders. It is suggested however that functional abrasion may reduce resorption of underlying bone, the energy expended being taken up by the tooth rather than the residual alveolar ridge.

Porcelain teeth

Porcelain teeth are used less readily for partial dentures, partly as a result of their cost and partly from technical problems in denture construction related to their form and properties. Such teeth are extremely resistant to abrasion and their surface hardness means that they are not subject to surface scratches and consequent staining from foodstuffs and the oral fluids. They maintain well their anatomical contour and their interocclusal relationship. The main disadvantages of porcelain teeth are the fact that their form cannot easily be altered and repolished, and since they require mechanical retention to the acrylic resin they cannot be reduced in size where there is limited inter-ridge distance. In addition many patients report that they are noisy during function.

When considering normal stock teeth from the manufacturer there is little difference in aesthetics between the best quality acrylic or porcelain teeth. In the lower price ranges however, acrylic teeth are usually aesthetically superior.

References

ANDERSON J.N. (1976) *Applied dental materials*. 5th ed. Blackwell Scientific Publications, Oxford.

APPLEGATE O.C. (1960) The selection of alloys. *D. Clin. N.A.* Nov., 595.

BAHRANI A.S., BLAIR G.A.S. and CROSSLAND B. (1965) Slow rate hydraulic forming of stainless steel dentures. *Brit. dent. J.* **118**, 425.

B.S. 3366 (1961) *Dental Cobalt Chromium Casting Alloy*. British Standards Institution, London.

COMBE E.C. (1977) *Notes on dental materials*. 3rd ed. Churchill Livingstone, Edinburgh.

DAVY K.W.M. and CAUSTON B.E. (1982) Radio-opaque dentures base: a new acrylic co-polymer. *J. Dent.* **10**, 254.

DINGER E.J. and PEYTON F.A. (1951) Distortion of gold partial denture castings. *J. pros. Dent.* **1**, 443.

EARNSHAW R. (1956) Cobalt-chromium alloys in dentistry. *Brit. dent. J.* **101**, 67–75.

EARNSHAW R. (1956) Research on dental cobalt-chromium casting alloys. *Proc. Brit. Soc. pros. Dent.* 1956.

EARNSHAW R. (1961) Fatigue tests on a dental cobalt-chromium alloy. *Brit. dent. J.* **110**, 341.

ELLIOT R.W. (1963) The effects of heat on gold partial denture castings. *J. pros. Dent.* **13**, 688.

HARCOURT H.J. (1961) Fracture of cobalt chromium castings. *Brit. dent. J.*, **110**, 43.

JOHNSON W. (1956) A comparison of cobalt-chromium alloys and yellow and white gold alloys. *Proc. Brit. Soc. pros. Dent.* 1956.

JOHNSON W. (1957) Gold alloys for casting dentures. *Brit. dent. J.* **102**, 41–49.

MCCABE J.F. and WILSON H.J. (1976) A radio-opaque denture material. *J. Dent.* **4**, 211.

OSBORNE J. and WILSON H.J. (1970) *Dental mechanics for students*, 6th ed. Staples Press, London.

OSBORNE J. and LAMMIE G.A. (1953) Some observations concerning chrome-cobalt denture bases. *Brit. dent. J.* **94**, 55.

SKINNER E.W. and PHILLIPS R.W. (1967) *The science of dental materials*, 6th ed. W.B. Saunders Co., Philadelphia.

TSAO D.H., GUILFORD H.J., KAZANOGLU A. and BELL D.H. (1984) Clinical evaluation of a radiopaque denture base resin. *J. pros. Dent.* **51**, 456.

WOOD J.F.L. (1974) Mucosal reaction to cobalt-chromium alloy. *Brit. dent. J.* **136**, 423.

10

THE COMPONENT PARTS OF A PARTIAL DENTURE

Many decisions regarding the design of a partial denture are necessarily taken at the treatment planning stage in order to prepare the mouth suitably for the reception of the proposed appliance. For instance, decisions regarding the position of occlusal rests must be made at an early stage so that rest seats may be prepared before taking the final impression. Similarly, decisions to modify tooth contours to allow either better clasp retention, easier insertion, or a more hygienic relationship of the denture to the proximal gingivae, must be taken following the examination and surveying of the study casts.

It is, therefore, somewhat artificial to describe a system of denture designing undertaken when the working cast has already been obtained. There are, however, many detailed decisions on design that can only be settled after the working cast is available; these include the particular types and exact position of the clasps to be used and the position of connecting bars. Hence, in considering the system of developing the denture design described below it should be appreciated that many of the decisions will have been taken in principle before the working casts are available for the final decisions to be made. In practice the steps described should be followed as completely as possible at the treatment planning stage and the process repeated in the light of the more exact information that becomes available when the working casts are obtained.

The designing of the denture is described here as a laboratory exercise, but this does not mean that a denture can be designed purely on technical criteria. In fact, the information that can be gained from the cast must be subservient to that which has already been obtained from a full clinical examination. It is essential at this stage to have available the case notes and relevant X-rays. The working casts must then be surveyed following the principles laid down in Chapter 8. Further, some decisions will require a study of the occlusion and consequently the casts may have to be mounted on an articulator.

A System of Partial Denture Design

The general principles which must be followed when designing any denture will be discussed in the order in which they should normally be considered. However, it may often be appropriate to take decisions regarding the connectors prior to making a final choice of retainers since if it is decided, for example, to have a large area of palatal coverage then the necessity for clasp retention may be decreased.

First stage—outlining the saddle areas

The first step is to outline the saddle areas. As a general rule, maximal coverage of the edentulous ridge is desirable. In this way a greater area of bone is called upon to resist the vertical and horizontal loads which fall on the saddle during mastication. In consequence, the pressure falling on any unit area of edentulous ridge is reduced, and this assists in keeping the forces acting on the bone within its physiological limit.

In practice this means that the buccal flange should extend to the mucosal reflection indicated on the cast. It is assumed that the cast has been obtained from a correctly peripherally adapted impression and, therefore, in extending the buccal flange to this reflection it does not impinge upon moving muscle. Anteriorly, the labial flange should be extended to the mucosal reflection, but aesthetics make a primary demand in this region and occasionally the labial flange, which might be effective in stabilizing the denture against a posterior displacement, has to be omitted in order that a natural appearance can be obtained. Extension of upper saddles on to the hard palate should be liberal, as this helps the underlying bone to resist horizontal and vertical components of stress. Lingual extension in the lower should be to the full depth permitted by muscle function.

The antero-posterior dimension of a bounded saddle is determined by the abutment teeth, but regard must be paid to tooth undercuts revealed in surveying. When a free-end saddle is considered, maximal coverage posteriorly is desirable since this ensures reduced loading of the underlying bone. However, posterior extension has added significance when resistance to antero-posterior displacement is considered. The tendency in the lower is for the saddle to be displaced backwards as a result of the inclined plane action of the cusps in protrusive movement. An extension of the saddle over the retromolar pad, where its direction changes from horizontal to more nearly vertical, helps to prevent the posterior movement of such a saddle. Conversely in the upper, an extension behind a well-developed tuberosity helps to prevent a forward movement of the saddle.

Whereas the writers advocate maximal extension in all cases, this principle does not receive universal support. For instance, Beckett agrees with this axiom only when it has been decided that the saddle is to be mucosa borne. He claims that, whereas in theory a denture may be both tooth and mucosa supported, in practice it is expedient to make it either tooth *or* mucosa supported. When Beckett makes a saddle entirely tooth borne he reduces its size in order to allow freedom of tongue and cheek movements.

To avoid pressure falling on the gingivae of the abutment teeth Nevin and others have advocated freeing the saddle entirely from the mucosal area and simply providing a metal span between the teeth. This principle can be applied only to bounded saddles in the posterior part of the mouth.

Second stage—planning the support of the saddles

Supporting a saddle means arranging for the vertical load falling on it to be adequately resisted during function. This load may be borne by the mucosa or by the teeth or by both. In the lower, only the edentulous ridge is available for mucosal support while in the upper the whole of the hard palate may also be used. From the point of view of bony area available, therefore, the upper is more suitable than the lower for mucosal support. This is further enhanced by the different kinds of bone that are found in the maxilla and mandible. Maxillary bone, displaying a thin cortex and diffuse thin trabeculae in its spongiosum, stands up to pressure from a denture saddle better than the typical mandibular bone. This latter is characterized by a thicker cortex, the spongiosum containing less numerous but thicker trabeculae than are found in the maxilla. It must be borne in mind, therefore, when deciding upon design, that there is less possibility of satisfactory mucosal support for the lower denture than for the upper. As pointed out earlier an assessment of the bone factor is necessary to decide upon the extent to which additional tooth support is required.

Tooth support is effective through occlusal rests, incisal rests, onlays, or embrasure hooks which bear on the occlusal or prepared surfaces of the standing teeth. When possible, wide distribution of load should be effected by placing occlusal rests on a large number of standing teeth. With the exception of Class I dentures, a minimum of three occlusal rests should be used since if they are widely separated a tripod principle of support will apply. When the roots lie vertically and, therefore, in the same axis as the load being considered, the natural teeth can readily accept increased load without danger of breakdown. Even a tooth that is to some extent periodontally involved will generally accept additional stress in the direction of its long axis.

Tooth support is always possible with bounded saddles whereas with free-end saddles part of the load must be borne by the mucosa.

Third stage—planning the bracing of the saddles

Bracing means providing resistance to lateral movement and it may be effected by the mucosa and by the teeth. The lateral component is the force most likely to be destructive to both the ridge and the supporting structures of the teeth and its wide distribution is a principle to be commended.

The structures described in Table 10.1 aid in the distribution of lateral load.

Table 10.1

	Resisting structures in upper	Resisting structures in lower
On the working side	**Acting on mucosa:** Palatal surface of saddle Palatal bars	**Acting on mucosa:** Buccal surface of saddle
	Acting on teeth: Palatal clasp arms Occlusal rests Onlays Continuous clasps	**Acting on teeth:** Buccal clasp arms Occlusal rests Onlays Embrasure hooks
On the balancing side	**Acting on mucosa:** Buccal surface of saddle	**Acting on mucosa:** Lingual surface of saddle Lingual plate
	Acting on teeth: Buccal clasp arms Occlusal rests Onlays Embrasure hooks	**Acting on teeth:** Lingual clasp arms Occlusal rests Onlays Embrasure hooks Continuous clasps

Two approaches to the control of lateral load should be considered. First, it is often practicable to reduce the magnitude of the lateral component of force by reducing the size of the occlusal table and by selecting teeth with sharp efficient cusps. The proportion of the total force that is resolved as a lateral component can be decreased by reducing the cusp angle. This may be achieved by stoning both natural and artificial teeth, using onlays, or crowning.

The second method of reducing the lateral load falling on teeth and mucosa is by distributing it widely. A large number of patients who require dentures show some evidence of periodontal disease, and treatment by an appliance giving mutual support to the teeth would appear logical. This wide distribution of lateral load is largely effected against the standing teeth, and onlaying and special clasping methods are available to this end.

Fourth stage—planning the resistance of the saddle to antero-posterior movement

These movements may be prevented by resistance at the end of the saddle towards which the movement takes place. In the upper this is by structures in the anterior part of the mouth and in the lower by structures posteriorly placed. The best resistance to this displacement is provided by a healthy standing tooth, or better still, a row of such teeth with good contact points. The shape of tooth roots in general indicates that they can resist antero-posterior forces better than they can resist lateral forces.

In a previous paragraph it has been described how posterior extension of a lower free-end saddle over the retromolar pad might act as a resistance to backward movement, but this measure can only go a small way to overcoming the problem of providing a stable denture. As another example, in a Class IV upper saddle there is no tooth resistance in the direction of displacement, but the position here is more favourable since the anterior part of the hard palate can be covered by the denture base. A large steep vaulted palate is necessarily more effective in this respect than a small shallow palate.

Resistance to antero-posterior displacement may also be effected at the end of the saddle away from which movement tends to take place. Clasp arms which encircle the mesio-distal convexity of one or more teeth are the components most commonly used for this purpose, but continuous clasps, onlays, and embrasure hooks can also be employed. The amount of resistance required from such methods depends upon the condition present at the other end of the saddle. Where only mucosal resistance is available, such as in free-end saddles, extra resistance will be needed by clasping teeth from which the saddle tends to move. Where premolars are standing this does not present any difficulty. However, the problem is not capable of easy solution when the abutment teeth are flat-surfaced canines whose mesio-distal axis may be placed antero-posteriorly; in these cases incisal embrasure hooks or rests provide the only solution.

Figure 10.1 illustrates three possible methods of securing lower free-end saddles against this movement. In the first method care must be taken to ensure that the clasp arms, particularly the more rigid arms, encircle the mesio-distal convexity of the abutment teeth. The second method is, without doubt, the most effective but may have aesthetic disadvantages and may also necessitate grinding opposing teeth to provide clearance in the occlusion. When canines are the abutment teeth, as in the third method illustrated, incisal rests must be employed resting on an effective preparation (see p. 167). Again, there are aesthetic disadvantages.

Fifth stage—planning the retention

The retention of full dentures depends on the forces of adhesion and cohesion, the use of a peripheral seal, the action of muscle forces on suitably shaped polished surfaces, and good occlusion. Some of these factors are of considerable importance in the retention of partial dentures and, where possible, full use must always be made of them. The application of the forces of adhesion and cohesion demands accurately fitting denture bases, whether these be made in acrylic resin, cast, or swaged metal. Broad palatal coverage must always be considered in those

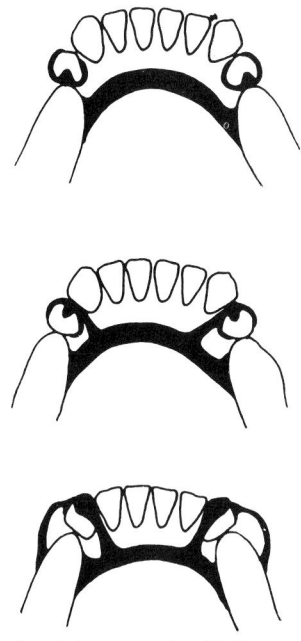

Fig. 10.1. Three methods of resisting posterior displacement of a lower free-end saddle denture.

cases where retention by clasping presents a problem owing to the shape of the teeth involved, the condition of their supporting structures, or owing to aesthetics. Peripheral seal is not such a practical retentive aid with partial dentures, since the periphery is not everywhere in contact with a compressible tissue. However, considerable use can be made of the polished surfaces so that the cheek and tongue muscles can assist retention. As a rule this is easily accomplished since the presence of natural teeth define the position of the artificial teeth on the saddle and thus ensure that the normal range of movement of either lingual or buccal muscles will not be encroached upon.

It is evident that the retentive forces acting in the case of full dentures do not apply to the same extent in partials. Extra retention, therefore, is provided by direct or indirect retainers.

The usual method of retaining partial dentures is by clasps. The various types available are discussed later in this chapter. In some cases problems will arise concerning how many clasps are required to retain a denture and on which teeth they should be placed. Obviously, Class I dentures will normally only have two clasps and the only decision to be made will be which particular type of clasp is most appropriate. When bounded saddles are present it will be necessary to decide if they require clasp retention both anteriorly and posteriorly. Certainly, short bounded saddles are often only clasp retained at one end. Retentive clasp arms on the buccal aspect of canines and first premolars are often contraindicated, particularly in the upper jaw, on account of their objectionable aesthetic effect. However, in the upper jaw it is often possible to supplement retention by the use of increased palatal coverage by the connector, thus offsetting the possible disadvantage of not being able to clasp upper canines.

It has been stated with a good deal of truth that good clasp retention at three widely separated points will make a denture difficult to dislodge. Certainly, multiple clasping for the purposes of retention is rarely needed; the use of clasps for bracing may need to be more widespread.

Sixth stage—joining the saddles and retainer units

When the saddles are adequately supported, braced, stabilized against antero-posterior movement, and retained, they are finally joined by rigid connectors to form the partial denture. When the appliance is constructed in metal the joining of the saddles is by metal bars or plates. These have the advantage of minimal encroachment on the oral muscles as they function in talking, eating, and swallowing. They must always be *rigid* so that mutual support, bracing, and resistance to antero-posterior movement is achieved between the individual saddles, and consequently load is widely distributed. That dimension where a bar ends and a plate begins is not finite, but the latter is characterized by its broader coverage, often, but not always, extending over the gingival margins. When metal is used a plate may be preferred to a bar on the grounds of better tolerance, or broader distribution of load. When acrylic resin is used a plate connector is imperative to give the necessary strength and rigidity.

The rule laid down for rigid connection between saddles and retainer units needs modification when a stress-broken principle is used in the design. It is then necessary to discriminate between saddles that are largely mucosa borne and those that are largely tooth borne. In these cases saddles of the same type are joined by rigid connectors, as are isolated retainer elements and tooth-borne saddles, whereas connectors used between saddles of dissimilar type, or between a mucosa-borne saddle and an isolated retainer unit, must always be flexible. The significance of this procedure will become more apparent when stress breaking is considered in more detail.

The General Problem in Designing a Partial Denture

The forces to which a partial denture is subjected cannot be measured accurately. A dentist can only gauge the power of the musculature by clinical assessment. The general musculature of the patient, the presence of marked faceting and/or attrition on the remaining teeth, the presence of natural teeth as antagonists to the denture, the previous prosthetic history of the patient, and the general health of the individual are significant points for observation. Nor is it possible to ascertain, more than approximately, the extent to which damaging continuous forces, developed during clenching or grinding will require to be resisted.

The problem is further complicated when the materials used in denture construction are considered. Accurate information on their physical properties is available, but even so, the dentist cannot design or plan his denture as would a civil engineer plan a bridge. The dentist still thinks of a long or short, thin or thick, clasp arm; he cannot measure with accuracy in definable units.

Lastly, there is no method of assessing accurately the reactions to be expected in the living tissues that support the partial denture. Even after the most thorough clinical examination with every modern aid, the dentist cannot say which tissues will react favourably to a given load. In addition there is no assurance that the general health of the patient will remain at a constant level. Any dentist knows that unfavourable reactions—bony, gingival, or periodontal—are liable to appear under a partial denture during a period when the patient is unwell.

It must, therefore, be admitted that partial denture prosthetics is not an accurate science, and, like dentistry as a whole, is still a science and an art. However, this should not deter the dentist from using his observations, approximate though they may be, when planning partial dentures. For instance, it is known that a short rooted, slightly periodontally involved tooth will resist lateral load less favourably than a multi-rooted tooth in healthy condition. It is known, too, that a wrought gold clasp arm, having a lower modulus of elasticity than a cast cobalt chromium arm of similar dimensions, will throw less lateral load on to a clasped tooth. Consequently, wise denture planning would suggest that the lateral load acting on the periodontally involved tooth should be reduced by using a wrought gold wire clasp instead of one of cast chrome cobalt.

However, there is evidence that the designing of partial dentures is becoming more scientific. For instance, Wilson gives this information regarding the dimension of a stress-breaker wire used in a Class 1 lower:

'A 17 gauge tapered to about a 19 gauge is desirable, the heavier end being attached to the denture base or saddle connector and the tapered end is soldered to the retainer. About three-quarters of an inch length is sufficient although this is modified according to the conditions prevailing.'

This specification, based on clinical experience, could not be described as vague. Another example is the work of Warr, who has measured the coefficient of static friction between teeth and denture alloys, in the presence of saliva, and has shown wide variations to exist depending upon the cleanliness of the surfaces and the roughness of the alloy. The same author has indicated a mathematical method by which the undercut to be engaged by a clasp arm can be determined, knowing the length, taper, section and material. Anderson has measured the dimensions most appropriate for lingual bars, plates and other types of connectors.

For the present the main problem to be faced is the control of the muscular forces acting on the partial denture and their distribution to those tissues most fitted to accept them. Although in planning an appliance, accurate measurements of muscular force and tissue reaction cannot be made, every use should be made of the information available to design an appliance which will not damage any particular tissue by throwing too great a stress upon it.

In order to do this it is necessary to consider in greater detail the components of partial dentures. These may be listed as:
1 saddles
2 occlusal rests and similar components
3 direct retainers
4 indirect retainers
5 connectors.

The Saddles

The saddle is the part of a partial denture that replaces lost alveolar tissue and carries artificial teeth. The fitting surface of a saddle can be made of acrylic resin or metal; both have advantages and disadvantages, but the majority are made in acrylic resin, and certainly this material should be used exclusively for free-end saddles. In a few cases it may be necessary to use soft lining materials to form the fitting surface of free-end saddles. Such materials may be the only solution to the problems of the atrophic mucosa, the prominent mylohyoid ridge, or an irregular bone surface which for good reasons cannot be modified surgically.

Acrylic resin has the advantages of cheapness, low specific gravity, good aesthetic appearance, and the ease with which it can be rebased. The last factor accounts for its choice for largely mucosa-borne free-end saddles, under which the rate of alveolar resorption is greater than under tooth-borne saddles, and consequently rebasing must be carried out routinely. Using acrylic resin this process can be accomplished quickly and economically.

However, a saddle with a metal fitting surface has some advantages. When they are used, they are normally cast.

The condition of the underlying mucosa is often better under metal than under acrylic. In the first place, the fitting surface of a cast saddle can be polished to give a smooth finish without any appreciable loss of tissue adaptation; this is not so with acrylic resin. The smooth metal surface is less abrasive to the underlying mucosa than the rougher acrylic surface and consequently chronic inflammatory reaction is less likely under metal. The surface of acrylic resin will be much improved if the model is covered with thin gauge tin-foil and the resin is processed against it. Since metal does not absorb water and has a dense surface it is easily kept clean and free from deposits. Such deposits may be calcareous, rough, and consequently irritant through mechanical action, or infective by providing a nutritive plaque for the proliferation of pathogenic bacteria, which in high local concentration may involve a slightly abraded mucosa in a low grade inflammatory process. If a metal surface is left in the 'as cast' condition it is liable to be more traumatic than acrylic, and to favour the formation of soft and hard deposits. The better thermal conductivity of metal has often been suggested as a further reason for the better tissue health found under such surfaces. Applegate has pointed out that an additional mechanism might be in 'aiding the escape of body heat' which is facilitated by the metal base with its higher thermal conductivity.

Apart from the increased cost of production, the most serious disadvantage of the metal base saddle is the fact that it is more difficult to rebase it, when ridge resorption makes this desirable. However, it is the opinion of some writers that alveolar resorption under metal saddles is less than under acrylic resin saddles, other factors being equal. This is said to be due to the increased thermal stimulation to the underlying tissues which maintains a more efficient circulation.

It is the opinion of Applegate that if teeth have been missing for a long time from an area that is to support a free-end saddle, the alveolar bone may have undergone structural change due to lack of functional stimulus. In these cases, until there has been some trabecular rearrangement in response to the new functional stimulus provided by the saddle, further loss of alveolar bone may be expected. This type of case, then, is one which should always have an acrylic resin saddle. However, a metal base may more safely be used when there is a history of a previous saddle having received stable support.

Some claim that a cast metal surface, even after a light polishing, has better tissue adaptation than acrylic resin. This is largely a matter of personal opinion, and will further depend on the technical ability applied to the making of the appliance. Applegate's contention that resin 'even under ideal conditions of processing, is not entirely free from volumetric change and later warpage' must be supported. Also, much research has been applied to the production of investment materials which compensate accurately for alloy contraction on solidification from casting to room temperature. Consequently, it would not be surprising if, in fact, the cast metal displayed better surface adaptation than acrylic.

The desirability of maximal saddle extension was discussed at the beginning of this chapter, and it now remains to consider the relationship of the saddle to the abutment tooth and its gingival margin. Contact between the saddle and the proximal surface of the abutment is necessary to prevent food packing between saddle and abutment. Further, the gingival margin should be relieved from saddle pressure during function. A number of workers who have undertaken clinical surveys of partial denture wearers have all noted that when a saddle was adequately tooth supported and when the saddle made close contact with the proximal surface of the abutment tooth the underlying gingiva was in good condition. When, owing to the proximal undercuts, there was a small space between the saddle and the neck of the tooth this predisposed to a chronic hypertrophic gingivitis and pocket formation. However, if this space was enlarged deliberately by angulating the saddle away from the tooth below the contact point and so creating a self cleansing space, the gingival reaction was much better.

Hence it appears that the situation shown in Fig. 10.2a should not be permitted. If possible the proximal undercuts should be eliminated by grinding or by the construction of full coverage crowns or by inlays, thus producing the situation shown in Fig. 10.2b. Alternatively the saddle should be designed as shown in Fig. 10.2c. A clinical example of this situation is shown in Fig. 10.3.

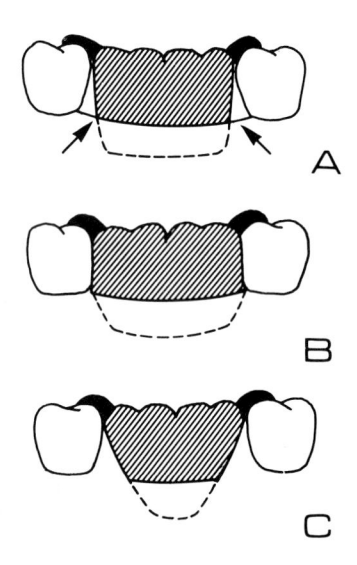

Fig. 10.2. A Undesirable small proximal spaces between the saddle and the abutment teeth.
B An ideal saddle–abutment tooth relationship.
C Enlarged spaces which can be self-cleansing.

Irrespective of whether it is practical to have close saddle contact with the abutment tooth or whether a large self-cleansing space has to be provided, it is most important that the contact between the abutment tooth and the saddle occurs at the natural 'contact point' of the abutment tooth. If contact is made above the natural contact point, pressure applied to the saddle may tend to move the tooth away from the saddle. Should the contact be below the natural point then there is a potential space into which food may be packed. Surveying the cast with the occlusal plane at right angles to the carbon marker will ensure this desirable saddle–abutment tooth contact relationship.

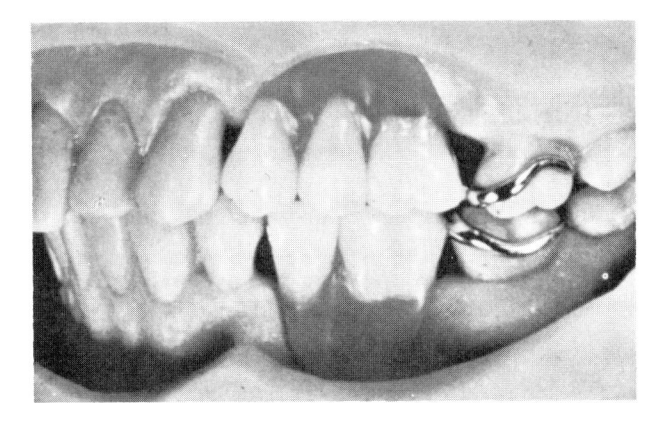

Fig. 10.3. Saddles designed to produce self-cleansing spaces adjacent to the abutment teeth.

In the case of posterior bounded saddles where aesthetics does not have to be considered, a modified construction may be employed, as shown in Fig. 10.4. A bar of metal attached directly to the connector forms the occlusal surface and there is no mucosal contact at all. This allows the gingivae to be free of pressure and to be readily self-cleansing. Pressure is also removed from the mucosa overlying the ridge which may be advantageous if this is atrophic. The possible disadvantages of this type of saddle are the facts that some patients may not

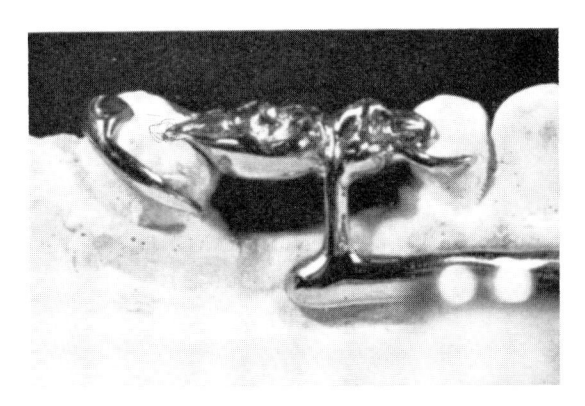

Fig. 10.4. Bar type saddle allowing the gingivae to be free of pressure and self-cleansing.

tolerate the connecting strut between the lingual bar and the occlusal area, and that food may not always be readily removed by the tongue. Moving the strut forwards to lie nearer the premolar may be helpful to both these factors.

The methods of attaching the teeth to the saddle vary according to whether acrylic or porcelain is selected. Acrylic teeth are always fixed to the saddle through a bond with resin. The saddle may have a fitting surface of cast metal on to which acrylic resin base material is attached by retention tags. In these cases the union of tooth to the resin, being of a physico-chemical nature, is always sufficiently strong. In some cases of close anterior occlusion a small saddle may display a weakness of the union between metallic base and intervening resin.

Porcelain teeth may be preferred to acrylic teeth in the anterior or posterior parts of the mouth. Anterior porcelain replacements are either pin teeth, facings, or tube teeth. When the anterior occlusion is close facings and metal backings can be used. If a gold base is being used the backing may be cast integrally with the base or soldered to it afterwards. Cobalt chromium backings must be cast with the base. A porcelain or acrylic facing is subsequently cemented in position.

In the posterior part of the mouth diatoric, tube, or true pontic porcelain teeth may be used. The first type are mechanically held in acrylic resin while tubes are held in position by cementing to a metal post which is accommodated accurately in a round channel centrally placed in the long axis of the tooth.

Occlusal Rests and Similar Components

An occlusal rest is a metal projection attached to a partial denture, extending over and bearing on the occlusal or prepared surface of a standing tooth (Fig. 10.5). It must fit the surface accurately and must be cast and not made from wrought metal.

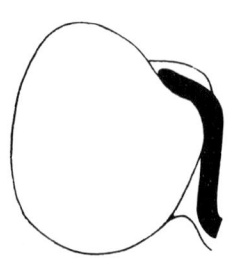

Fig. 10.5. The occlusal rest.

An occlusal rest serves these purposes:
1 It transmits vertical load to the tooth.
2 It transmits some lateral load to the tooth.
3 It deflects food.

The Component Parts of a Partial Denture 211

4   It may improve occlusion.
5   It may act as an indirect retainer.

Transmission of vertical load

When vertical load is applied to a bounded saddle which is supported at both ends by occlusal rests, pressure is exerted against the rested teeth. This results in a stretching of the periodontal fibres and an eventual stressing of the bone that surrounds the teeth.

Presuming the saddle to have been constructed on a cast from a mucostatic impression and with its fitting surface, therefore, conforming to the form of the alveolar tissues at rest, only a small proportion of the stress bears directly on the alveolar bone owing to the compressible nature of the covering mucosa. The proportion of force that does act on the ridge depends on the comparative compressibilities of the particular teeth and the particular mucosa. Where a marked difference in compressibility exists, as when the mucosa is of loose consistency, then the proportion of load falling on the ridge is very small. The desirability of loading a healthy tooth rather than the edentulous ridge has already been discussed; the large bony support of the former may be expected to react more favourably by bone deposition.

The proportion of the magnitude of load that will be transmitted to the teeth on which the rests are placed can be varied, as discussed by Chick. For example, rests placed at equal distances from the middle of the saddle will, assuming the load to be applied to the middle of the saddle, transmit an equal load to the teeth on which they are placed. However, in the example illustrated (Fig. 10.6) the load on the premolar can be reduced and that on the molar increased by moving the rest to the mesial aspect of the premolar and this may be desirable since,

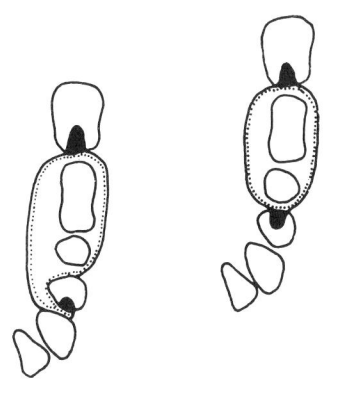

Fig. 10.6. Altering the magnitude of the load transmitted by an occlusal rest by moving it away from the saddle.

normally, molar teeth can accept greater loads than premolars. The strict truth of this depends on the assumption that the load acts through the middle of the saddle, and certainly this will not always be so. However, it can be stated as a general principle that if it is necessary to decrease the magnitude of the load on a tooth, then the rest should be moved away from the saddle; concurrently this will increase the load on the other tooth by an equal amount.

If the saddle concerned is not rested at either end, then the vertical load falling upon it must be resisted entirely by the bone of the edentulous ridge. The area of bone stressed is therefore reduced and also the particular bone to which pressure is applied is that least likely to withstand extra loading without resorbing. In such conditions it is most likely that alveolar resorption will take place, bringing in its wake several undesirable sequelae.

As the saddle sinks, damage to the related gingival margin and periodontal membrane ensues. The pressure of the saddle on the gingival margin has two effects. In the first place, a gingivitis is initiated, which is liable to develop into a periodontal involvement of the abutment tooth and hasten its loss. Quite apart from this, as the saddle sinks it effects a mechanical stripping of the gingiva and periodontal membrane from its tooth attachment, and again this is a complication likely to lead to early loss of the tooth. Because of these two processes a partial denture which has no occlusal rests in its design has become known as a 'gum stripper'.

As the edentulous ridge is resorbed the occlusal relationships are affected. In addition, the positions of the clasp arms are altered and their functions of retention and bracing are therefore impaired. If resorption is excessive, or if originally the arm lay in close approximation to the gingival margin, pressure is applied to this delicate tissue and inflammation ensues.

It is therefore apparent that the transmission of the vertical load to the teeth, preserving as it does the bone of the edentulous ridge consequently helps to prevent these harmful sequelae:
1 breakdown of the periodontal membrane
2 loss of correct occlusal relationships
3 loss of correct position of clasp arms.

Transmission of lateral load

When a saddle carries occlusal rests at each end they may aid in the distribution of lateral load to the abutment teeth. If the occlusal surface of the abutment is flat, then no lateral stress is communicated to it, whereas if the rest fits accurately into a box-shaped preparation the lateral load is transmitted entirely to the tooth. Where the occlusal rest is placed in contact with the sloping walls of the cusps of the tooth, an intermediate condition exists and some of the lateral force is conveyed as a lateral stress to the tooth.

The Component Parts of a Partial Denture

It is rarely desirable to use an occlusal rest to convey lateral stress to an abutment tooth. It is only when it is not possible to use bracing arms of clasps for this purpose that a box-shaped preparation should be used. Aesthetics, for example, may preclude the use of a bracing arm on the buccal aspect of a lingually inclined lower premolar.

It is more usual to provide saucer-shaped rest seat preparations which allow a very slight lateral movement of the rests over the teeth. This allows the flanges of the saddles to compress the mucosal tissues and transfer a proportion of stress to the underlying bone, thus sharing the load between the ridge and the abutment teeth.

Deflection of food

The occlusal rest covers a space which might otherwise exist between the saddle and the abutment. A free-end lower saddle lightly clasped to its abutment tends, in function, to be displaced backwards, opening up the potential space between saddle and tooth, into which food is liable to be packed. This may be a cause of caries on the proximal surface of the tooth or more often result in a traumatic gingivitis. When an occlusal rest covers this space, entrance of food is prevented since it is deflected bucally or lingually.

It is not uncommon for posterior teeth to be separated interstitially by a small space, particularly following extraction of one tooth and forward drifting of its neighbour. Such spaces are potential food traps and if they can be covered by occlusal rests much damage can be prevented (Fig. 10.7).

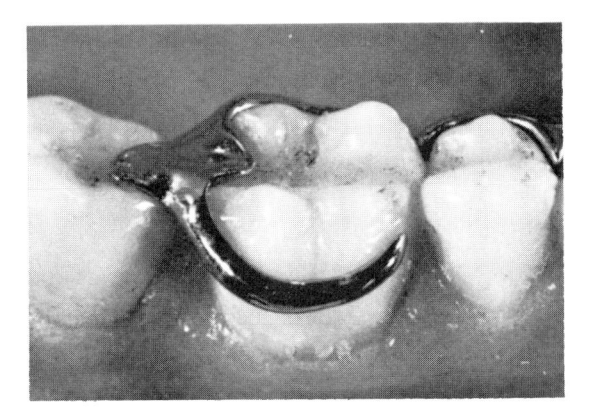

Fig. 10.7. Occlusal rest extended to cover potential food trap between two lower molars.

Improvement of occlusion

Very often an occlusal rest can be shaped to improve the existing occlusion. A common example of this is when a rest placed on a tilted tooth is built up to give a larger contact with opposing teeth. When the area of the rest is extended to cover a large proportion of the occlusal surface it is termed an onlay.

The effect of the occlusal rest on the tooth

For purposes of discussion a tooth may be likened to a section of a cone with a curved surface and two parallel flat circular surfaces. The circular surface of greater size may be taken as representing the occlusal surface of the tooth and that of less area the apical area of the root. (Exceptions to this are the upper first and second molars where the roots are often very divergent.) If vertical pressure is applied over the whole of the occlusal surface an uncomplicated downward movement of the diagrammatic tooth takes place in its socket (Fig. 10.8). If, however, a vertical pressure is applied at the periphery of the occlusal surface the downward movement is complicated by a torque being placed on the tooth and a rotatory effect is introduced (Fig. 10.9). Such a rotatory effect should always be minimized as far as is practicable and three methods are available for this purpose.

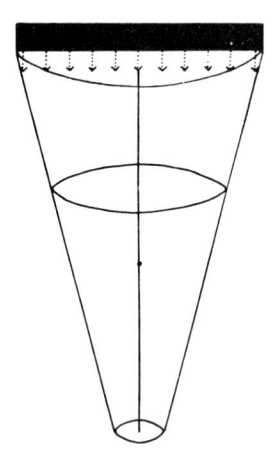

Fig. 10.8. Shows that the application of a vertical load over the whole occlusal surface results in the uncomplicated downward movement of the tooth.

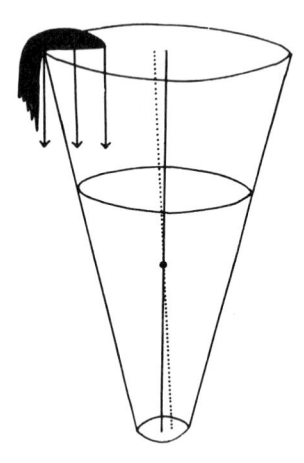

Fig. 10.9. Shows that a torque acts under vertical loading when the occlusal rest is placed at the periphery of the occlusal surface.

In the first place a large mesio-distal coverage of the tooth may be used, the tip of the rest preferably extending to the centre of the mesiodistal fissure (Fig. 10.10). A second possibility is by reciprocation, two shorter rests being placed diametrically opposite, one on the mesial part of the occlusal surface and one on the distal (Fig. 10.11). The third possibility is to place the rest on the surface of

Fig. 10.10. Shows a reduction of torque under vertical load when the occlusal rest extends over the centre of the mesio-distal fissure.

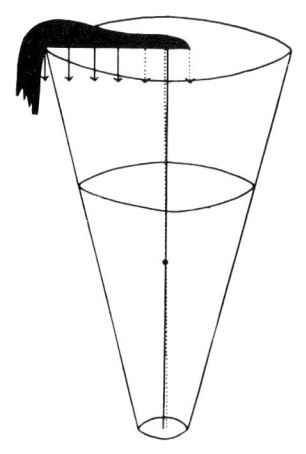

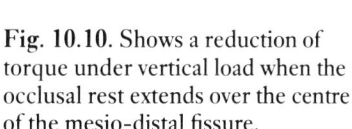

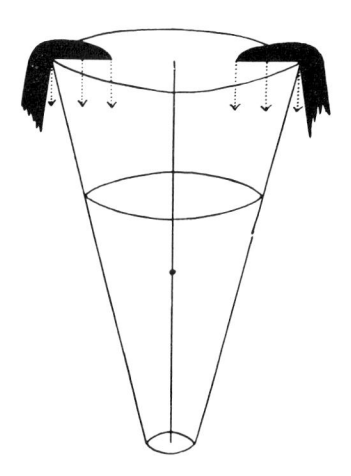

Fig. 10.11. Shows the reciprocating effect of occlusal rests placed diametrically opposite and the uncomplicated downward force that results.

the tooth further removed from the saddle so that contiguous standing teeth help to resist the rotatory movement (Fig. 10.12).

In the majority of cases this torque can be resisted by the bony support of the natural tooth, if the tooth is vertically placed in the same axis as the force under consideration. When, however, the tooth is tilted and its long axis lies at an angle

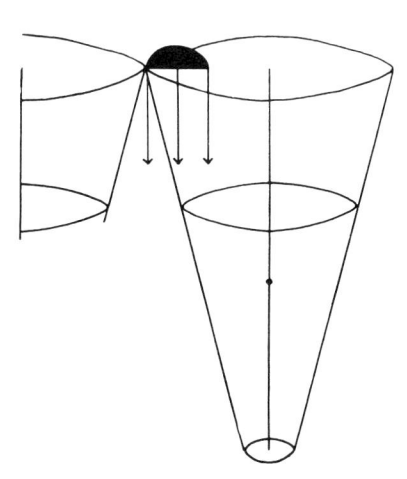

Fig. 10.12. Shows the effect of a contacting contiguous tooth in resisting a torque which results from an occlusal rest placed at the periphery of the occlusal surface.

216 Chapter 10

to the vertical force, a complication is introduced. This commonly happens where a tilted lower molar is the posterior abutment of a bounded saddle. In effect, the force is farther removed from the centre of rotation in the root, its moment is correspondingly increased, and consequently a further tilting of the tooth is liable to occur. If a rest is placed on such a tooth next to the saddle, a good contact point with the saddle is necessary to mitigate the tendency to further tilting. In such cases there is some merit in placing the occlusal rest over the distal part of the tilted tooth; in this situation the line of application of the force lies closer to the centre of rotation, as a result of which the torque is decreased.

When the rest seat is horizontal the entire vertical force has the same direction as the long axis of the tooth. When, however, the rested surface lies at an angle to the vertical an inclined plane effect comes into operation as illustrated in Fig. 10.13. When the rest lies directly above the centre of rotation, the crown of the tooth, supposing it to be an incisor, may be displaced labially.

Rested surfaces may lie at an angle to the vertical in the following cases:
- A tilted tooth, in particular a tilted lower molar.
- When a rest is placed on the palatal or lingual surface of an incisor or canine.
- When a rest seat has been prepared in a posterior tooth and where, instead of the surface being horizontal, it slopes down towards the saddle.

Reference has already been made to the first case of the tilted lower molar. Here the tendency of the denture to move backwards counteracts in some

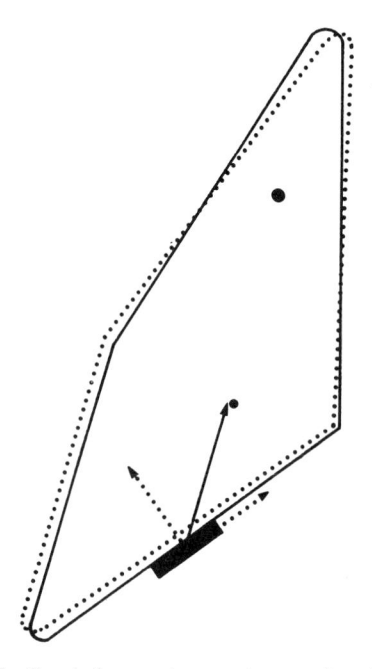

Fig. 10.13. Inclined plane action causing rotation of rested tooth.

measure the rotatory effect of the load being applied at a point far removed in a horizontal plane from the centre of rotation in the root. Here no preparation of the tooth is required, but good contact points at both ends of the saddle are essential. The possibility of placing the rest distally rather than mesially has already been mentioned.

In the second case, when a rest is placed on the palatal or lingual surface of an incisor or canine, one component of force tends to displace the tooth anteriorly. In the lower the effect may be resisted by the overbite of an upper tooth, but in the upper the force is entirely unopposed and therefore tilting of the tooth is more likely to take place. In this type of case, the preparation of a rest seat is always necessary to produce a horizontal surface to receive the rest. Various methods of accomplishing this have been discussed in Chapter 7.

The third case where the rest seat slopes towards the saddle arises accidentally during rest seat preparation.

The dimension of the occlusal rest

An occlusal rest must be of sufficient bulk not to deform either permanently or elastically in function. If permanent deformation takes place the rest no longer bears on the tooth, and in consequence the saddle becomes entirely mucosa borne. When the rest is too thin and is deformed elastically, a proportion of the load is transferred to the ridge and fracture will occur as a result of fatigue.

The actual thickness of the rest depends on the alloy used. Since cobalt chromium has a higher modulus of elasticity than gold, occlusal rests made of the former may be thinner. This has the advantage of necessitating less deep rest seat preparation.

The importance of the mesio-distal length of the rest has already been mentioned, and the advisability of extending it over the centre of the mesio-distal fissure emphasized.

The width of the rest where it covers the marginal ridge should be as great as possible, so that the line of action of the occlusal force on the saddle lies within, or at the most only slightly outside, this dimension. Such a condition ensures stability of the denture and is particularly important in the case of a unilateral appliance.

Lastly, the thickness of the rest where it passes over the marginal ridge must be adequate. This is a point of stress concentration and consequently should be the region of greatest thickness. Unfortunately, the marginal ridge encroaches on the rest in this situation and tends to make it thinner. It is therefore usually necessary, during rest seat preparation, to reduce the enamel in this area to ensure adequate thickness at this part of the rest. The proximal edge of the enamel should be rounded rather than square, as this prevents a weak edge on the tooth and thickens the rest where this is required.

Rest seat preparation

This is one of the most necessary steps in partial denture technique, and a description of the procedure was given in Chapter 7.

Onlays

When an occlusal rest is extended to cover the greater proportion of the occlusal surface of a tooth it is called an onlay (Fig. 10.14). Onlays may be cast in gold or cobalt chromium alloy, but when made of gold the appliance is unnecessarily heavy and costly. It has been suggested that the hardness of cobalt chromium alloy would have an excessive abrasive action upon the enamel of opposing natural teeth, but in practice this does not seem to occur. It is possible that, in some cases, there may be more marked faceting than usual, but the degree is slight.

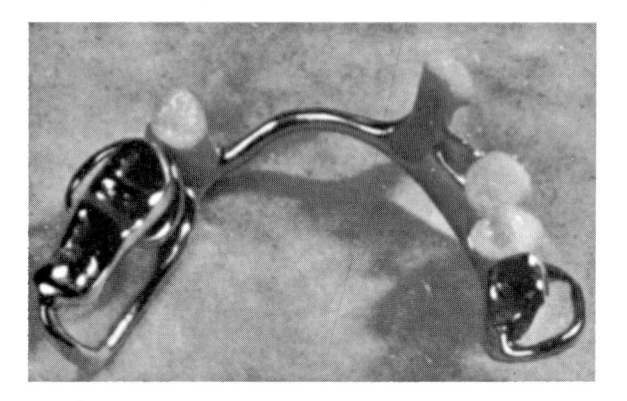

Fig. 10.14. Lower denture showing onlays.

Another method of constructing onlays is to cast the fitting surface in metal and to attach acrylic resin to form the occlusal surface. The metal casting fits over the occlusal surfaces of the teeth and to this the acrylic resin is attached by means of retention tags (Fig. 10.15). This combination onlay has the following advantages:
- The weight of the appliance is reduced (Fig. 10.16).
- The appearance may be improved if the buccal edge of the metal is flared to a thin edge and care is taken to obtain a good colour match between the acrylic and the natural teeth. The presence of the underlying metal makes this difficult but the result can be improved by highly polishing the surface of the metal in contact with the resin, or by using an opacifier, which is painted on to the metal.

The Component Parts of a Partial Denture

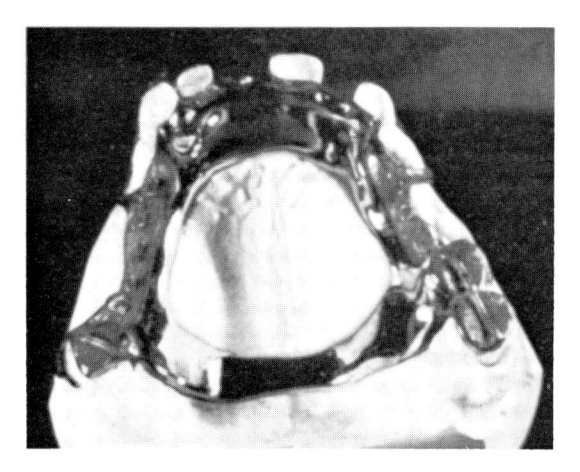

Fig. 10.15. Metal onlays which are to have acrylic resin added to them to increase their thickness.

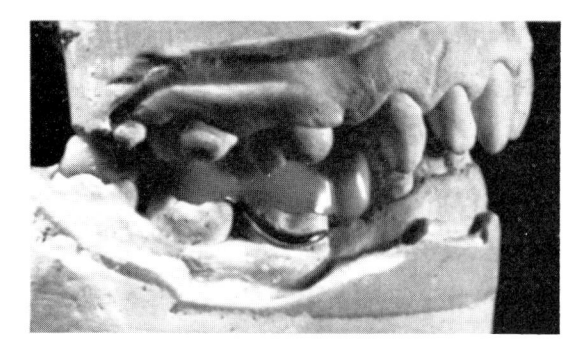

Fig. 10.16. A case showing excessive interocclusal clearance and requiring unusually thick onlays. Acrylic resin is supported by cobalt chromium.

- Final grinding-in for correct occlusion is facilitated. Whereas this is easily done with acrylic resin, it is difficult when the onlays are made entirely in cobalt chromium alloy.

The disadvantages of combination onlays are the facts that they are more liable to abrasion and require a large inter-occlusal space to find a practical application. In some instances use may be made of entire acrylic resin onlays. Certainly, diagnostic appliances are always made of acrylic resin.

One of the hazards of onlay appliances is the development of widespread caries in the underlying teeth. For this reason their use in young patients should be minimal and preferably only for diagnostic purposes, any permanent changes required in the occlusal surfaces being achieved by fixed restorations. Even during the temporary period of wear for diagnosis, extreme emphasis must be placed upon oral hygiene and frequent clinical examinations carried out.

Whether, in older patients, onlay appliances should be permanent depends upon the particular circumstances of each case. If the onlays form part of a partial denture, replacement of which by fixed bridge-work is not practical, then obviously the onlays are a permanent part of the treatment. When clinical conditions are satisfactory for fixed restorations and tolerance of the appliance is poor or its retention is less than adequate, then fixed appliances are the method of choice.

When it is decided that an onlay appliance is to be worn permanently, it is generally found that the majority of patients are more comfortable with acrylic resin than alloy occlusal surfaces. Franks has shown that the electrical output of the masseters is reduced significantly when cobalt chromium occlusal surfaces are used in comparison with identical appliances with acrylic resin surfaces. This may be a protective mechanism initiated by the proprioceptors of the periodontal membranes in response to the extreme hardness of the alloy. The main disadvantage of the acrylic resin surface is its relatively rapid abrasion which necessitates frequent replacement, or resurfacing, of the appliance.

In shaping an onlay buccally and lingually it is necessary to continue the convexity of the lateral surfaces of the tooth, thus ensuring that a convex self-cleansing surface is maintained (Fig. 10.17). Failure to do this results in an area of enamel situated just below the margin of the onlay where food and mucus stagnate; caries may readily be produced in such locations.

Onlays serve the following functions:
1 They may support a partial denture.
2 They may correct an overclosed occlusion.
3 They may improve the occlusion.

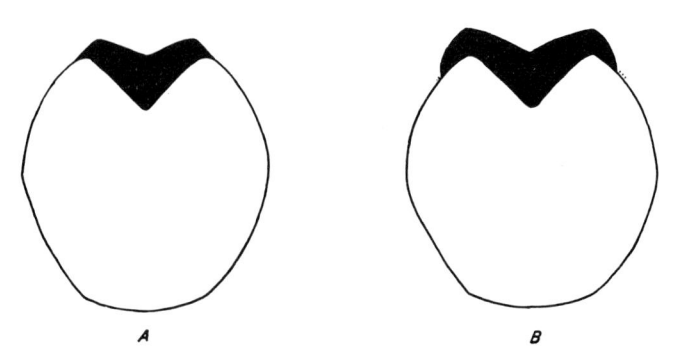

Fig. 10.17. A, the correct, and B, the incorrect method of shaping an onlay. It will be noted in A, that the whole buccal and lingual surfaces of the tooth are self-cleansing, whereas in B, a shelf exists on those surfaces immediately beneath the onlay which harbours food debris.

4   They may effect a reduction in cusp angle and therefore reduce lateral stress on the teeth.
5   They may splint the natural teeth.

1   *Partial denture support.* For this purpose onlays function in exactly the same way as occlusal rests, but there is no danger of their bending or breaking. If the tooth lies in the same axis as the vertical force, the onlay has the advantage over the occlusal rest of covering the entire tooth surface, and hence there is no danger of tilting the tooth through the load being applied at a distance from the central axis of the root (Fig. 10.8). There is generally no need to prepare the tooth to receive an onlay; the cusps present several different inclined planes but, on balance, horizontal components cancel out and only the vertical components act.

2   *Correction of an overclosed occlusion.* By the use of onlays occlusion can be obtained at an increased vertical dimension. The indications for this are considered in Chapters 7 and 16.

3   *Improvement of the occlusion.* The use of onlays in a partial denture may be a helpful method of improving occlusion. It can be particularly useful in cases showing periodontal involvement when it is necessary to distribute occlusal loading as widely as possible, and also when a full upper denture opposes a partial lower, good, widely distributed occlusion being helpful for the stability and retention of the full denture.

4   *Reduction of cusp angle.* A reduction of the cusp angle effects a reduction in the lateral component of force acting during mastication. This may be accomplished by the use of onlays which may be indicated in the treatment or prevention of periodontal disease.

5   *Splinting.* Onlays splint together the teeth over the occlusal surfaces of which they are constructed. In this way mutual support is afforded to these teeth, and may prove a useful adjunct in the treatment of periodontal disease. Onlaying provides one of the simplest means of splinting the teeth, but is less effective than fixed restorations.

It remains to be emphasized that the use of onlays may necessitate an increase in the vertical dimension, and this step should only be taken after thorough diagnosis.

Embrasure Hooks

These are metal attachments to a partial denture which are placed in the embrasure between two contiguous natural teeth. They cover the occlusal or incisal surfaces of the teeth and continue over to the labial or buccal surfaces (Fig. 10.18), but never extend below the survey line, and consequently play no part in direct retention.

An embrasure hook may serve the following purposes:
1 Support the denture.
2 Brace the denture.
3 Resist antero-posterior stress.
4 Splint natural teeth.
5 Act as an indirect retainer.

1 *Support.* Since embrasure hooks cover the occlusal or incisal surfaces they support the appliances in the same way as do occlusal rests. They find application where it is desirable to distribute the support of a denture over more teeth than the abutments. Since they are often placed at the mesial or distal angles of the teeth, their line of action is outside the root axis and leverage may be applied to the teeth. The use of the incisal edge for support is more common in the lower jaw than the upper since the lingual surfaces of the lower anterior teeth do not permit cingulum preparations being made in them so readily. Generally such support is required for the connector between two posterior free-end or bounded saddles when the anterior abutments are canines, but may be required when there is an anterior saddle in the incisor region. It is sometimes possible to provide support for such a connector by means of embrasure hooks fitted over the incisal edge without any previous preparation of the teeth concerned. If this method is used, hooks may be aesthetically displeasing owing to their relative prominence in relation to the incisal edge level of the natural teeth. In such a position they will also be poorly tolerated by the patient and may interfere with the occlusion of the anterior teeth.

Certain cases may appear to offer suitable conditions for the placing of embrasure hooks without any previous tooth preparation (Fig. 10.18). Particularly the configuration of the incisal edge between the lower canine and lateral

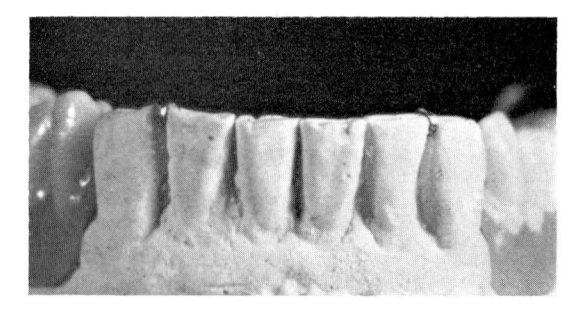

Fig. 10.18. Embrasure hooks in lower incisor region.

The Component Parts of a Partial Denture 223

incisor may suggest an ideal site for an embrasure hook. If such a condition is present, associated with two free-end saddles, there is a strong likelihood that the hooks may apply a 'wedging' action leading to separation of the canine and the lateral, and loss of denture support. Since the tendency of lower partial dentures is to move backward there is a distinct possibility of this occurring with a free-end saddle denture (Fig. 10.19). However, if posterior teeth are present this form of support may be used successfully. In most cases it is possible to make such hooks aesthetically hardly noticeable. When such favourable conditions do not exist some form of preparation must be made as described in Chapter 7.

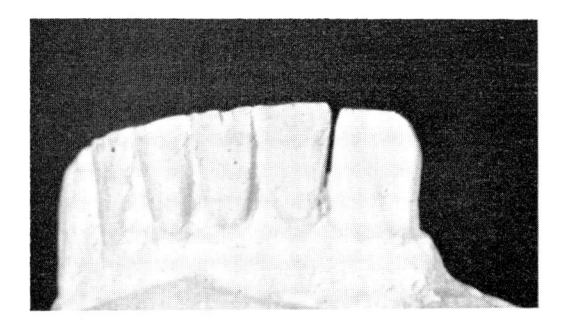

Fig. 10.19. Separation of canine and lateral caused by the wedging action of an embrasure hook.

The preparation shown in Fig. 7.22 may be used on canine abutment teeth. Such a preparation accommodates what is more truly an incisal rest rather than an embrasure hook. Such rests may be extended directly from a lingual plate, carried on a separate strut from a lingual bar, or extended from a broad coverage of the canine cingulum (Fig. 10.20). The latter method has the better tolerance factor if a lingual bar connector is used.

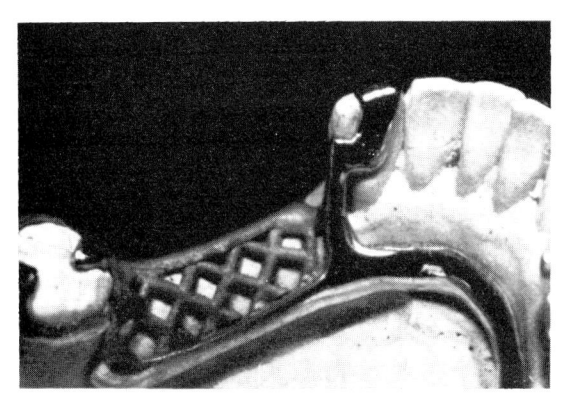

Fig. 10.20. Incisal rest carried from broad cingulum coverage of lower canine. The preparation for this rest is shown in Fig. 7.22.

2 *Bracing.* Embrasure hooks make contact with both the lingual or palatal and labial or buccal surfaces of the teeth. As a result they distribute the lateral load acting on the saddles to these teeth, both on the working and balancing side of the mouth. They may be included in a design where broad distribution of the lateral stress is indicated.

3 *Resistance to antero-posterior stress.* Where embrasure hooks are used on anterior teeth they may be useful in resisting antero-posterior movements of the denture. In particular their use may be indicated with Class I lower dentures when the abutment teeth are canines, which are so rotated mesiodistally that little resistance to posterior movement can be gained from clasps. In such cases the use of incisal rests rather than embrasure hooks is recommended for the reason given above. Only an abutment tooth in good periodontal condition can be relied upon to resist the 'wedging' action of narrow embrasure hooks in these circumstances.

4 *Splinting the natural teeth.* When these hooks are placed in all the embrasures a simple splinting of the natural teeth is effected. A lateral load falling on the saddles or on any standing tooth is immediately shared by all the teeth and mutual support is afforded. In this way multiple embrasure hooks may find application in cases where the teeth show periodontal involvement.

5 *Indirect retention.* Embrasure hooks may be used on anterior teeth to assist indirect retention. They may be attached to a continuous clasp when this is included in the design but if such a component is contra-indicated they may arise from a lingual plate.

As with occlusal rests embrasure hooks may be made in either cobalt chromium or gold. Since they are often used anteriorly aesthetics is a prime consideration, and in this respect the cobalt chromium hook is to be preferred. As a result of its physical properties its bulk can be less than one made of gold and it can often be inconspicuously concealed behind a rotated lateral or canine. Further, the highly finished silver coloured surface of the chrome alloy reflects the white enamel colour much more effectively than does yellow gold, thus aiding considerably in the aesthetic result.

Direct Retainers

Direct retention is effected by precision attachments or by clasps.

Clasps

A clasp is a metal component of a partial denture which fits against the vertical enamel surface of a standing tooth, aiding in the bracing and retention of the appliance. Although it is necessary to retain partial dentures this is not the only factor to be considered in designing appliances intended to conserve the remaining mouth structures. The control of lateral load is of paramount importance and its distribution between standing teeth and ridges by means of clasp arms is one of the most successful methods of preserving the alveolar bone and the remaining teeth.

Clasps considered as retaining devices

The retentive arm of a clasp provides resistance to a displacing force directed occlusally, because its terminal end rests on an undercut surface of a standing tooth. In order that the denture may be displaced the clasp arm must be moved over the most bulbous contour on to the non-undercut zone of the tooth. The aim in designing clasps must be to ensure that the forces tending to dislodge the denture are less than the force required to displace the clasp arms in this manner.

As with the masticatory stress, the magnitude of the vertical displacing force acting on a partial denture is not capable of accurate measurement. Amongst other factors it depends on the nature of the food, the position of the saddles, the size of the denture occlusal table, and the weight of the appliance. The magnitude of the force required to displace a clasp over the maximal bulge of the tooth depends on the following:

1 depth of the undercut engaged
2 modulus of elasticity of the alloy used in its construction
3 section of the clasp arm
4 length of the clasp arm
5 angle of approach of the clasp arm
6 the position of the clasp in relation to a fulcrum axis.

1 *Depth of undercut engaged.* The efficiency of clasps in relation to the undercut engagement depends jointly upon the degree of both vertical and horizontal engagement. When describing the procedure for surveying it was shown that, depending upon the shape of the tooth, the distance below the survey line at which the same amount of horizontal undercut is engaged will vary. It is obvious that the greater the horizontal undercut engaged, the greater must be the deflection of the clasp arm necessary to remove the denture. However, the vertical distance of engagement is also of significance. It will be seen from Fig. 10.21 that to be removed the clasp has to be forced over an inclined plane. The steeper this inclined plane the greater is the force required to move the clasp out of the undercut. Consequently the shorter the vertical degree of engagement for a given degree of horizontal engagement (which is measured by the undercut gauge) the more efficient will be the clasp, all other factors being equal. For

example, if a 0.25 mm undercut gauge is used to locate the position of the clasp arm on two teeth and on the one tooth the clasp is 4 mm below the survey line, and on the other it is 2 mm below, then, other factors being equal, the latter clasp will provide more retention. There is an optimal degree of horizontal undercut which should be engaged by any particular clasp, which depends on the other five factors listed above. Should this optimal value be exceeded there is a danger of traumatizing the tooth on insertion and removal and every likelihood of early fatigue fracture of the arm. Further, particularly with cobalt chromium alloy, there is a danger of the stress required to seat the denture exceeding the elastic limit of the clasp arm. This results in a permanent deformation of the clasp, so that its terminal section positioned in the undercut lies away from the enamel; such a situation fails to retain the denture when a displacing force is applied and may also predispose to caries or ulceration of the cheek. On the other hand, when insufficient undercut is engaged the clasp is ineffective in retaining the denture.

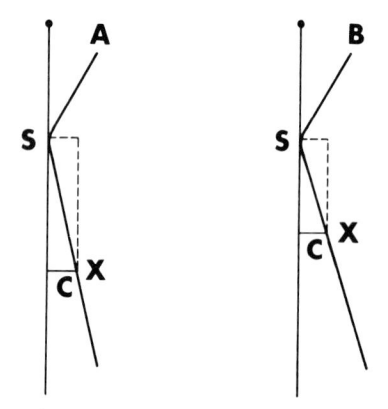

Fig. 10.21. S is the position of the survey line on two teeth, A and B. Although the degree of horizontal engagement, C, is the same on both teeth, the vertical distance, SX, is less on tooth B and hence the inclined plane over which the clasp arm must pass is steeper, thus indicating more efficient retention.

2 *Modulus of elasticity of the alloy used.* The modulus of elasticity of cobalt chromium alloys is higher than that of casting golds, and the latter have a higher modulus than wrought gold wires. Therefore a clasp of the same cross-section is stiffer in cobalt chromium than in cast gold and one in cast gold is stiffer than one in wrought gold. Consequently, to obtain similar results, clasps made in different alloys must have different lengths and sections. For instance, the high modulus of cobalt chromium alloy can be overcome by using longer clasps of thinner section, and by engaging the undercut to a less degree.

3 *Section of the clasp arm.* The thicker the clasp arm the greater is the force

required to effect its displacement over the greatest contour of the tooth. Obviously an optimal section exists for each type of clasp, taking into account its design, alloy used, and degree of undercut engaged. It is therefore, desirable to use preformed wax or plastic patterns when waxing up a partial denture, since these patterns are made with cross-sections suitable to the alloy being used and to the degree of undercut engagement stipulated. Clasp arms that are too thick require too much seating force, whilst arms that are too thin, as well as providing insufficient retention, are liable to accidental displacement or fracture.

Wrought wires, normally of round section, are more flexible, not only on account of their metallurgical structure but also because their round section is more favourable to flexibility than the usual half round section of cast clasps.

4 *Length of clasp arm.* The longer the clasp arm the less is the force required to displace it sufficiently to disengage the tooth. Consider a rod of metal AB (Fig. 10.22) rigidly supported at point A. If a fixed load is placed at point B it will effect a deflection in the rod through the distance BC. Now let us substitute a shorter rod of length AD but of the same section, and apply the same load at its extremity; the deflection of the rod will be reduced to DE. If a similar deflection to BC were required, a greater load would need to be applied to point D. Thus the length of the arm is an important factor in controlling the retentive capacity of a clasp.

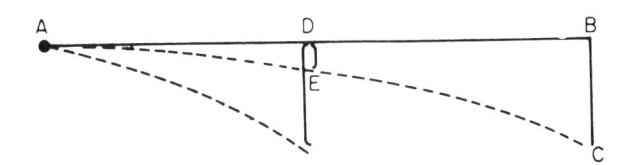

Fig. 10.22. The deflection of a rod fixed at A when weights are applied at the points B and D (see text).

Bates has pointed out that cobalt chromium clasp arms of short length, or marked curvature, have insufficient deflection at the proportional limit to be of practical value as retaining devices; in addition they will exert high forces on the tooth concerned. Gold alloys, with their lower modulus, have twice the deflection for the same load and hence give better retention if the arm has to be short, as will be the case with an occlusally approaching clasp on a premolar.

5 *Angle of approach of the clasp arm.* The clasp arm may approach the undercut areas of the tooth from an occlusal or gingival direction (Fig. 10.23). The force required to displace a clasp arm from the tooth is dependent on the angle of approach of the tip to the plane of the undercut. In general a gingivally approaching clasp arm displays better retentive action than an occlusally

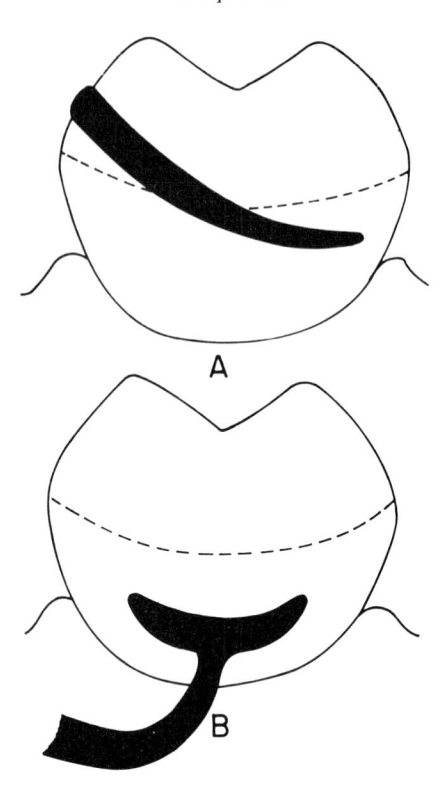

Fig. 10.23. A, the occlusal and B, the gingival approaches of a clasp arm into a tooth undercut.

approaching arm and this is explained by the trip action taking place with the gingivally approaching arm, an effect first noted by Stone.

A good method of demonstrating trip action is described by De Van who advises pushing and pulling 'a fountain pen having a short blunt nib across a supported writing pad. As the angle of the pen to the pad approaches a right angle we receive a tactile sensation of tripping during the action of pushing. This vibratory trip is entirely absent when the pen is pulled across the pad. The foregoing experiment is most valuable, for we not only feel and see tripping action, but also our pad bears a graphic chart of it. The push lines will reveal at regular periodic intervals heavier markings indicative of periodic flexions of the shoulders of the pen's nib. The lighter lines uniting these dashes indicate the intervals of release when the pent up energy in these resilient flexions is suddenly made available to effect motion. The result of pulling the pen across the pad regardless of angulation will be an unbroken line of like intensity. This clasp and pen analogy is a happy one, for they possess similar metal parts; resilient shoulders or arms, tips or bearing points.'

The Component Parts of a Partial Denture   229

When a vertical displacing force acts on a gingivally approaching arm, the clasp itself is stressed in such a way as to increase its angle of approach to the plane of the undercut. This torsion of the clasp arm, therefore, makes more force necessary to displace it over the tooth. The angle of approach of such a clasp arm is determined by the inclination of the buccal or labial alveolar mucosa as it slopes away from the gingival margin. The clasp arm must not impinge upon this tissue, but at the same time its angle of approach cannot be increased to such a degree as to interfere with the action of the cheek musculature or to trap food between its connecting bar and the ridge. However, an increase of the angulation of the connecting bar just before the head of the clasp makes contact with the tooth is a practical method of increasing the retentive effect without altering the optimal bar position in the sulcus (Fig. 10.24). It will be noted that with this type of clasp there is no trip action upon insertion. At this stage the angle of incidence of the clasp to the non-undercut plane increases as the seating pressure is applied, thus facilitating the insertion of the denture.

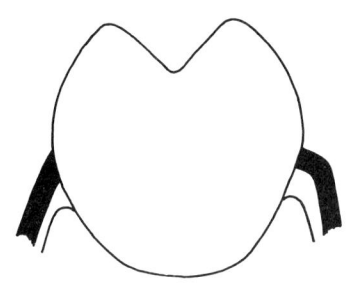

Fig. 10.24. The effect of increasing the angle of approach of a gingivally approaching clasp arm by a bend near the contacting surface of the tooth.

An opposite state of affairs exists in the occlusally approaching clasp arm. Here the trip action is effective on insertion, thus making the denture more difficult to seat. However, on removal, as the clasp arm is pulled out of the undercut it thus provides less resistance to displacement than the gingivally approaching clasp, all other factors being equal.

6   *Position of clasp in relation to displacing force and fulcrum axis.* To illustrate the principle involved, consider the hypothetical situation of an anterior saddle replacing the six front teeth with rests placed mesially on the first premolars. When food is incised the saddle tends to rotate about the axis of the occlusal rests. Displacement of the saddle can be resisted by forces which act on the opposite side of the fulcrum axis and it is pertinent to review the effect of the clasp placed on the last molar tooth of one side of the dental arch (Fig. 10.25).

The appliance might be considered as a lever of the first class, and the system

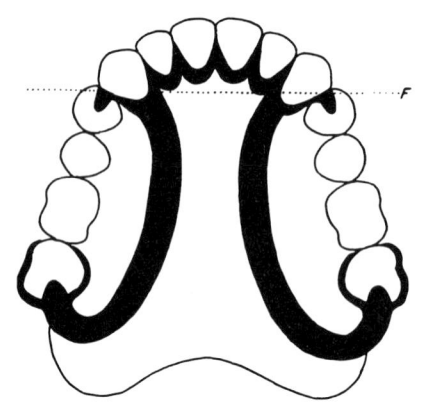

Fig. 10.25. A hypothetical case considered to show the position of the clasp in relation to the displacing force and the fulcrum axis.

of forces act as illustrated in Fig. 10.26a. It has been assumed that the displacing force on the anterior saddle has a value w, and that this acts at a distance d from the fulcrum or rest on the first premolar. To give balance in the system (or produce a stable appliance) a reaction in the clasp of value W would be required. But let us suppose this acts at a distance $2d$ from the fulcrum point, a condition that might well arise if a second molar were the clasped tooth. In this event we have:

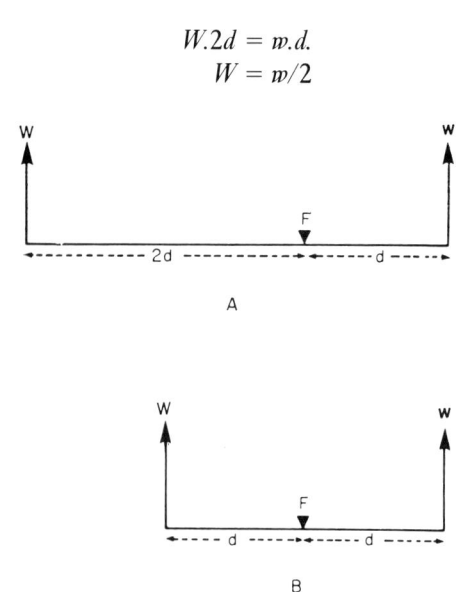

$$W.2d = w.d.$$
$$W = w/2$$

Fig. 10.26. The system of forces acting when the fulcrum axis is placed at different distances from the displacing force.

The Component Parts of a Partial Denture 231

In other words, the position of the clasp has been advantageously chosen so that the reaction in the clasp need be only half the magnitude of the displacing force.

If, however, the clasp were situated at a distance d (Fig. 10.26b) from the fulcrum, by placing it on a more anterior tooth, a force of the same magnitude to the displacing force would need to be resisted by the clasp.

This situation illustrates the manner in which the position of the clasp in relation to the fulcrum axis affects the magnitude of the functional force required to effect its displacement.

In function clasps are required to resist rotational movements of the denture rather than its vertical displacement as a whole. Forces causing such movements may act unilaterally so that one side of the denture tends to be displaced, or they may be applied to cause antero-posterior rotational displacement.

An example of the latter condition may be found in the lower bilateral free-end saddle denture. When a force is applied which tends to displace the saddles away from the mucosa, rotation of the denture will take place. The axis of this rotation is somewhat indeterminate, but most likely will be in the region of the tips of the clasp arms (Fig. 10.27). Obviously, since the tips of the clasp arms will move farther into the undercut area, they do nothing to prevent the movement of the denture. In such cases the retention by clasping can be improved by reversing the conventional position of the rest and clasp arms as shown in Fig. 10.28. Now the centre of rotational displacement is moved to the occlusal rests,

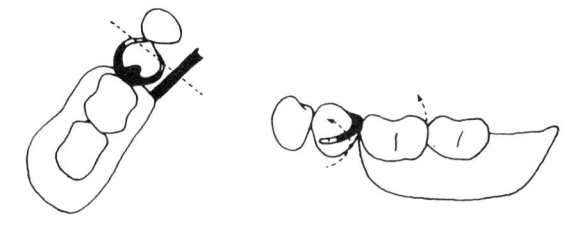

Fig. 10.27. Rotational displacement of a free-end saddle inadequately resisted by conventional rest and clasp arm position.

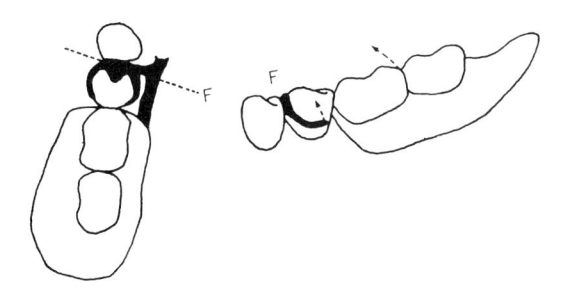

Fig. 10.28. The effect on resistance to displacement of reversing the rest and clasp arm position in the case of a free-end saddle.

and hence the movement of the tips of the clasp arms is upwards towards the survey line. Hence rotational displacement is more likely to be resisted. The only disadvantage of this procedure is one of aesthetics, particularly if the clasped tooth is a first premolar.

When the antero-posterior rotational movement of a bounded saddle is considered, any rotational effect at one end of the saddle is resisted by the clasp placed at the opposite end. However, it will be noted that if the position of the rest and clasp arm is reversed from that conventionally used, two clasps resist the rotation (Fig. 10.29). The disadvantage of this approach is the tooth preparation often necessary to accommodate such an arrangement.

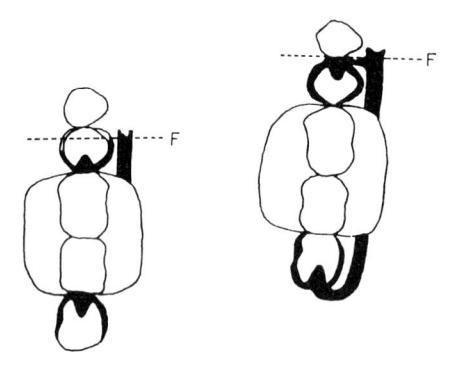

Fig. 10.29. The effect of reversing the occlusal rest and clasp arm positions in a bounded saddle.

Passive placement and spring tension. It has so far been assumed that when the clasp is in position the whole retentive arm lies passively against the tooth without exerting any pressure against it. Such a condition has been described by Blatterfein as 'passive placement', but should the clasp arm exert a continuous spring force against the tooth, the term 'spring tension' is used. In this case when a displacing force acts on the denture, additional force is developed between the tooth and clasp, in addition to the force necessary to lift the clasp over the survey line.

The use of spring tension is to be deplored. It is known that continuous pressures, even of small magnitude, are effective in producing tooth movement. When spring tension is used, forces act continuously on the clasped tooth; the effect of such forces is more harmful in the older group of patients than in the younger, since the potentiality to lay down new bone decreases with age. The only method of preventing movement of abutment teeth is by ensuring that equal and opposite forces act on each side of the clasped tooth. However, it is impossible to control the amount of stress that is placed on a tooth as a result of spring tension, and consequently it is almost certain that the force developed in one direction will be greater than in the other; hence a displacing force acts continuously on the clasped tooth. Even assuming that it were possible to develop equal spring forces in the clasp arms, they would have to lie in the same horizontal plane on either side of the tooth, otherwise a torque would cause rotation about a centre somewhere in its root (Fig. 10.30).

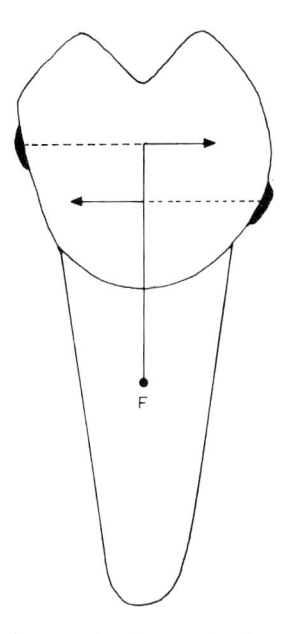

Fig. 10.30. A system of spring forces acting in opposite clasp arms when these do not lie in the same horizontal plane. It should be noted that there is not a balance of moments about the fulcrum axis.

Clasp arm reciprocation. Reciprocation has to be considered in the horizontal and vertical planes. Horizontal reciprocation demands that a clasp arm be balanced by another on the opposite surface of the tooth. When a clasp arm is displaced over the survey line there is a tendency for the tooth to be rotated away from the arm, but this can be prevented by a clasp arm on the opposite side of the tooth. This reciprocating arm may be of two kinds, either a retentive arm that exerts a balancing force in the opposite direction, or a rigid bracing arm that plays only a passive part in resisting any tendency of the tooth to tilt. In order to be completely effective such a bracing arm should act on a vertical surface rather than on one that is convex so that contact with the surface can be maintained as it moves in an occlusal direction. Suitable grinding of the enamel can often improve the surface of a clasped tooth from this point of view. Reciprocation of a retentive clasp arm can also be achieved, if other considerations permit, by the preparation of a deep square rest seat.

234   *Chapter 10*

Considering reciprocation in the vertical plane it is evident that the reciprocating clasp arm should lie, as far as possible, on the same horizontal level, otherwise it may have moved above the occlusal surface before the undercut of the tooth is completely traversed by the retentive arm (Fig. 10.31). The insertion of inlays or grinding the enamel are approaches sometimes employed to allow reciprocating clasp arms to be placed on the same horizontal level.

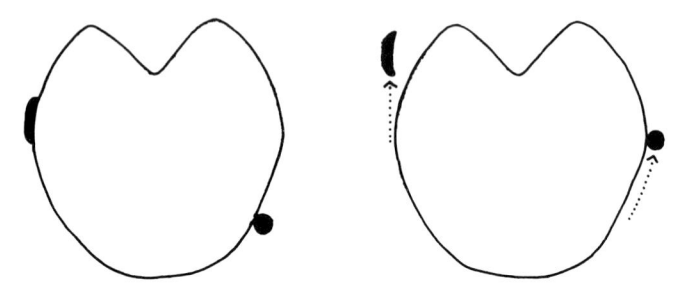

Fig. 10.31. The effect on denture removal of placing a bracing arm above the retaining arm. Note that the retaining arm still acts on the tooth when the bracing arm has ceased to be in contact.

When the principle of passive placement is observed the only occasions when a stress requires to be reciprocated are during insertion or removal of the denture and on those occasions when it tends to be displaced. The incidence of the latter stresses is infrequent, being confined to meal times. In addition, their magnitude is small in comparison to those of the lateral component of mastication. Hence it might be thought that reciprocation need not be considered when designing a clasp, provided passive placement was observed. However, this is not so since clasp arms, particularly of the more resilient type, may become displaced and exert some spring tension. Consequently, the principles of reciprocation should always be observed although some latitude from placing opposite arms in the same horizontal plane can be allowed.

Enamel abrasion. There are two ways in which a clasp might abrade the enamel; first, by wear on the tooth during removal and insertion of the denture by the patient, and second, by continual friction of the clasp during masticatory stresses. Phillips and Leonard studied both these phenomena by laboratory experiments and came to the conclusion that 'the partial denture clasp, regardless of the type of alloy used, does not produce abrasion on enamel'. Severe abrasion was noted, however, when amalgam was the bearing surface for either gold or chrome alloy clasps. They state that *apparent* abrasion, sometimes seen clinically under clasps, must be attributed to other causes. However, Warr has stated that, whilst roughening the contacting surface of chrome cobalt clasps may produce an increase in retention of 50%, it will 'almost certainly be at the expense of tooth attrition'. The experience of the authors is that abrasion of enamel is a clinical rarity, a view further supported by the laboratory experiments of Bates.

As with decalcification and caries, sometimes seen adjacent to a clasp, lack of oral hygiene by the patient leading to plaque and bacterial accumulations is considered to be the most significant factor.

Clasps considered as bracing devices

It has already been mentioned that the lateral stress acting on a denture can be resisted by either the edentulous ridge, the remaining teeth, or both. Clasp arms are one of the components which may be used to distribute the lateral load to the standing teeth.

To illustrate the principle involved it is helpful to consider the bracing action of an arm of the conventional 'cast three-arm clasp'. The condition at either end of the bounded saddle illustrated in Fig. 10.32 will be considered.

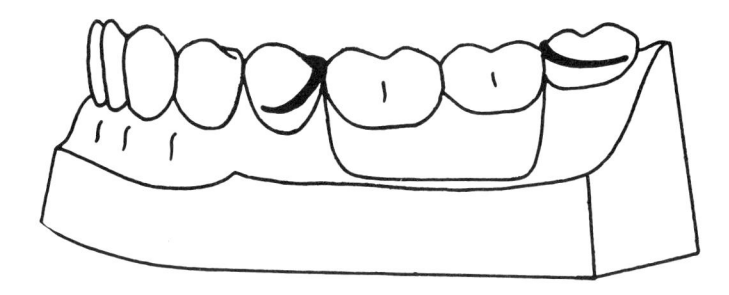

Fig. 10.32. The bracing action of clasps at either end of a bounded saddle.

Such a clasp arm can be divided into three positions (Fig. 10.33). The first lies above the survey line and is the rigid portion and consequently its cross-section is considerably greater than the other parts. The second portion of the clasp is that part which crosses the survey line, and its function is to connect the first bracing portion with the resilient retaining portion. In section it is intermediate between the parts into which it merges. The third or terminal portion of the clasp is the resilient part that lies in the undercut zone of the tooth. To ensure flexibility in this part of the clasp its cross-section is greatly reduced. It should be noted that the decrease in section from the bracing portion to the retaining portion is gradual; in other words, the arm tapers evenly, so that there is no sudden change in section. This ensures that there is no point of stress concentration that might lead to fracture as the arm is opened over the maximum convexity of the tooth.

It is the first portion of the clasp that is the bracing element and transmits the lateral load to the tooth. The relative amounts of load that fall on the tooth and on

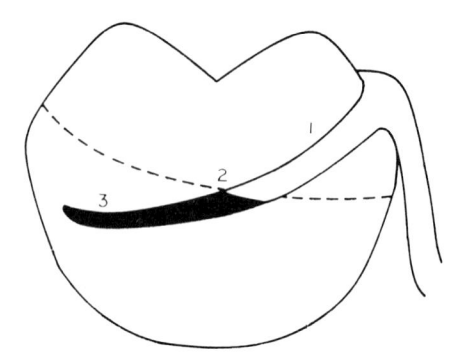

Fig. 10.33. The three parts of an occlusally approaching clasp arm in relation to the survey line.

the ridge depend on the rigidity of the clasp arm, the relative compressibility of the tooth in its socket, and the particular mucosa that covers the edentulous ridge.

The greatest amount of load falls on the tooth when the clasp arm is rigid. However, a very small amount of clasp arm opening may take place under lateral load, but the thicker the section of the clasp arm the less will be its liability to displacement. Thick clasp arms, however, have some disadvantages. In the first place, a very thick bracing portion does not allow a sufficiently resilient clasp tip in the undercut, even if a high degree of taper is incorporated. Second, increasing the section of the clasp arm increases the susceptibility to caries by covering the enamel of the tooth more extensively. Third, the natural contour of the tooth is grossly altered by a thick clasp and this has the effect of interfering with the stimulation of the gingival margin which lies in relationship to the clasp (Fig. 10.34). A thick clasp arm forms a shelf above the gingival margin and prevents the movement of food over this tissue and, in the absence of meticulous oral hygiene, a gingivitis is liable to occur. Again, the occlusion sometimes limits the vertical height of a clasp arm, little space existing between the survey line and the

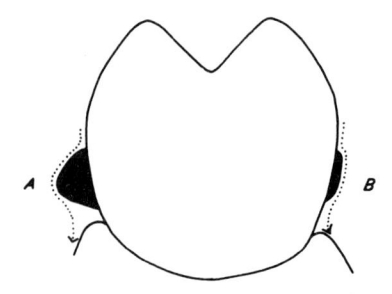

Fig. 10.34. Illustrates in *A* how a thick clasp arm prevents food stimulation of the gingival margin, whereas the thinner arm *B* allows movement of food over the entire gingiva.

opposing tooth. There is, therefore, a limit to the thickness of a clasp arm to provide rigidity.

The modulus of elasticity of the alloy is important in its effect on the rigidity of the bracing section, the higher the modulus the more rigid the arm and the less opening that will occur under lateral stress. Consequently, a chrome alloy clasp will transmit more lateral load to the tooth than one made of gold, if both are of equal section.

The relative compressibilities of the tooth in its socket and the mucosa covering the adjacent edentulous ridge are the last factors controlling the relative pressures which fall on tooth and ridge when the saddle receives a lateral thrust. When the covering soft tissue has a thin tough fibrous submucosa the load to which it is subjected is increased. In this case, as the clasp arm opens, the pressure is directed down to the alveolar bone; conversely, when the mucosa is very compressible and thick, little pressure is directed to the ridge and the teeth must accept the load.

It is impossible to measure the variables involved in finite units but general assessments can be made as regards relative tooth and tissue compressibility and their anticipated reaction to lateral loading. Accordingly, clasp design can be modified and the distribution of load between tooth and saddle controlled approximately. This is effected by selecting a material and clasp arm section in keeping with the clinical situation.

When wrought gold wire is used the bracing effect is reduced, but it can be varied by selecting different wire gauges. Some clasps that are occlusally approaching are characterized by having a single arm which completely embraces the tooth on three sides; this class includes the back action, the reverse back action, and the ring clasps. On one side of the tooth the arm lies above the survey line, and hence can be made extremely rigid if desired, while on the opposite side the arm lies below the survey line and is necessarily much more resilient. Such clasps are said to provide unilateral bracing. It must be borne in mind, however, that the retentive arm does provide some bracing, although this is less than that provided by the rigid reciprocating arm. It must also be appreciated that the three arm type of clasp may often consist of one arm which is solely bracing and lies totally above the survey line, whilst the other arm is almost completely retentive in its function.

So far only the occlusally approaching cast clasp arm has been considered. The bracing supplied by a gingivally approaching arm is always less than that provided by an occlusally approaching arm, being of the same order as that given by the retentive arm of the back action clasp. The bracing of these gingivally approaching clasps can be controlled by varying the length, section, and modulus of elasticity of their connecting bar. It is obvious, however, that a reduction in the bracing property also implies a reduction in the retentive capacity.

As a general principle the lateral load on a denture should be borne by as large a number of teeth as possible, the load falling on any one being thereby reduced, and the likelihood of exceeding the physiological limit of stress, minimized. It is not necessary to limit the clasping to the abutment teeth only, since it may be used as a method of splinting, affording mutual support to the teeth. Other methods of splinting exist and these may have some advantage aesthetically or in simplicity of construction; clasping, however, offers a possible line of treatment.

Particular clasping methods

Clasps generally make use of the undercuts on the buccal and lingual surfaces of the standing teeth to obtain retention, but Roach and De Van have pointed out some advantages in using the undercuts on the proximal surfaces of the teeth. It is proposed first to present a classification of survey lines found on the buccal and lingual surfaces and to consider some clasping methods available in each case. Occlusally and gingivally approaching varieties of clasps are described whenever possible.

It should be appreciated that the survey line is not the only consideration when deciding how to clasp a tooth. The root size and form, as well as the clinical condition of the supporting structures, must be taken into account, since upon these depend the amount of lateral load that should be placed on the tooth. In particular, the short rooted tooth, the tooth supported by atrophic bone, and the periodontally involved tooth, are less able to accept high bracing forces; suitable clasp design and material of construction are necessary in these instances to keep the lateral load falling on the tooth within the physiological range.

Blatterfein's classification of buccal and lingual survey lines. Blatterfein has put forward a simple comprehensive classification of survey lines which has proved helpful and practical in resolving clasping problems.

It is necessary to define the terms *near zone* and *far zone* introduced by Blatterfein to divide the buccal and lingual tooth surfaces into two halves by a vertical line through the long axis of the tooth. The near zone is that half which lies nearer to the saddle and the far zone that half which is more remote from the saddle (Fig. 10.35). Similarly the mesial and distal tooth surfaces are described as near or far depending on their proximity to the saddle.

The medium survey line. This survey line appears on the buccal or lingual surface of the tooth, approximately equidistant from the occlusal surface and gingival margin in the near zone and slightly nearer the gingival margin in the far zone (Fig. 10.36).

This class of survey line often indicates the use of an occlusally approaching arm, sometimes described as a circumferential arm. Depending on the bracing effect required this may be made of cobalt chromium, cast gold, or wrought gold wire, appropriate sections being used (Fig. 10.37). When both arms of this clasp are similar and are associated with an occlusal rest, the whole is known as a three arm clasp.

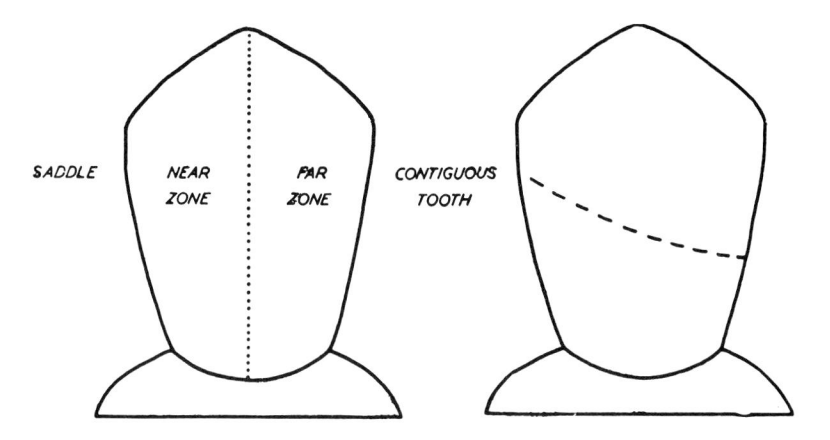

Fig. 10.35. The near and far zones described by Blatterfein.

Fig. 10.36. The medium survey line.

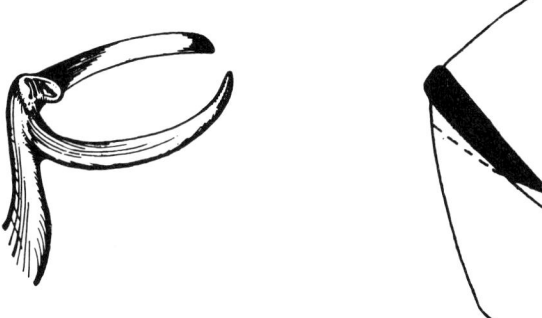

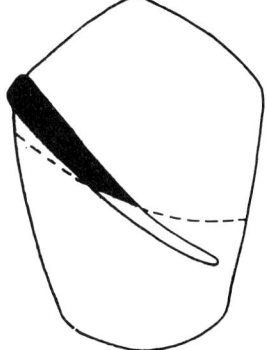

Fig. 10.37. The circumferential clasp arm. The bracing area is shaded and the retentive area unshaded.

A gingivally approaching arm may be used on a tooth having a medium survey line. The various forms of bar clasps are appropriate, the length of the bar used depending upon the resilience required in the arm. If a larger degree of undercut is to be engaged more resilience is required and the length of the bar is increased. It is often necessary on aesthetic grounds to engage the undercut more deeply so that the end of the clasp may be placed nearer to the gingival margin. The more resilient the arm in these cases the less the bracing effect; this factor, too, makes its separate demand on bar length.

The diagonal survey line. This survey line lies nearer the occlusal surface than the gingival margin in the near zone of the tooth, but in the far zone the opposite condition exists and little under-cut is present (Fig. 10.38). Such survey lines are most commonly found on the buccal surfaces of canines and premolars.

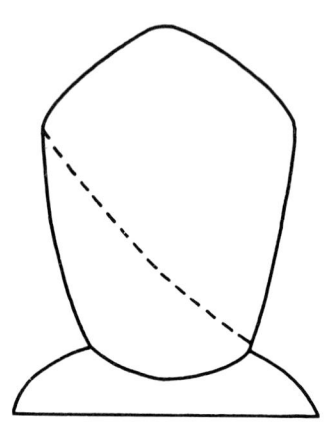

Fig. 10.38. The diagonal survey line.

If an occlusally approaching arm is preferred, there are two possible clasps that can be used. In the first the rigid part of the clasp arm crosses from the near zone to the far zone above the survey line and sweeps round to return into the undercut of the near zone, tapering suitably towards its extremity (Fig. 10.39). One disadvantage of this clasp is that it has no application where there is a short clinical crown, as insufficient space exists to accommodate the double clasp arm. Also, since the diagonal survey line is often found on the buccal or labial surfaces of teeth that are shown in smiling, the conspicuous double arm may constitute a serious disadvantage. Owing to the short length of the arm and the curvature involved such arms cannot be made in cobalt chromium alloy.

The second occlusal approach into the undercut is by a clasp arm that encircles the tooth on three surfaces. It first traverses the opposite surface of the tooth, then runs in the embrasure between the clasped tooth and its continuous tooth in the arch, and finally crosses the surface from far to near zones (Fig. 10.40). Such a clasp is always cast and provides unilateral retention. Unless the tooth is single standing, such as a second molar, it may require quite extensive preparation of the marginal ridges of the clasped tooth and its contacting tooth.

This type of diagonal survey line may be found on the lingual surface of lower molars or the buccal surface of upper molars, and may be associated with a low survey line on the opposite surface of the tooth. In these circumstances the most useful form of clasp is the ring clasp, described below, which enables the retentive arm to enter the undercut area from the far zone.

The Component Parts of a Partial Denture 241

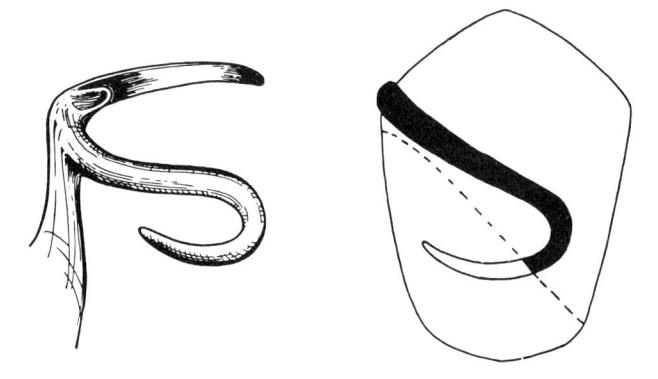

Fig. 10.39. The first occlusally approaching type of clasp possible with the diagonal survey line. The bracing area is shaded and the retentive area unshaded.

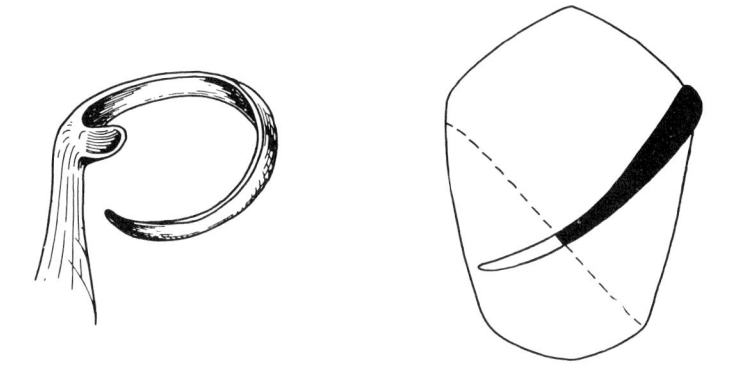

Fig. 10.40. The second occlusally approaching type of clasp possible with the diagonal survey line. The bracing area is shaded and the retentive area unshaded.

When the survey line is this combination of diagonal and high, the ring clasp is always preferable to the circumferential or three arm clasp.

When a gingival approach is preferred the L or T bar clasps are useful, usually having an aesthetic advantage over the occlusally approaching types. The near portion of the head of the L form lies in the undercut while the far portion is situated above the survey line. If the latter section is thickened an additional bracing effect can be secured (Fig. 10.41a). The head of the T form lies entirely in the undercut (Fig. 10.41b). Chrome cobalt alloy or cast gold alloy may be used. If there is rather more undercut available than is shown in Fig. 10.41 a 'U' shaped bar may be used (Fig. 10.42). As there are now two bars effectively engaging the undercut, retention will be improved.

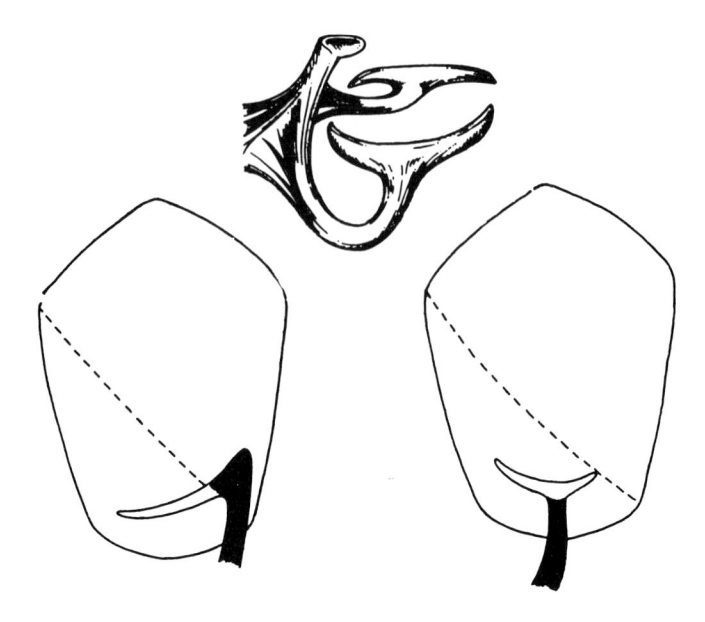

Fig. 10.41. The L and T bar clasp arms. The bracing area is shaded and the retentive area unshaded.

The high survey line. This survey line appears much nearer to the occlusal than the gingival of the tooth in both near and far zones (Fig. 10.43). It may arise as a result of abnormal tooth form where the occlusal surface has a considerably larger perimeter than the amelo-cemental junction and where only a small degree of convexity is present on the tooth surface. More commonly, however, it results from inclination of the tooth. Consequently, it is frequently found on the lingual surfaces of lower teeth and on the buccal surfaces of uppers.

Once again, if an occlusally approaching arm is required, one that encompasses three surfaces of the tooth may be used, but if the arm is to cover only one surface of the tooth, wrought wire is generally to be preferred (Fig. 10.44). Such an arm is brought immediately below the survey line and the greater part of its length engages in the undercut. Often the undercut is deep and to get sufficient flexibility in the arm near its point of attachment it is necessary to use wrought gold wire, which is characterized by its high resilience. It should be emphasized that the bracing action of this arm is low. Generally insufficient space exists between the survey line and the occlusal surface of the tooth to accommodate the rigid bracing portion of a cast clasp, since it may interfere with the occlusion. Further, even if space does exist it is sometimes doubtful if the tooth can be expected to react favourably to a rigid clasp arm located so high on its

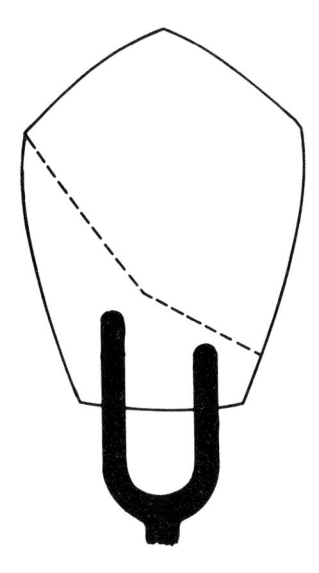

Fig. 10.42. The U-shaped bar clasp arm.

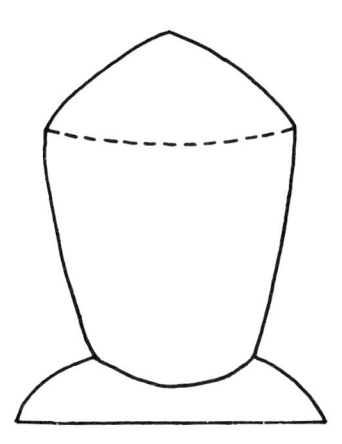

Fig. 10.43. The high survey line.

crown. Such a position increases considerably the moment of the force acting on the tooth under lateral load.

When a high survey line results from an inclined tooth it is generally found that the opposite surface of the tooth has little or no undercut. In these cases it is often desirable to use a clasp arm encircling in turn the non-undercut surface, the near or far proximal surface, and the surface with the high survey line. The portion of the arm lying on the non-undercut surface is above the survey line and

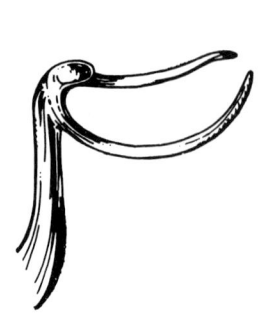

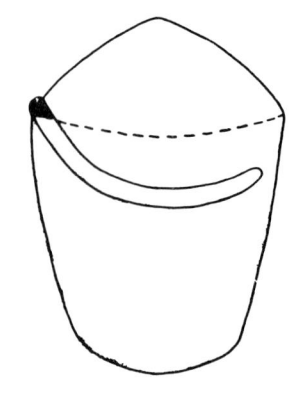

Fig. 10.44. The wrought wire clasp arm. The bracing area is shaded and the retentive area unshaded.

is rigid by virtue of its thickness. The portion contacting the proximal surface is variable in position, lying either in or out of the undercut. The arm tapers gradually towards the terminal part which contacts the third surface and is resilient, lying below the survey line throughout its whole length. Such a clasp gives unilateral retention and the bracing is considerably more effective on the non-retentive side. Attachment to the denture may be by a strut which is joined to the thicker extremity of the arm. When this strut is buccally placed, as is frequently the case with a lower denture, the clasp is described as a reverse back action (Fig. 10.45a). Conversely, when the strut is palatally or lingually placed it is called a back action clasp (Fig. 10.45b); because of the curve of Monson this variety is more common with an upper denture. Upon the length, thickness, and alloy of this strut depends the bracing quality of the clasp. Even with a short, thick strut, there is always more displacement of the saddle permitted than with the circumferential clasp and consequently more lateral load falls on the ridge.

The ring clasp (Fig. 10.46) is very similar to the back action clasps and is used on single standing molar teeth which, because of a severe tilt have a high and/or diagonal survey line, and almost completely encircles the tooth, its termination being in the near zone of the undercut surface. The attachment of the clasp to the denture is more direct than in the case of the back action clasp, being by a strut similar to that used with the circumferential clasp. Sometimes a buccal or palatal reinforcing arm is placed against the mucosa as shown in Fig. 10.46 to give extra rigidity. The bracing action of the rigid portion of this clasp is high, but is greatly reduced in the retentive part.

Gingivally approaching clasp arms find little application with high survey lines that result from tilted teeth. In these circumstances the supporting ridge generally conforms in its slope to that of the tooth. Assuming a vertical path of insertion this means that a large tissue undercut exists and it is necessary to keep

The Component Parts of a Partial Denture 245

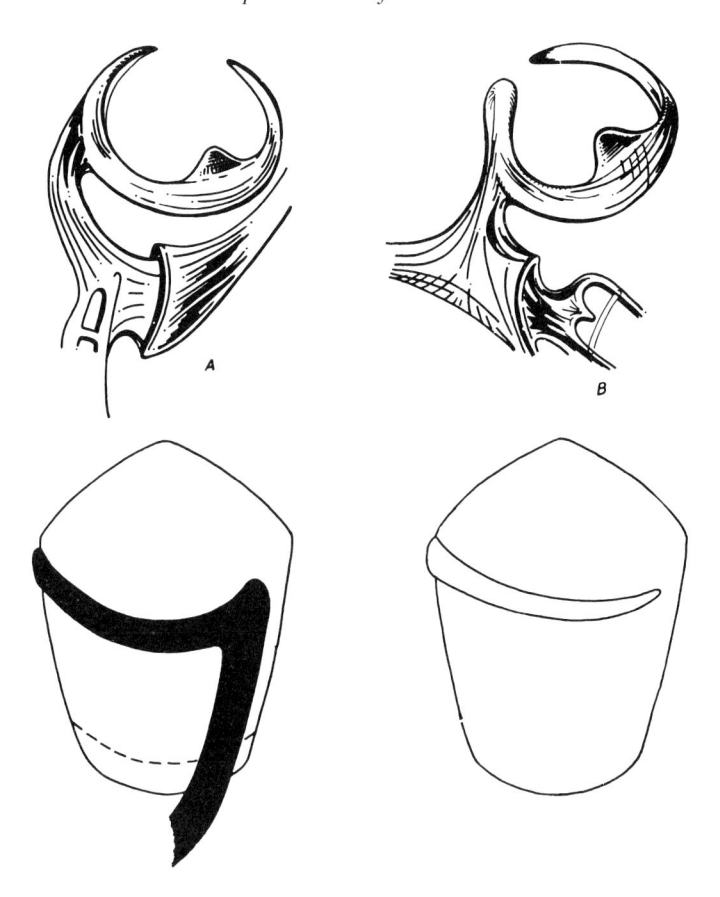

Fig. 10.45. Reverse back action (A), and back action (B), clasps. The bracing areas are shaded and the retentive areas unshaded.

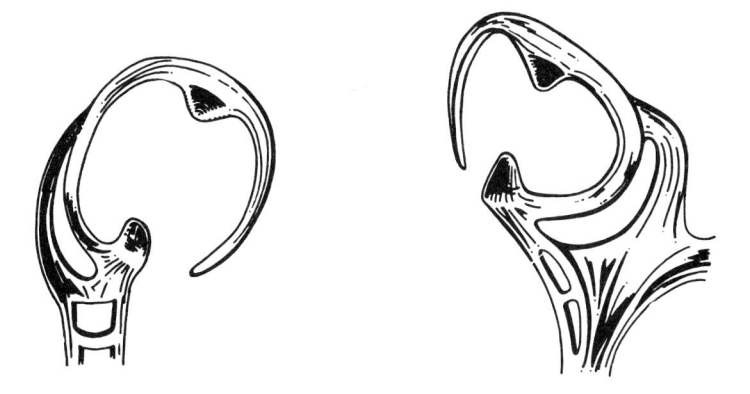

Fig. 10.46. The ring clasps.

the bar of the clasp far removed from the mucosa. This may be a disadvantage since food is liable to be trapped between the strut and ridge, and the muscle action of the tongue or cheek may be impaired.

The low survey line. This survey line is traced very low on the buccal or lingual aspect of a tooth (Fig. 10.47). It frequently occurs as a result of marked inclination of the tooth, when it is associated with a high survey line on the opposite surface and the possibilities in this case have been discussed above. It is also found on the conically shaped tooth, when the opposite surface has a similar survey line.

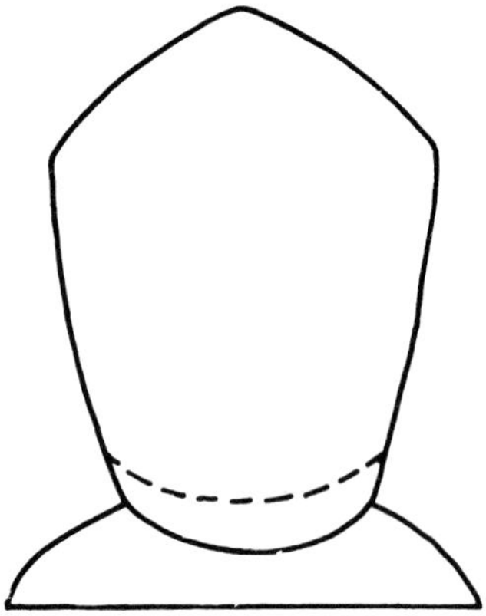

Fig. 10.47. The low survey line.

A tooth surface having a low survey line cannot bear a retentive clasp arm. In the first place insufficient undercut exists to be effective in retaining the denture, and second, a clasp arm placed in such an undercut will be situated dangerously near the gingival margin. When a clasp arm on a denture that is poorly tooth-supported is brought into the proximity of the gingival margin, this tissue will be traumatized as the ridge is resorbed and the saddle sinks. If tooth support is adequate, however, it is possible to place a clasp arm within 1 mm of the gingiva with the assurance that the health of this tissue will be maintained. Two dangers do exist, however, in bringing the arm too near the gingival margin. First, if the arm is thick a non-self-cleansing area is liable to exist immediately adjacent to its gingival edge (Fig. 10.34). Second, if there has been gingival recession or if gingivectomy has been done, it is necessary to keep the clasp arm well above the amelo-cemental junction. Cementum is very liable to caries and should never lie in a non-self-cleansing zone.

The tooth surface with a low survey line can always bear a bracing arm and this may be of two kinds. It may be part of a clasp arm that encircles three sides of the tooth, as found in the reverse back action and ring clasps, or it may be a rigid arm confined to the one surface of the tooth. In this latter case if the tooth is tilted, a wrought wire is usually placed on the opposite side.

If additional retention is required, and this is particularly likely to be so when the tooth is conical, three methods exist for obtaining it:
1   Using the near proximal undercut of the tooth.
2   Using the extended arm clasp.
3   Crowning the tooth and developing suitable contours.

1   *Using the proximal undercut.* Even where no undercut exists lingually or buccally it is rare to find none on the near proximal surface of the tooth. By the use of a De Van clasp, which will be described later, some degree of retention can often be obtained.

2   *Using the extended arm clasp.* An extended arm clasp is depicted in Fig. 10.48. The arm is similar to a cast circumferential arm but it covers two teeth. It remains above the survey line of the first tooth, which in this case is low, and crosses into the undercut of the adjacent tooth. The arm must be placed sufficiently near the occlusal surface of the first tooth to avoid contact with the interdental papilla as it crosses to the surface of the second. This type of clasp has a splinting action and distributes the lateral load over two teeth. If made in gold its use is restricted to two premolars, but with cobalt chromium alloy a longer arm can be used and two molars may be clasped.

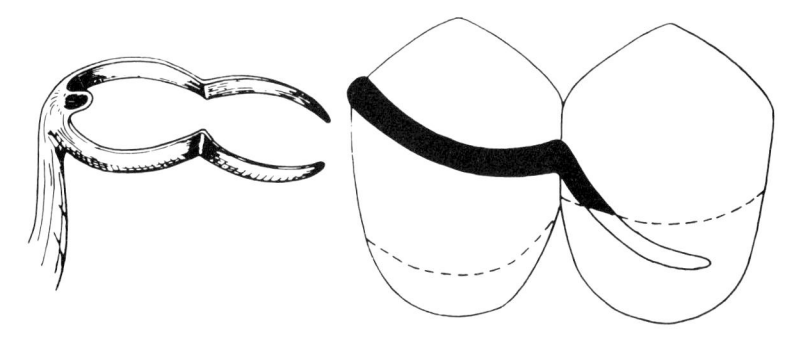

Fig. 10.48. The extended arm clasp. The bracing area is shaded and the retentive area unshaded.

3   *Crowning the tooth.* Where the abutment teeth are all conically shaped it may be necessary to crown them, at the same time developing desirable undercut surfaces. However, the occasions when this procedure is essential are extremely few.

Combination clasps

The various types of clasp arms discussed are often combined on the same tooth, for example, a cast arm being placed on one surface and a wrought wire on another (Figs 10.49 and 10.50). Such clasps are known as combination clasps. A common application of this principle is for clasping premolar abutment teeth of lower Class I dentures. A lingual bracing arm made of chrome cobalt is cast as an integral part of the denture framework, but the buccal retentive arm consists of a wrought gold wire embedded into the acrylic resin of the saddle. The more resilient wrought arm may be desirable on account of the periodontal health of the abutment tooth, and certainly is preferable to a short cobalt chromium arm on the grounds of efficiency.

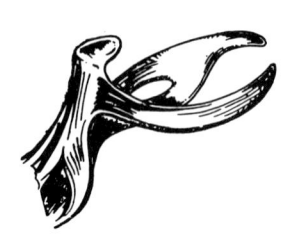

Fig. 10.49. A combination clasp having a rigid bracing arm and a non-flexible gingivally approaching retentive arm.

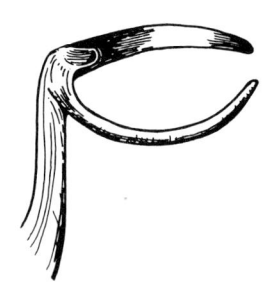

Fig. 10.50. A combination clasp having a rigid bracing arm and a wrought retentive arm.

Clasps utilizing proximal undercuts

There are two clasps that use proximal undercuts.

The first is the mesio-distal clasp which may be used when clasping canines. It often happens that there is little undercut on the buccal surface of a canine or that it is aesthetically displeasing to clasp this surface. Bar clasps can be used, but occasionally the mesio-distal clasp offers a better solution. Such a clasp is always cast in gold and embraces the canine on the mesial, palatal, and distal sides, having the form shown in Fig. 10.51. If a diastema exists between the canine and the lateral incisor then this space provides accommodation for the mesial part of the clasp. More often, however, it is necessary to cut the mesial surface of the canine to create the necessary space and this may be carried out with one-sided abrasive disks and strips. Needless to say, a contact point with the lateral is restored when the clasp is in position. This clasp is aesthetically acceptable since the metal on the distal surface of the canine is not obvious and that showing on the mesial margin resembles a discreet inlay. It gives good retention and grips the tooth rigidly, thereby conveying to it a large proportion of the antero-posterior and lateral load. Consequently, in free-end saddle cases, it must never be employed without also using a stress breaker. For this reason, although it is a useful clasp on occasion, it does not find frequent application.

The De Van clasp makes use of the near proximal undercut and has a small head which bears on the tooth entirely below the survey line. The bar of the clasp arises from, and generally lies closely against, the periphery of the saddle. It is a wise precaution to under-extend the saddle slightly in the region of these arms in case it requires adjustment. The De Van clasp should be reciprocated by a lingual or palatal strut which contacts the tooth at the junction of its lingual or palatal and far proximal surfaces. This strut ends in a lingually or palatally placed occlusal rest, the primary occlusal rest being placed on the near proximal part of the occlusal surface (Fig. 10.52); this reciprocating arm may be replaced by an embrasure hook. The De Van arm gives little bracing effect, and, if this is required, some other means, such as a deep square rest seat preparation or an embrasure hook, must be used.

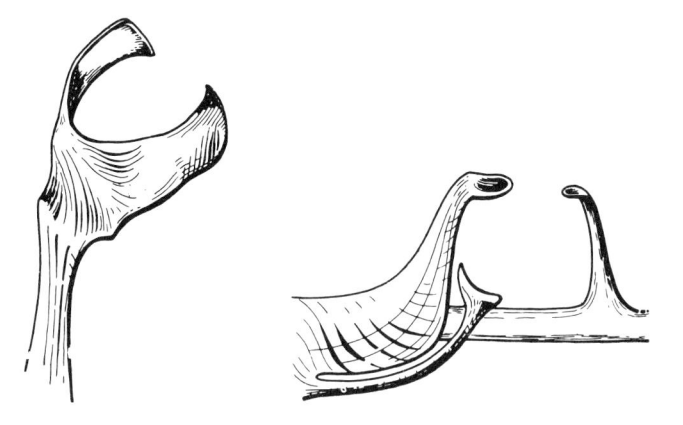

Fig. 10.51. The mesio-distal clasp.

Fig. 10.52. The De Van clasp.

The following advantages have been claimed for this type of clasp:
- It can be used when buccal and lingual survey lines are unfavourable.
- Since it can be hidden discreetly behind the buccal convexity of the tooth, it often has a distinct aesthetic advantage when used on premolars or canines.
- The angle of approach of the clasp to the undercut gives a marked trip action and hence increases retention.
- The distribution of stress during insertion and removal or resulting from a displacement of the clasp arm is resisted by the clasped and adjacent teeth. The application of this stress is therefore in a favourable direction and tends to be resisted by a number of teeth.
- Its compact design in relation to the saddle periphery helps to prevent its accidental displacement.

The relative merits of occlusally and gingivally approaching clasps

1 *Retention.* Due to trip action the gingivally approaching clasps give better retention than the occlusally approaching types. Consequently, in cases where the degree of undercut is small and some doubt exists about retention, the former clasps, with a wide angle of approach to the plane of the tooth surface, are preferred.

2 *Bracing.* Since the occlusally approaching clasp arm generally has a rigid portion lying in contact with the non-undercut zone of the tooth, its bracing effect is greater than the gingivally approaching arm, where only a resilient component of the clasp makes contact with the enamel. The bracing effect in the latter case varies with the length, section, and alloy of the bar of the clasp, a situation which likewise applies to the back action clasps.

3 *Caries susceptibility.* The incidence of caries under clasp arms may be said to be inversely proportional to the efficiency of the patient's oral hygiene. Well designed, well fitting, and well cared-for dentures rarely produce enamel caries under clasp arms. However, if cementum is exposed there is some risk of cemental caries with gingivally approaching arms.

4 *Gingival health.* When properly designed clasps are used in combination with adequate tooth support of the denture, gingival health is rarely affected. Traumatic gingivitis is, however, more often seen with gingivally approaching clasps, either as a result of inadequate relief of the clasp bar, or through its accidental displacement.

5 *Aesthetics.* The gingivally approaching clasp has sometimes to be preferred to the other type, as it can be less conspicuous in those cases where part of the buccal or labial surface of the tooth is exposed in smiling. In cases where gum is shown, however, the gingivally approaching clasp is even more noticeable than the occlusally approaching variety.

6 *Tolerance.* Occlusally approaching arms are always well tolerated, but gingivally approaching arms may not be. When a tissue undercut exists, a gingivally approaching bar must be kept well away from contact with the mucosa so that there is no trauma upon insertion and removal (Fig. 10.53). This necessarily creates a space and some patients complain of food retention in this site. A gingivally approaching clasp, especially one well displaced from the tissue, is least well tolerated with a lower denture where the clasped tooth lies anterior to the second premolar.

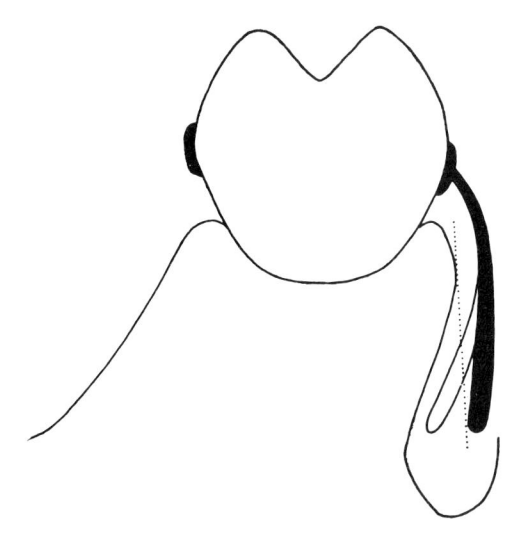

Fig. 10.53. Illustrates the necessity of keeping a gingivally approaching clasp arm out of a tissue undercut.

7 *Compactness.* This term was first applied by De Van, who stated that 'a clasp is compact when its parts are few and close to the main body of the denture'. The De Van clasp is the best example of compact design. The occlusally approaching clasps are, in general, more compact than the gingivally approaching types, the arms of which are liable to displacement, particularly if they are flexible. A compact design renders the clasp less liable to distortion by accident or in cleaning.

Unilateral and Bilateral Bracing and Retention

It is often necessary, owing to absence of suitable undercuts, to use a clasp that displays unilateral retention; by this is meant engaging the undercut surface of the tooth on one side only, and consequently there is reduced bracing on this surface. An argument can, however, sometimes be advanced for using unilateral bracing and retention, even where suitable undercuts exist on both buccal and lingual tooth surfaces.

An analysis of the different clasps described reveals that unilateral bracing and retention may be obtained in two ways. First, a single arm clasp may be employed which encircles three surfaces of the tooth; the back action, the reverse back action, and the ring clasps are examples of this type, as also is the occlusally approaching clasp used for a diagonal survey line. The second way in which unilateral bracing and retention can be obtained is by using separate arms on the buccal and lingual tooth surfaces. On one side a rigid bracing arm lies wholly above the survey line, while on the opposite side a flexible retaining arm, occlusally or gingivally approaching, is used. The bracing arm in this case may be placed on a tooth surface which shows any of the classes of survey line other than the high.

Some points regarding this latter method warrant further consideration. A very resilient clasp arm, such as a wrought gold wire or a long arm bar, is liable to be displaced if the patient uses it as a lever in removing the denture, or when the denture is being cleaned or is accidentally dropped. Such displacement, if towards the tooth, causes a continuous lateral pressure which might well go unnoticed or unheeded. It is difficult, too, when readjusting such a displaced arm, to make sure that a truly passive state has been secured. It may therefore be wise, when using resilient clasping, to presuppose that some clasp deformation is inevitable and to place a rigid reciprocating arm lying in the non-undercut zone of the opposite surface, which will effectively resist the lateral force on the tooth.

It is apparent, when the Class I denture is considered, that a resilient clasp arm, which moves readily over the tooth surface when a rotation takes place about the occlusal rest, has some advantage. Also since the reciprocating rigid arm lies above the survey line it, too, is able to rotate freely.

The disadvantage of a clasp which shows unilateral bracing and retention is that the lateral load cannot, when desired, be evenly distributed over the clasped teeth of both sides of the mouth without additional components being used in the denture design. Hence, if such clasps are preferred, the bracing arms on *both* sides of the mouth should be placed either lingually or buccally. Where inclined teeth make this type of clasping necessary, the survey lines indicate this condition (Fig. 10.54) since the teeth always slope in opposite directions on each side of the jaw. Where there is no marked inclination this arrangement must still be used, otherwise the denture is well braced by teeth against a lateral force in one direction but is very poorly braced in the opposite. In the latter instance the edentulous ridge is asked to accept much more lateral load than in the former.

A Comparison of Cast Gold and Cobalt Chromium Clasps

Owing to its higher modulus of elasticity cobalt chromium alloy transfers a greater part of the lateral load to the abutment tooth than does a similar arm constructed in gold. Therefore, if the same conditions of load distribution are to apply when cobalt chromium alloy is preferred to gold, differences in clasp design are required. This can be achieved by reducing the sections of the cobalt chromium arms, particularly with cast three arm clasps, but not, of course, to the extent that fracture may occur. In other cases the lateral load may be reduced to

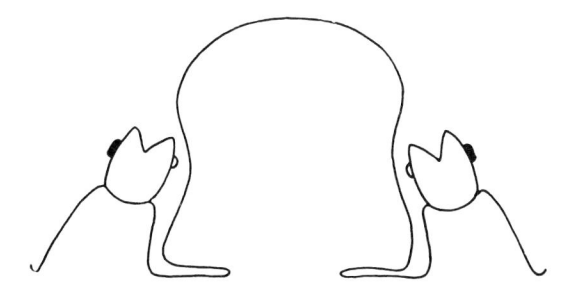

Fig. 10.54. Illustrates the use of bilaterally placed reverse back action clasps on lower premolars. The shaded area represents the bracing arm and the unshaded area the retentive arm.

the order of that transferred by gold by using a bar type clasp, whose gingivally approaching arm has less bracing action than the shorter arm of the three arm clasp.

The ideal amount of retention can be secured with cobalt chromium by reducing the section of the arms and by engaging to a less extent into the undercut. As a general principle cobalt chromium clasps need engage approximately half the depth of undercut that is necessary for gold. In practice this means that cobalt chromium alloy clasps should have a horizontal undercut engagement of 0.25 mm whilst gold alloys usually require 0.50 mm.

This constitutes a distinct advantage for cobalt chromium alloy, as it is often found that on many teeth an insufficient amount of undercut exists to accommodate a 0.50 mm gauge, but a much larger number have the necessary depth of undercut for a cobalt chromium clasp. Thus it would appear, from the point of view of retention, that a larger number of teeth can be adequately clasped with cobalt chromium.

From the retentive points of view it is wise with cobalt chromium clasps to place the retentive portion at some distance from the point of attachment to the denture, to allow greater flexibility. Such long arm clasps as the bar, De Van, back action, ring, and extended arm varieties are useful in this respect. On molar teeth the arms of the three arm clasp are sufficiently long to give adequate resilience in the retentive tip, but this is not so with premolars. Therefore it is advisable that retentive arms on premolars should be either gingivally approaching cobalt chromium, or occlusally approaching wrought gold alloy.

Again, the higher modulus of elasticity of the cobalt chromium alloy results in excessive force being required during insertion and removal of the denture if gold clasp dimensions are used. In addition, since the proportional limits of the cobalt chromium alloys are similar to those of cast gold there is the possibility of permanently prising open a cobalt chromium clasp that has been deeply engaged into an undercut.

There is also the danger of displacement of clasp arms if the patient does not remove the denture in the planned path of insertion and removal.

Rotation of a denture during removal may result in ultimate fracture of clasp arms, particularly those made in cobalt chromium which can be stressed beyond their limit. This careless method of removal also applies undue stress to clasped abutment teeth.

When the abutment teeth are either short rooted or periodontally involved they cannot accept a large lateral force and in these cases it is suggested that cobalt chromium has too high a modulus of elasticity to be used. Such abutment teeth should always be clasped using either wrought gold wire or cast gold bar clasps, if the pressure on them is not to exceed the physiological limit.

Clasps with splinting action

It has already been stated that clasps may be utilized as one means of splinting teeth. This may be achieved through several clasps each independently attached to the saddles or bars of a denture, or through a single clasp which arises from one point of attachment.

Two clasps come into this latter category. The extended arm clasp, splinting a maximum of two teeth and constructed preferably in cobalt chromium alloy, has already been described. The compound clasp is one which has application in partial dentures of all classes. It takes the form of two circumferential clasps arising from a common body situated in the embrasure between the two clasped teeth (Fig. 10.55). Generally only two teeth are splinted by such a clasp, but it is possible to increase this number by combining the compound and extended arm design (Fig. 10.56).

Precision Attachments

These attachments are normally supplied to the dentist prefabricated by a manufacturer. They consist of two parts, commonly designated male and female, that are matched to interlock together. One of these parts is attached to the abutment tooth and the other to the saddle of the denture. Their function is to provide positive direct retention for a partial denture. In this respect they may prove more efficient than clasps, but the clinical situations in which they are used require careful assessment, and, although in all cases the patient's standard of oral hygiene must be good, this factor is of even greater importance to the success of a precision attachment partial denture.

Preiskel has sensibly classified the types of precision attachments as follows:
1. intracoronal
2. extracoronal

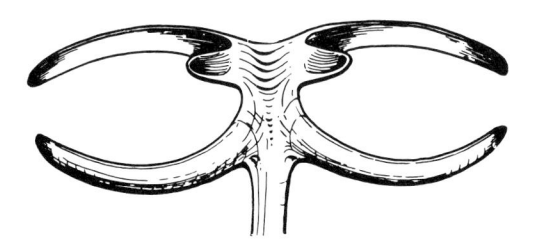

Fig. 10.55. The compound clasp.

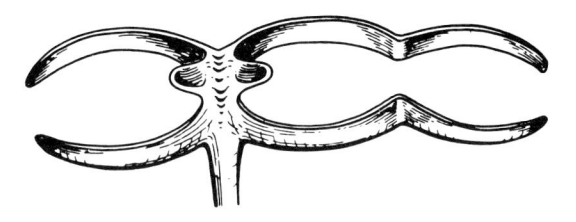

Fig. 10.56. Combination of the compound and extended arm clasps.

3   stud
4   bar.

Advantages of precision attachments

- Labial or buccal clasp arms on canines or premolars are not required so aesthetics can be better.
- Vertical and horizontal loads are applied more directly to the abutment teeth than by clasps or rests. This is advantageous only if the supporting structure of these teeth are perfect.
- The efficiency of retention is not affected by the contours of the abutment teeth.
- The number of components of the denture is reduced and hence tolerance should be better.
- When used with lower free end saddles posterior movement of the denture is prevented.
- Their use may be indicated when retentive clasp arm reciprocation cannot be achieved.

Disadvantages of precision attachments

- Extensive preparation of all abutment teeth is necessary, together with construction of the necessary crowns or inlays.

- When the crowns of the abutment teeth are small or short, these attachments cannot be used.
- Teeth with large pulps are at risk owing to the relatively deep preparations that will be required for intracoronal attachments.
- Intracoronal attachments are not normally advised for free end saddle dentures owing to the rigidity of the union between tooth and saddle. An extracoronal attachment incorporating some type of stress breaker should be used in these cases.
- Owing to the chairside and laboratory time involved and the high cost of the attachments themselves, a precision attachment denture becomes expensive.

Intracoronal

The female part of an intracoronal attachment is some form of slot and it is embedded into some type of restoration, such as an inlay or crown, which is attached to the abutment tooth. The male portion of the attachment is a flange which fits accurately into the slot and is attached to the saddle of the denture.

This type of attachment provides rigid connection between the saddle and the abutment tooth and provides retention by the frictional contact between the parallel surfaces of the flange and slot. By the nature of its construction and the position in which it is placed it also provides bracing and support for the denture. Hence it serves the purpose of a retentive clasp arm, a bracing clasp arm, and an occlusal rest all in one unit.

Modern attachments utilize an H-shaped flange which is stronger and has nearly double the frictional surface area of the earlier T-shaped flanges. At least two, but sometimes three or four, of these attachments are included in a denture and they have to be aligned so that all the slots (and hence the flanges) are parallel to each other to ensure insertion and removal. A heavier and more precision-built type of surveyor is essential for the paralleling of the wax patterns of the inlays into which the attachments must be placed.

The main problem encountered in the use of intracoronal attachments is providing sufficient room within the contour of the abutment tooth to accommodate the female part. It is essential that this part does not project over the gingival margin, nor interfere with occlusal contacts. Hence adequate depth of preparation is required antero-posteriorly to avoid the gingiva, and sufficient height must be available to provide as large an area of frictional contact as possible between slot and flange.

Most manufacturers' attachments are provided in varying sizes; the McCollum attachment comes in two sizes and the Crismani 699 in three. Various devices are incorporated in some attachments to provide additional retention for a given frictional area. In the Schatzmann attachment a spring-loaded piston in the male portion engages a socket in the female portion (Figs 10.57 and 10.58).

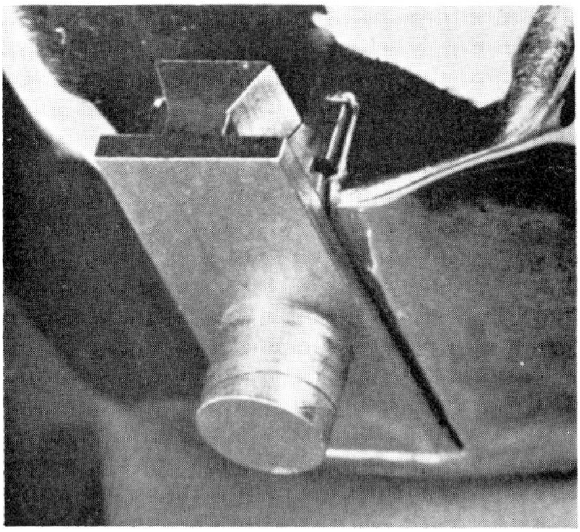

The Component Parts of a Partial Denture 257

Fig. 10.57. The Schatzmann attachment.

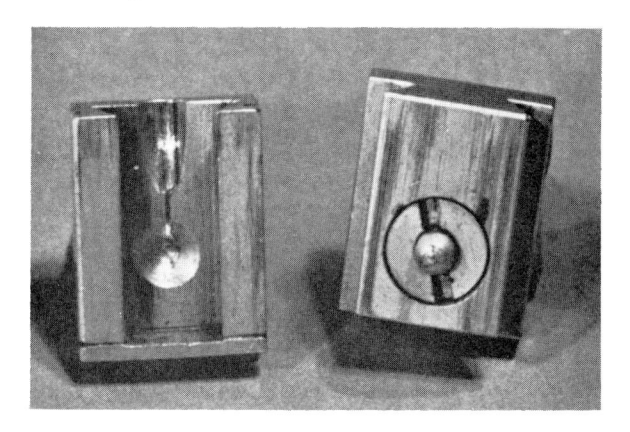

Fig. 10.58. The male and female parts of the Schatzmann attachment.

Replacement of the spring that activates the piston is necessary in these devices, possibly as frequently as every six months. The McCollum attachment has a split sectional H flange which can be carefully opened a little, by inserting a fine blade, to increase the frictional pressure (Fig. 10.59). The Crismani attachment has a retaining clip in the male portion that engages a retaining groove within the female slot. Access to replace this clip when necessary is obtained by a countersunk screw in the face of the flange (Fig. 10.60).

All these additional retentive devices are supplied so that the inevitable wear that takes place in these attachments can be compensated. However, there are limits to which these adjustments can be made, and wear, and consequent

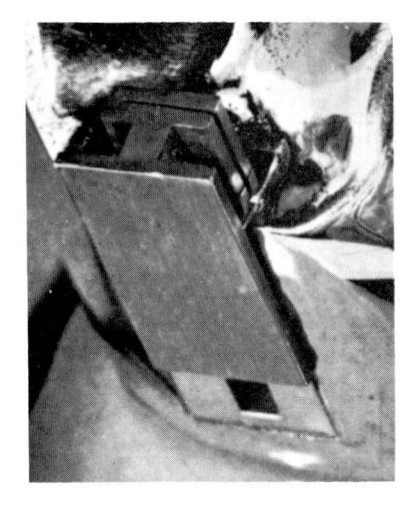

Fig. 10.59. The McCollum attachment.

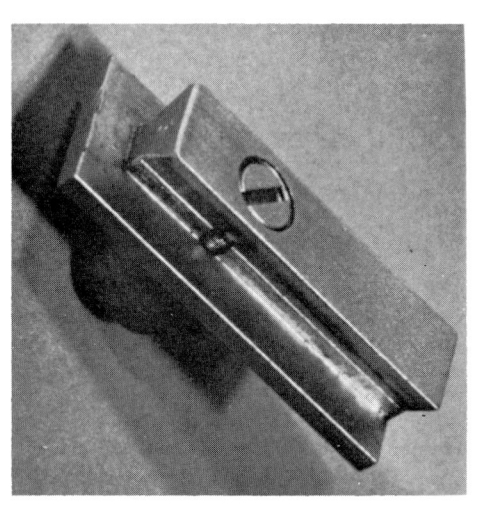

Fig. 10.60. The Crismani attachment.

loosening of the denture, are unavoidable disadvantages of the longterm use of these appliances.

As stated earlier, intracoronal attachments are best used for bounded saddles and may prove particularly useful for unilateral dentures in Class III cases when tooth contours are unsuitable for clasps. If it should be decided to use them for free-end saddle dentures the rigid connection between the denture and the abutment teeth means that at least two teeth must be splinted together on either side to form double abutments and if only six anterior teeth remain they should all be splinted together to form one abutment. To reduce the loads to which the attachments may be subjected it is desirable to incorporate into the denture a rigid lingual bracing arm fitted to the most distal abutment tooth. Such an arm will also add some stability to the denture and provide a guiding plane for its insertion.

Extracoronal

These attachments have all, or a part, of their mechanism lying outside the contour of the crown of the abutment tooth. As a result, loads falling on the tooth via the attachment are applied outside the long axis of the tooth. Consequently, well-supported abutment teeth are essential for the successful use of these attachments. If possible it is desirable to splint the abutment tooth to the adjacent tooth to provide a double abutment.

The most widely used attachment of this type is the Dalbo 669 which is supplied in two sizes. The male portion consists of an L-shaped bar carrying a ball joint at its lower end. The upright part of the bar is joined to an inlay or crown in the abutment tooth (Fig. 10.61). Fitting over the ball joint is the female portion which is placed in the saddle of the denture (Fig. 10.62). This portion contains a spring (Fig. 10.63) which allows vertical movement of the saddle, whilst the ball joint allows rotation in an antero-posterior axis (Fig. 10.64). Owing to the movement that is permitted by this type of attachment it is usually used for free-end saddle dentures, since a considerable degree of stress-breaking action is obtained. However, it should be appreciated that the amount of movement permitted must be minimal. One particular advantage of the Dalbo attachment is that because of the presence of the male portion, the free-end saddle cannot tilt upwards away from the mucosa.

Compared with intracoronal attachments they do not require space within the contour of the abutment tooth, and hence can be used when there is insufficient bucco-lingual width to accommodate an intracoronal attachment. In this respect they are well suited to use on lower canines when these teeth are the abutments for free end saddles; in addition better retention will be provided than can be obtained by the use of clasps on the usually conical-shaped lower canines. Posterior movement of lower dentures is also prevented effectively.

Owing to the projection of the ball joint of the attachment over the gingival margin there is considerable danger of irritation to this tissue or the creation of a 'dead space' below the ball joint with resultant proliferation of gingival tissues and inflammation. For this reason it is often better to align the attachment on the abutment tooth so that the male portion projects somewhat towards the lingual aspect of the lower ridge, and to ensure that light contact is made with the mucosa in the gingival area.

Since all lower free-end saddle dentures, at some period, will require

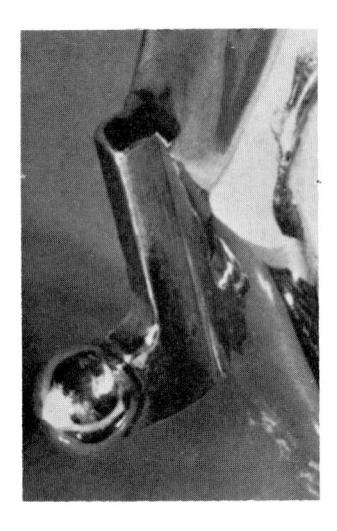

Fig. 10.61. The male portion of the Dalbo attachment joined to an inlay.

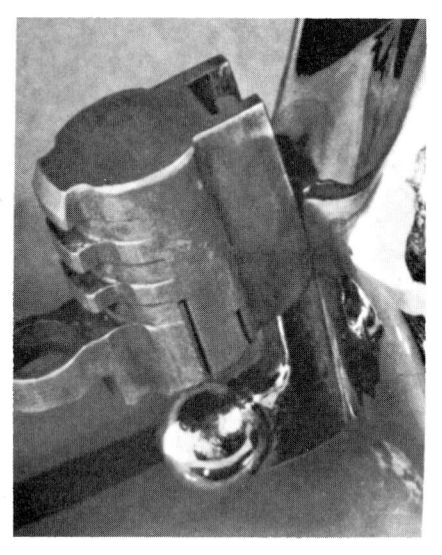

Fig. 10.62. The female portion of the Dalbo attachment being fitted to the male.

rebasing, a modification of the Dalbo attachment, the Pin Dalbo, has been produced (Fig. 10.65). This allows the attachment to be locked against movement by inserting the pin, thus allowing rebasing of the saddle without undue compression of the underlying mucosa.

Stud

These attachments are usually employed when a patient is nearly edentulous in

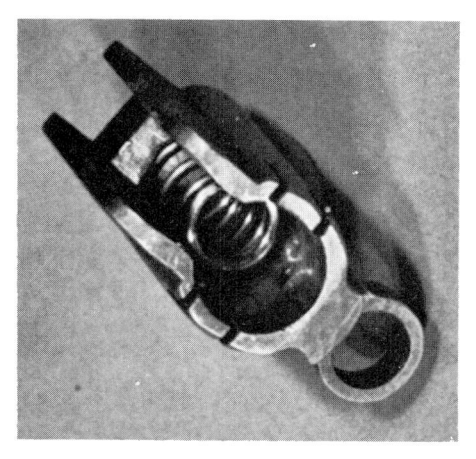

Fig. 10.63. Inferior view of the female portion of the Dalbo attachment showing the spring.

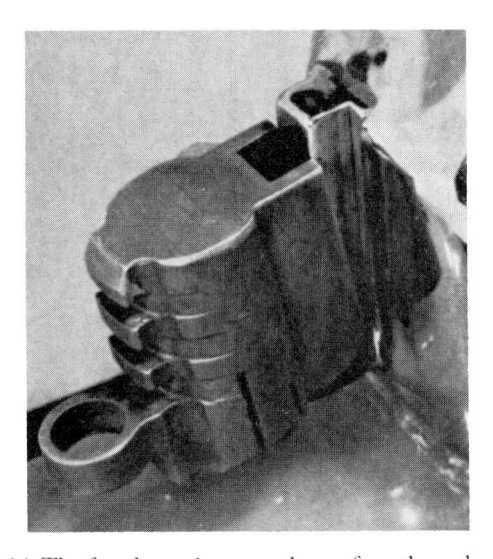

Fig. 10.64. The female portion rotated away from the male portion.

the lower jaw but two well-supported teeth, normally the canines, remain standing. The natural teeth have their pulps extirpated and the crowns cut off and the stud attachment fitted to the diaphragm of a post fitted to the root canal. The stud is slightly undercut and comprises the male portion of the attachment. The female portion is embedded in the body of what is virtually a full lower denture, and engages the male portion when the denture is fitted.

By this system improved retention and stability of the lower denture is assured. However, the number of patients who have two soundly supported lower

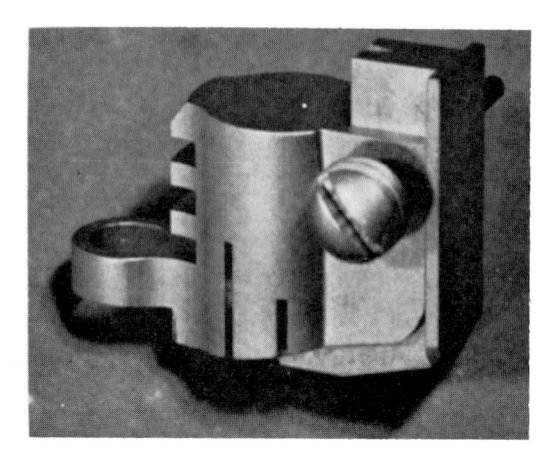

Fig. 10.65. The Pin Dalbo attachment.

canines and no other lower teeth, are few. Unless the roots to which the studs are attached are firmly supported this type of attachment should not be used.

One possible disadvantage of these attachments is the fact that the gingivae have to be covered completely and hence are likely to be irritated by any small movement of the denture. To minimize such movements the occlusion should be free of any cuspal interferences and the denture shaped to be as free from muscular interference as possible. The impression technique should allow the vertical loads to be resisted largely by the stud and less by the mucosal tissues.

Instead of using a prefabricated attachment the stud can be cast by a technician (Fig. 10.66) and the female portion replaced by using silicone soft lining material (Fig. 10.67). This is a simpler and cheaper approach, but the silicone will require replacement approximately every six months.

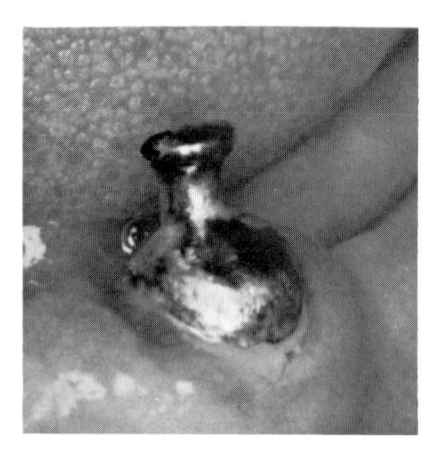

Fig. 10.66. Male stud attachment cast by a technician.

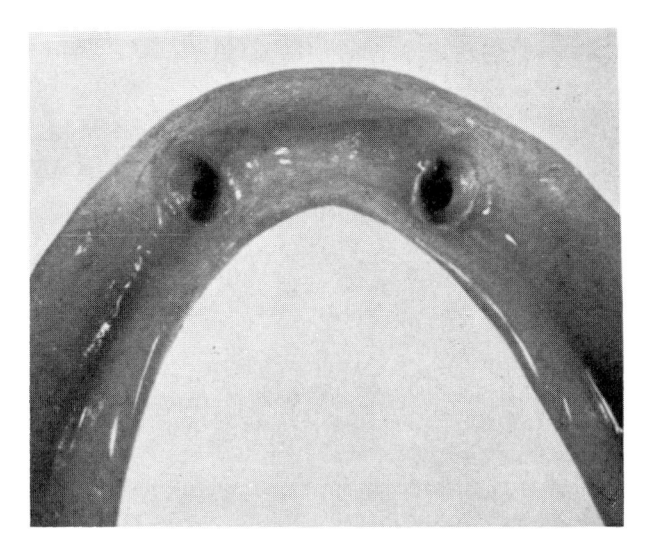

Fig. 10.67. Lower denture with soft silicone providing the female portion.

Bar

These attachments join together teeth or roots and in addition to providing retention for dentures, splint together the abutments to which they are fixed. These may be basically of two types, bar *joints* and bar *units*. Bar joints, of which the Dolder bar is the best example, allow some degree of movement between the attachment and the denture. They have their application when only a small number of teeth or roots remain and the appliance is virtually a full denture, usually in the lower jaw. Bar units are more rigid attachments and can be applied to provide retention, bracing, and support for partial dentures.

The commonest site for the use of a bar joint is when only two lower canines remain. Instead of using two stud attachments, the diaphragms on the root faces are united by a straight length of pear-shaped bar, approximately 3×2.2 mm in in cross section. This bar is positioned so that its lower border, the narrower part of the pear-shaped section, lies just in contact with the oral mucosa. An open-sided sleeve is placed into the fitting surface of the denture and engages the bar when the denture is inserted. Owing to the pear-shaped section of the bar retention is provided by the sleeve engaging the undercut areas of the bar.

Some degree of movement of the denture is permitted by this arrangement and this has a degree of stress-breaking effect which reduces the load transmitted to the supporting structures of the remaining roots.

Bar units, as distinct from bar joints, allow no movement between the sleeve and the bar. They may find application when there are four or more abutment teeth and when rigid splinting of these abutments is considered essential. The bars used are parallel sided and hence retention is purely frictional and no movement other than vertical is permitted.

Indirect Retainers

Although other factors participate, resistance to the displacement of partial dentures is largely effected by direct and indirect retainers. The principle of indirect retention can be discussed in relation to a Class I lower denture, having clasps and rests on the first premolars and the saddles connected by a lingual bar (Fig. 10.68). When a displacing force acts on one of the saddles of this denture, either through the action of a sticky bolus of food or through muscular action at the periphery of the saddle when the mouth is widely opened, the denture tends to rotate about an axis in the vicinity of the clasped teeth. Consequently, as the saddles rotate away from the ridge, the lingual bar moves downwards towards the floor of the mouth. If, however, resistance is offered to this downward movement of the lingual bar, a more stable appliance results and the principle of indirect retention is used.

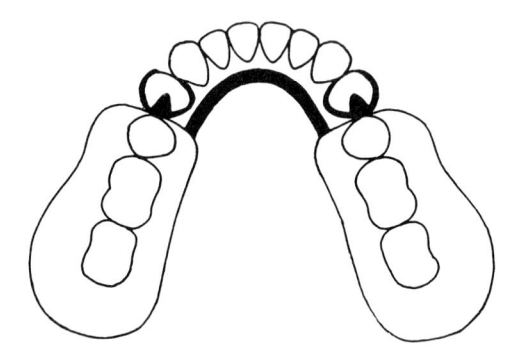

Fig. 10.68. The bilateral free-end saddle case under discussion.

Indirect retention, therefore, resists occlusally displacing forces acting on the saddle of a denture by creating a resistance on the opposite side of the fulcrum axis to that on which the displacing force is applied. If a continuous clasp is incorporated in the design (Fig. 10.69), when an occlusally displacing force acts on the saddles the lingual bar cannot rotate towards the floor of the mouth since the continuous clasp rests on the cingula of the standing teeth. Rotation is therefore prevented by a reaction in all the natural teeth upon which the continuous clasp presses. Alternatively the indirect retainer may be regarded as shifting the axis of rotation anteriorly from the premolars to the mesio-incisal point.

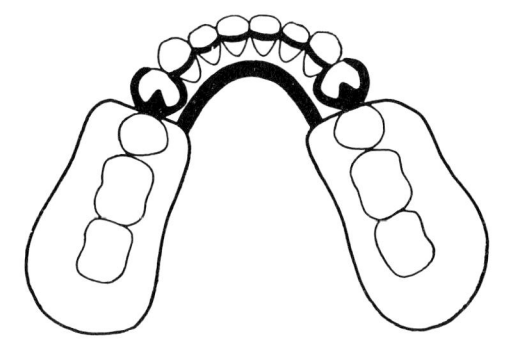

Fig. 10.69. The previous design with the addition of a continuous clasp.

The efficiency of the continuous clasp depends on the distance it extends anteriorly from the original fulcrum axis. The greater the distance of the mesio-incisal point from the place at which rotation takes place, the greater the effect since the moment of the force resisting the displacement is increased. This distance is dependent upon the number of standing teeth and the arch form. A square arch form tends to reduce this distance, whereas a tapering arch increases it (Fig. 10.70).

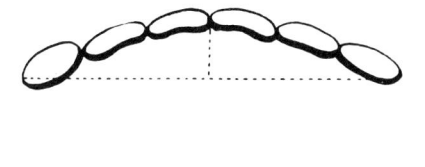

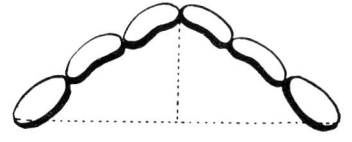

Fig. 10.70. Illustrates the effect of arch form on the efficiency of the continuous clasp as an indirect retainer.

The indirect retainer action of the continuous clasp has been described in the case of lower free-end saddles. When upper free-end saddles are considered its importance is even greater, since the weight of the appliance acts in addition to the displacing forces already discussed. If the saddles are bounded indirect retention is not required since clasps can be placed at the distal end of the saddles. The decision as to whether or not indirect retention should be used depends on other factors such as tolerance and occlusion, which will be discussed later. Moreover, some indirect retainers have additional beneficial actions as well as their primary function; for example, denture support and bracing, and these functions may, in some circumstances, be considered more important.

The continuous clasp

The continuous clasp is a metal band passing continuously over the cingula of the teeth from saddle to saddle, always lying above or on the survey line of the tooth. When it covers anterior teeth its shape is fluted so that it may rest on the cingulum, which is the most nearly horizontal surface of the tooth, and at the same time avoid impinging upon the interdental papilla (Fig. 10.71).

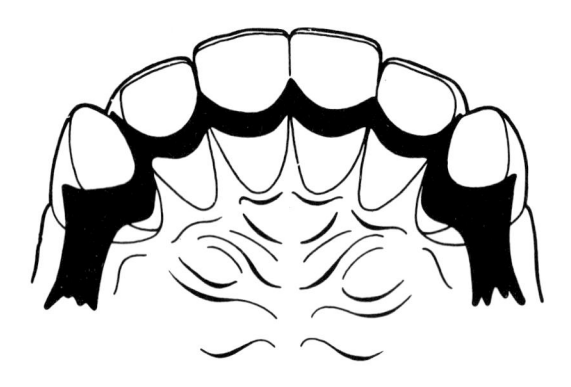

Fig. 10.71. Continuous clasp.

In addition to indirect retention the continuous clasp helps in the distribution of the load falling on the appliance. A small amount of the vertical load is borne by those teeth on which the continuous clasp fits and this action is most noticeable where their cingula are marked.

The continuous clasp distributes the lateral load to the teeth it covers, on the balancing side in the lower and the working side in the upper. This is an important function of the continuous clasp as the damaging lateral stress is thus shared over a larger number of teeth.

The continuous clasp gives strength and rigidity to the denture as a whole, particularly when it is used in conjunction with a lingual bar. If this latter component is lacking in rigidity the continuous clasp provides additional rigid connection between the saddles, a necessary feature if the lateral load is to be effectively distributed to tissues on the balancing side.

A continuous clasp can form a useful point of attachment for incisal rests or embrasure hooks when more direct tooth support than the continuous clasp itself provides, is required in the incisor region.

The continuous clasp does not have a universal application and there are contra-indications to its use, which are listed below.

Tolerance. The fact that continuous clasps are not well tolerated constitutes the most serious drawback to their use in both upper and lower jaws. Quite frequently patients are unable to accustom themselves to the presence of 'the wire' behind their front teeth, which is a continual source of annoyance to their tongue. This occurs most commonly in the nervous, often highly intelligent, type of patient, whereas the phlegmatic patient can generally tolerate the presence of the continuous clasp.

Phonetics. The presence of the conventionally designed continuous clasp in the upper jaw sometimes creates a temporary phonetic embarrassment, the patient finding difficulty in pronouncing the D and T, among other sounds, for a short period following fitting the denture.

Insufficient space. In many persons insufficient space exists when the teeth are in occlusion, between the gingival margins of the upper anteriors and the incisal edges of the lower teeth to accommodate a continuous clasp of a section compatible with strength. This is a limiting factor to the use of continuous clasps in upper dentures.

Palatally or lingually inclined teeth. These are more often a complicating factor in the lower jaw where the teeth tend to slope lingually, producing a survey line at the occlusal surfaces or incisal edges of the teeth. Hence there is no depth of non-undercut tooth surface for a continuous clasp.

Short clinical crowns. Here insufficient space exists between the gingival margins and the incisal edges to accommodate a sufficiently strong clasp.

Diastema. When a diastema exists the continuous clasp is visible between the teeth. The significance and acceptability of this depends entirely on the viewpoint of the patient. The continuous clasp may be divided as shown in Fig. 10.72.

Extreme length. Very long continuous clasps will have to be strengthened, either by increasing the section or supporting with subsidiary connectors.

Bearing in mind the high incidence of lack of tolerance and phonetic embarrassment, many attempts have been made to modify the original design. In the lower the alternative to a continuous clasp is generally a lingual plate, but in the upper modified designs of the clasp itself have some merit.

Three modifications warrant consideration. In the first the clasp is reduced in

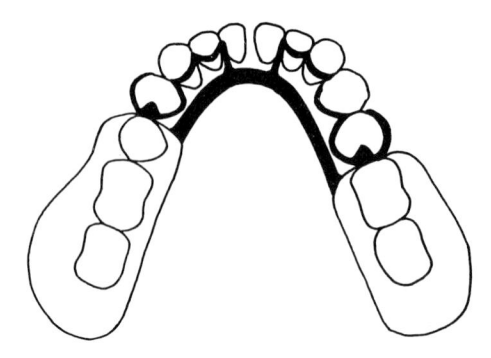

Fig. 10.72. Shows splitting of the continuous clasp to avoid poor aesthetic appearance where a diastema exists.

thickness but made to cover a greater area of tooth; in this case its gingival border is kept sufficiently far above the gingivae to exclude the possibility of its acting as a food trap. This design has some advantage but there is a limit to which the thickness can be reduced and at the same time successful casting and adequate strength assured. Often this modification presents phonetic and tolerance problems.

As a second modification the continuous clasp is extended so that its gingival edge makes contact with the mucosa at the point of junction of the free and attached gingivae (Figs 10.73 and 10.74) and there is little doubt that this type of clasp goes a long way to overcoming the tolerance and phonetic problems. Thirdly, the writers sometimes extend this modified continuous clasp further over the palatal mucosa, relieving the gingival margin (Figs 10.74 and 10.75).

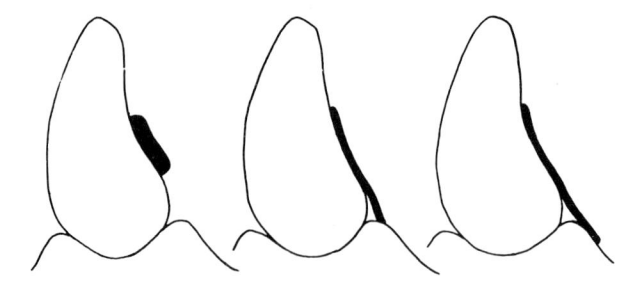

Fig. 10.73. Saggital sections through incisor teeth and continuous clasps to show different modifications.

However, this should only be done when the interstitial spaces between the teeth are not pronounced, otherwise the resultant food packing constitutes a serious disadvantage, as in the case of the lingual plate.

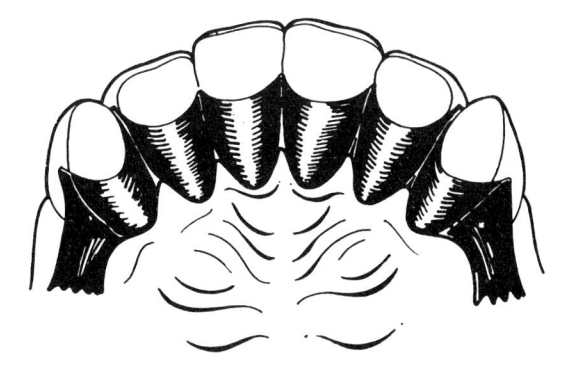

Fig. 10.74. A continuous clasp modification to make contact with the junction of the free and attached gingiva.

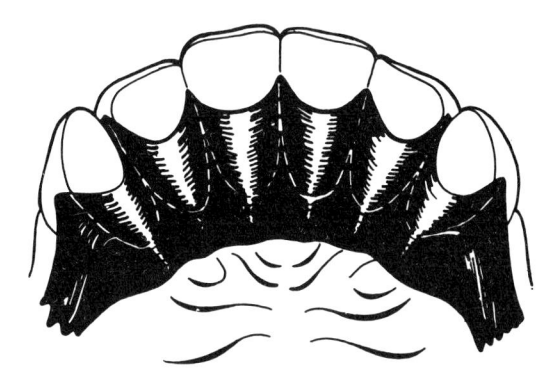

Fig. 10.75. Modified continuous clasp extended over the palatal mucosa.

Alternative methods of indirect retention

So far indirect retainers placed on the anterior part of the jaw have been considered. However, it will be apparent that Class IV dentures require an indirect retainer placed posteriorly to counteract a displacement of the anterior saddle away from the ridge. A Class III denture whose saddles cannot, for some reason, be clasped adequately may require anterior and posterior indirect retainers.

Consequently, indirect retainers may be divided into those placed in the anterior and those in the posterior part of the mouth. A further division occurs when it is realized that in the upper jaw either the teeth or the hard palate may be used as the tissue on which the retainer bears, whereas in the lower the teeth only can be used for this purpose.

The forms of indirect retention shown in Table 10.2 are available for upper dentures.

Table 10.2

Position	Tissue on which retainer rests	Type of indirect retainer
Anterior	Tooth	Cummer arm
		Anteriorly placed occlusal or incisal rest
		Continuous clasp and its modifications
	Palate	Palatal arm
		Anterior palatal bar
Posterior	Tooth	Posteriorly placed occlusal rest
	Palate	Posterior palatal bar or extension of palatal plate

The Cummer arm. This consists of an arm which extends forwards from the saddle or palatal bar to rest on an anterior tooth (Fig. 10.76). When compared with the continuous clasp it has two disadvantages. First, since it bears on a single tooth it is liable to apply an excessive load and tooth movement is thus possible, particularly if the arm is placed on a lateral incisor. Second, a long Cummer arm is liable to be distorted, resulting in either a continuous force being applied to the tooth, or, a space between the arm and the tooth.

The Cummer arm has the advantage over the continuous clasp that it may be used in cases where insufficient space exists for the latter. It is considered that these retainers should only be used on canines since these teeth, in contradistinction to the incisors, have long roots and a heavy bony support, and are not liable to be stressed excessively. In practice the number of dentures that require this type of retainer are very few. Lack of tolerance by the patient may also constitute a disadvantage of these arms.

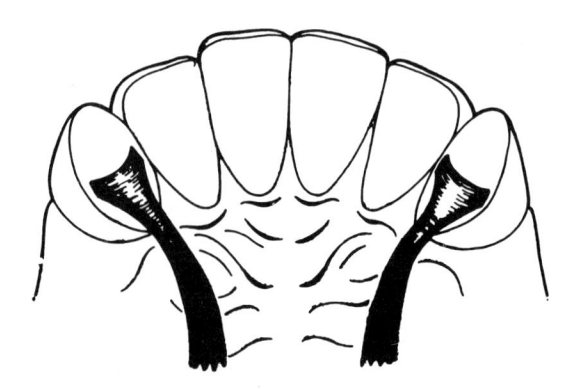

Fig. 10.76. The Cummer arm.

Anteriorly placed occlusal or incisal rest. The principle involved in this indirect retainer is similar to that employed in the Cummer arm (Fig. 10.77), but instead of bearing on an inclined surface it rests on a horizontal occlusal or incisal surface, thus reducing the possibility of tooth movement. Further, if the rest is placed on a premolar tooth the shorter arm is less liable to be displaced accidentally. The disadvantage of the anterior occlusal rest is that it cannot be placed any further forward than the mesial half of the first premolar, and its effectiveness as an indirect retainer is reduced accordingly. The occlusal rest, of course, helps to distribute the vertical load over a larger number of teeth and if the cusp angles are high, or if a square rest seat is considered suitable, the lateral load is also borne in part by the tooth in question. The disadvantage of the incisal edge rest is aesthetic and this factor means that in practice this is a rare type of indirect retainer.

Palatal arm. When a continuous clasp is contra-indicated a palatal arm may be used to give indirect retention in the anterior part of the maxilla. This is an extension from the saddle and palatal bar, covering an area of hard palate anterior to the fulcrum axis (Fig. 10.78). Such extensions are much broader than the Cummer arms and there is no danger of distortion. They may be made in acrylic resin or metal, according to the base material used. The more compressible the mucosa upon which they rest, the less efficient is their action.

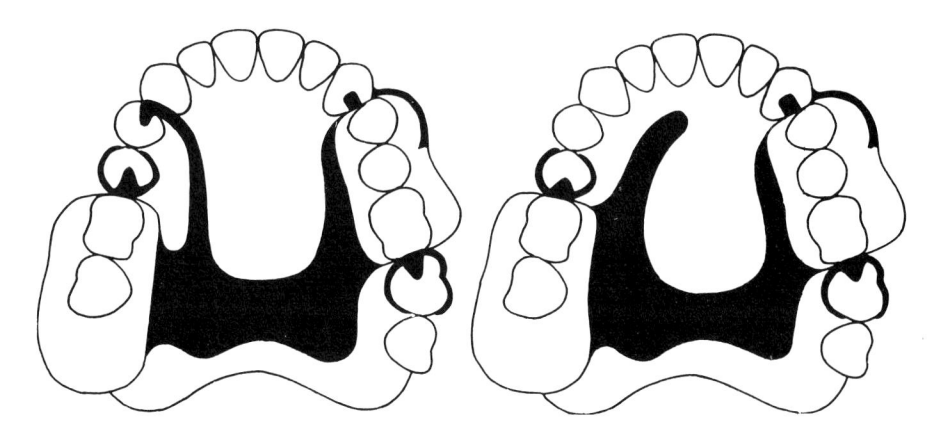

Fig. 10.77. Anteriorly placed occlusal rest.   **Fig. 10.78.** Extended palatal arm.

Anterior palatal bar. The anterior palatal bar may be formed by the union of two palatal arms in the mid-line (Fig. 10.79). Like the palatal arm it has the disadvantage of covering the rugae area and consequently is badly tolerated by some patients.

Posteriorly placed occlusal rest. This is the only tooth supported form of indirect retainer used in the posterior part of the mouth. It is most useful with a long Class IV saddle when it is placed bilaterally, bearing on the distal aspect of the occlusal surface, being carried on an arm which arises from the posterior edge of the palatal bar or plate (Fig. 10.80).

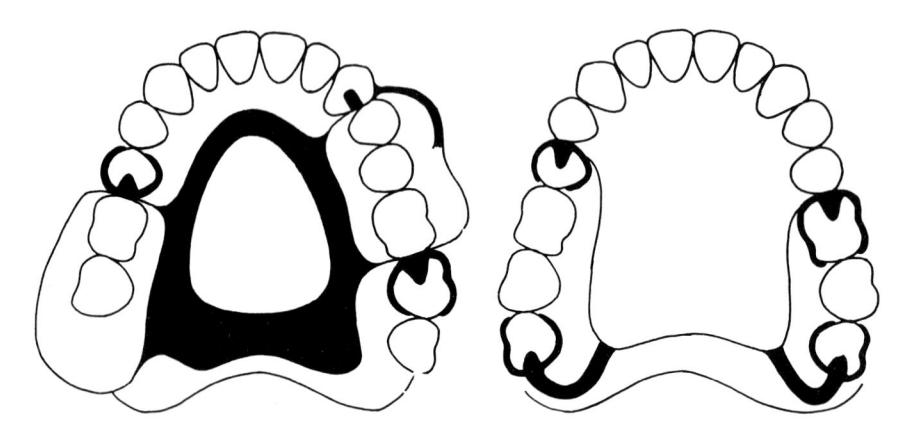

Fig. 10.79. Anterior palatal bar. **Fig. 10.80.** Posteriorly placed occlusal rest.

Posterior palatal bar. This is the only form of posterior retainer which bears on the hard palate and it will be discussed in detail in the next section. It is frequently used as the only means of posterior indirect retention but with a long Class IV saddle it may be combined with posteriorly placed occlusal rests.

Where the palate is covered with either an acrylic resin or metal plate in lieu of connecting bars, suitable shaping of the anterior or posterior margins of the plate can be used as equivalent measures to the palatal arm and the anterior and posterior palatal bars (Fig. 10.81).

In the lower jaw, only indirect retainers that bear on teeth have application. The occlusal rest and the continuous clasp, with or without embrasure hooks or incisal rests, are the methods commonly used anteriorly, and only seldom is posterior indirect retention necessary.

Connecting Bars and Plates

The saddles and retaining components of partial dentures are connected either by bars or plates. The difference between them is in the amount of tissue covered, the bar covering less than the plate. In the lower jaw the difference is clear cut, but

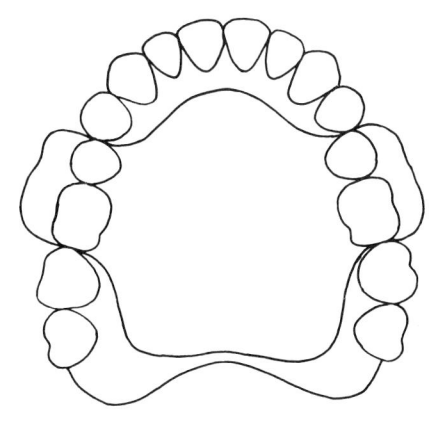

Fig. 10.81. Anterior and posterior extension of the palatal plate to give indirect retention.

in the upper there is no exact dividing line; what is described as a broad bar by one practitioner might be called a plate by another. Bars, however, must always be constructed in metal to give adequate strength and rigidity. A lingual plate used in the lower should, for similar reasons, ideally, always be made of metal, but in the upper a plate may be made in acrylic resin or metal.

All connecting bars and plates must be rigid if the lateral load of mastication is to be shared by the ridges and the standing teeth of the working and balancing sides. Therefore they must always be of such dimension as will ensure this, taking into account the physical properties of the material used. Acrylic resin requires a combination of thickness and broad coverage to give the necessary strength and rigidity.

It is necessary that, other factors being equal, the type of connector used should be the one that is most likely to be well tolerated by the patient. In this respect it should be realized that the palatal area behind the upper incisors is a highly sensitive contact area, as also is the tip of the tongue which is frequently in contact with that area. Consequently upper connectors should be designed, whenever possible, to leave this area of the palate uncovered. Although the contact sensation at the back of the mouth is less than at the front, too much posterior extension of an upper connector may give rise to nausea.

Hence the most desirable connector for the upper jaw from the aspect of tolerance is likely to be one that crosses the palate centrally. Experimental clinical work by Farrell confirmed this and also showed that if this area could not be used posterior connection was preferable to covering the area behind the incisors.

Table 10.3 lists the various plates and bars used to connect saddles and retainers in upper and lower dentures.

Table 10.3

	Connection possibilities
Upper	Posterior palatal bar
	Middle palatal bar
	Anterior palatal bar
	Palatal plate
Lower	Lingual bar
	Labial or buccal bar
	Lingual plate
	Modified continuous clasp

The posterior palatal bar

The posterior border of this bar lies in close relationship to the junction of the hard and soft palate in the mid-line (Figs 10.82 and 10.83). Laterally it comes forward in a smooth curve over the hard palate to join the saddles or retainers.

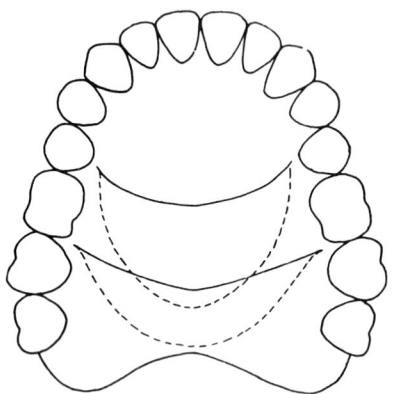

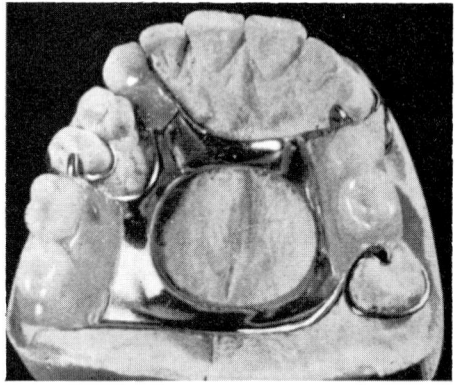

Fig. 10.82. The position of the middle and posterior palatal bars.

Fig. 10.83. A denture showing the anterior and posterior palatal bars.

The following advantages are claimed for a bar placed in this position:
- It acts as a posterior indirect retainer, helping to prevent rotational downward displacement of the denture anteriorly.
- It lies on a horizontal area of the palate and consequently is stable under vertical load.
- A maximum length of bar lies in contact with the lateral walls of the hard palate, thus resisting lateral load.
- It is well tolerated by the tongue.

Sometimes a denture with a posterior palatal bar displays an antero-posterior rock, and this can generally be attributed to one or both of two causes. In this region there is liable to be a preponderance of compressible tissue and if a mucostatic impression has been taken an antero-posterior rock occurs when pressure is applied to the bar. An impression technique that applies some degree of compression to the posterior border of the palate should overcome this problem. Second, if a steep vault exists it is not uncommon to find that, in casting, the long bar has drawn away from the model surface so that a slight space exists between the fitted denture and the mucosa of the palate.

The middle palatal bar

This bar is placed somewhat anterior to the previous bar and is generally broader. Its anterior border does not encroach upon the sloping rugae area, and therefore it is well tolerated and still lies on a horizontal part of the hard palate (Figs 10.82 and 10.84).

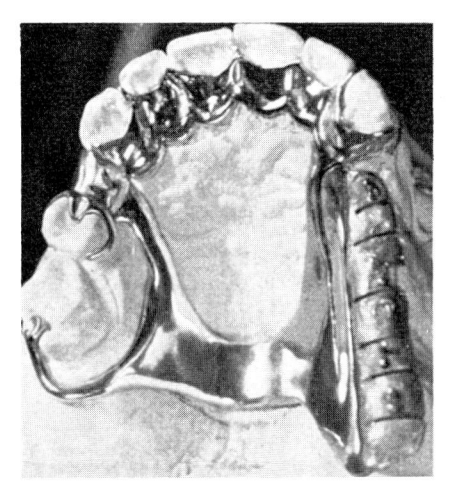

Fig. 10.84. A denture showing the middle palatal bar.

Dentures with this type of bar rarely show the antero-posterior rock occasionally found with the posterior bar. The tissue covering the palate in this area is less compressible and the bar is shorter; thus the causes of the rock are reduced. Moreover, this bar is more likely to lie within the limits of the palatal area defined by lines joining the occlusal rests and consequently instability is rare.

This type of bar does not act as an indirect retainer, but when bounded saddles are concerned, the retention of the denture is usually accomplished adequately by direct retainers. If indirect retention is considered necessary it can be secured by using posteriorly placed rests as described previously.

276   *Chapter 10*

Regardless of whether posterior or middle palatal bars are used it is preferable to make them broad and thin rather than narrow and thick. In this way the membranous bone of the palate is called upon to accept a share of lateral and vertical masticatory loads, and those falling on the ridges and standing teeth are reduced.

The anterior palatal bar

The anterior palatal bar (Fig. 10.83) is included in the design of a denture for one of two reasons. First, it may be used for its indirect retaining action, and to this end it is a useful alternative in those cases where the anterior occlusion contraindicates a continuous clasp. Second, it may be necessary when a posterior palatal bar is combined with a long saddle so that the design can be on the 'ring principle', giving adequate rigidity. However, if cobalt chromium alloy is used it is unlikely that this principle will have to be employed.

For example, the denture in Fig. 10.85 may not be a practical proposition if cast in yellow gold. During the masticatory cycle it might tend to distort because of its resilience, the points A and B tending to move farther apart to the detriment of the abutment teeth and the appliance. The presence of a continuous clasp between the points A and B (Fig. 10.86) would, of course, get over the difficulty by completing the metal ring in its design. There are, however, many cases where, because of insufficient space, the insertion of such a component is impossible. It is then necessary to complete the metal ring by placing an interior palatal bar between A and B (Fig. 10.87).

The necessity for an anterior bar is reduced when a middle bar is preferred to one placed posteriorly. However, the need for posterior indirect retention in

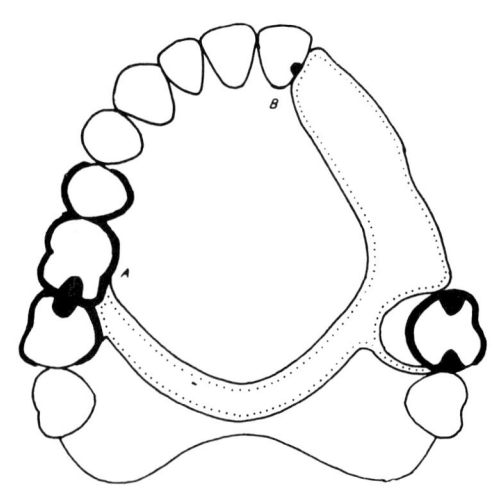

Fig. 10.85. A long saddle denture not constructed on the ring principle.

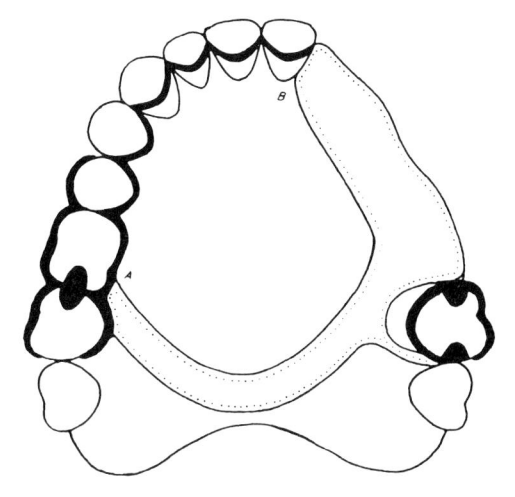

Fig. 10.86. The same denture with the ring completed by a continuous clasp.

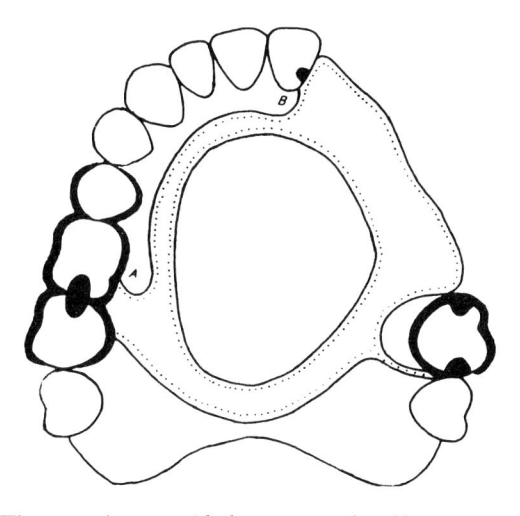

Fig. 10.87. The same denture with the ring completed by an anterior palatal bar.

cases such as the above, where anterior clasps may be contra-indicated for aesthetic reasons, must be remembered. Again, when the more rigid cobalt chromium alloy is preferred to gold, the need for the anterior palatal bar is reduced.

The great disadvantage of the anterior palatal bar is that it covers the rugae area of the palate where tongue activity is marked and as a result poor tolerance and phonetic embarrassment are highly probable. When the use of an anterior bar cannot be avoided it should be kept as thin as is practicable.

The palatal plate

The palatal plate, although it covers more tissue, has two distinct advantages over a design that employs bar connectors. In the first place, acrylic resin can be used and this is a big economic advantage. Second, the membranous bone of the palate accepts part of the masticatory load falling on the denture. Palatal plates of the 'horse-shoe' design find a useful application, when a number of small saddles, separated by single standing teeth, have to be connected. Connection of the saddles shown in Fig. 10.88 is better accomplished in this way than by bars.

When it is necessary for a palatal plate to cover the gingival margin the following conditions should be observed:
1 Unbroken contact of the margin of the denture with the palatal surface of the teeth on or above the survey line.
2 Relief of the gingival margins.
3 Adequate support of the denture on the teeth.

Figure 10.89 shows the fitting surface of a cast palatal plate which has not been relieved from the gingival margins. The traumatic effect of the rough cast metal surface impinging on the gingival tissue can be disastrous. Figure 10.90 shows another cast plate made for the same patient but in this case the gingival margins on the master model were relieved prior to duplication and the cast surface has been well polished. The effect of this plate upon the gingival tissues will be better than that shown in Fig. 10.89, but in both cases the provision of tooth support would be desirable. However, when only the six anterior teeth are standing this may not always be possible. To obtain adequate retention, full palatal coverage may be necessary, and hence the denture design cannot be as good as would be desirable.

The anterior and posterior borders of the plate may be shaped as in Fig. 10.81 to give indirect retention, and adequate relief may have to be provided in the midline should there be a marked difference in the displaceability of the mucosa between the lateral walls of the palate and the median area. Although acrylic resin may be used, a highly polished metal plate is preferable.

The lingual bar

The lingual bar (Fig. 10.91) is situated at least 1 mm, but preferably 2 mm, below the gingivae of the teeth. It must not impinge upon the musculature of the floor of the mouth so that there is no possibility of it traumatizing the thin mucosa in this area. However, from the point of view of tolerance it is preferable to keep the lingual bar as close as possible to the floor of the mouth. Patient tolerance of lingual bars will be better when they are fitted as close as possible to the mucosa covering the ridge. A tinfoil relief of minimal thickness is all that is required on the master cast prior to duplication. Owing to subsequent grinding and

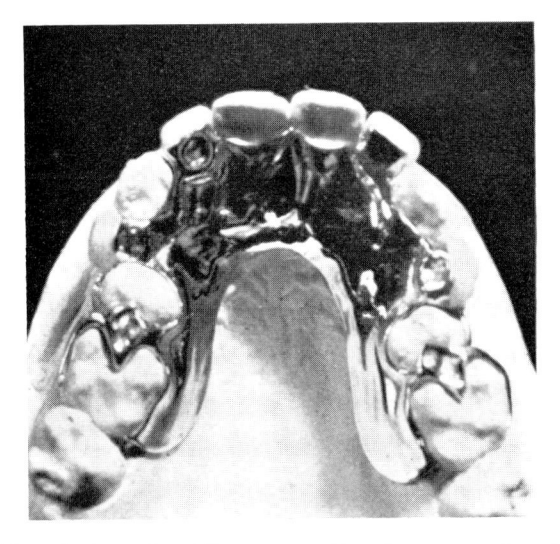

Fig. 10.88. Four single tooth saddles connected by a horse-shoe shaped palatal plate.

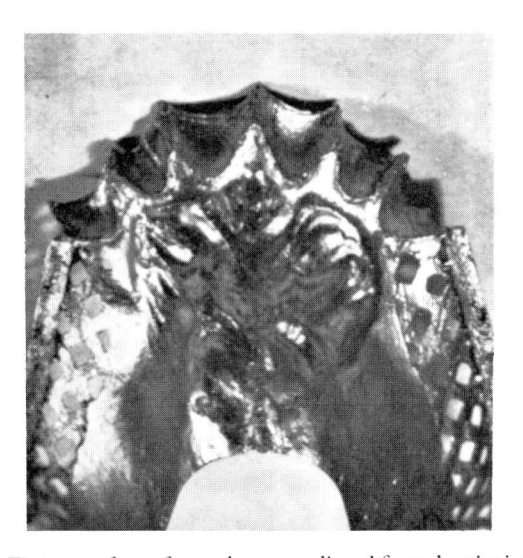

Fig. 10.89. Fitting surface of cast plate not relieved from the gingival margins.

polishing a slightly greater spacing will occur when the bar is fitted in the mouth. When it is anticipated that slight rotation of the denture may occur, then a somewhat greater spacing should be provided. The need for this space is greater when the inclination of the ridge (Fig. 10.92) is marked and when no indirect retainer is used.

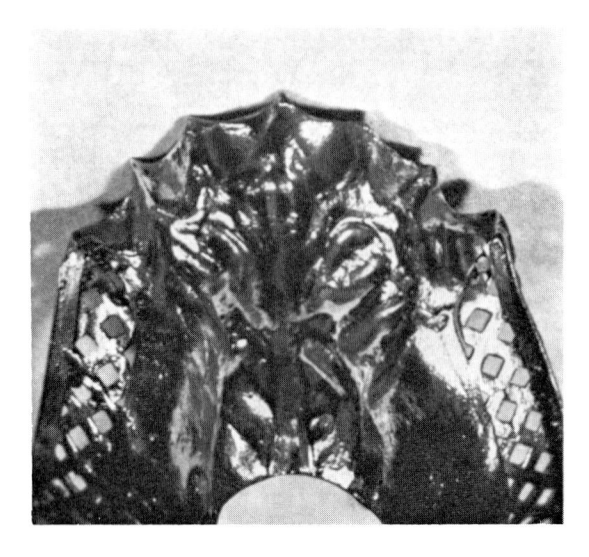

Fig. 10.90. Fitting surface of cast plate relieved from gingival margins and well polished in this region.

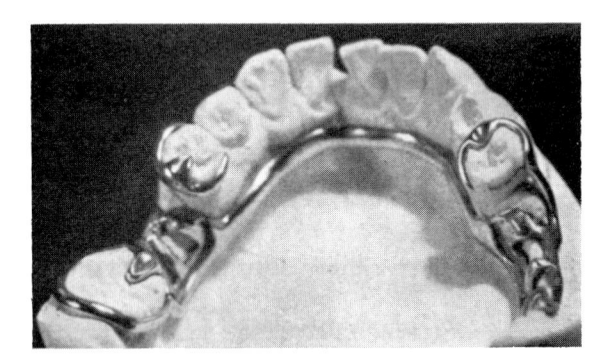

Fig. 10.91. A denture showing a cast lingual bar.

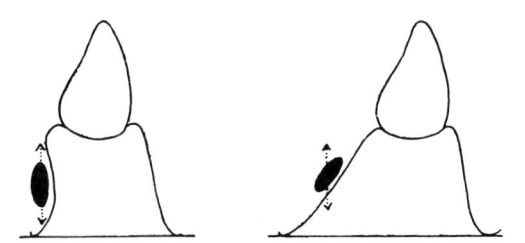

Fig. 10.92. Shows how the downward displacement of a lingual bar is more liable to cause trauma on a sloping ridge.

The Component Parts of a Partial Denture 281

Lingual bars must be cast in gold or cobalt chromium alloys. The section used depends on the length, the longer the bar the greater being the cross-section required. Cobalt chromium may be cast in thinner section than gold.

An oval section may be used, but a 'half-pear-shaped' bar has the advantage of being less irritating to the tongue (Fig. 10.93). This shape moulds against the ridge less conspicuously than does the oval section, and there is less possibility of food impaction on the top of the bar.

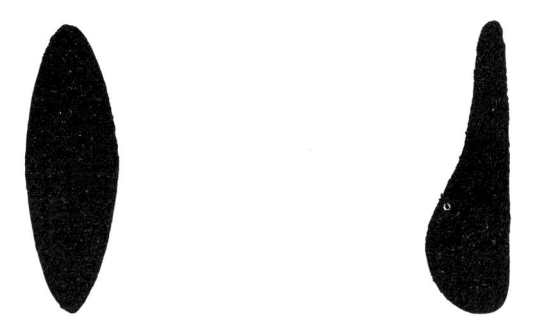

Fig. 10.93. Sections of oval and half-pear-shaped lingual bars.

Tryde and Brantenberg have described a modification of the lingual bar which they call the sublingual bar. It is positioned as low down in the mouth as possible without impinging upon the musculature and has the cross section shown in Fig. 10.94. The low position is an attempt to improve tolerance and in

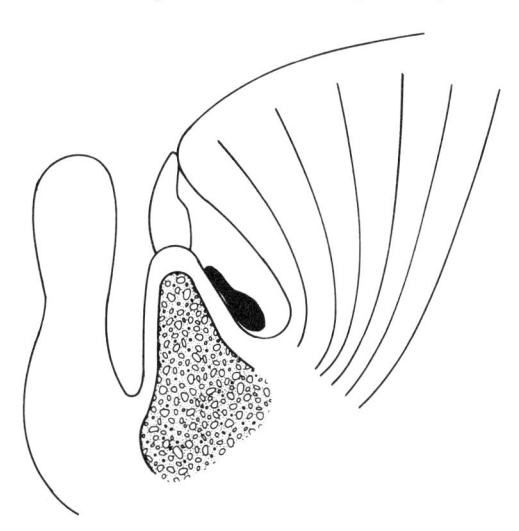

Fig. 10.94. Cross section of the lower jaw showing the shape and position of a sublingual bar.

this respect Derry and Bertram reporting on a clinical review of dentures of this type wrote 'not one patient complained of the sublingual bar type of major connector used in the present investigation. Most of them were surprised that something so voluminous could be worn so comfortably.' The writers' experience with sublingual bars confirms this statement. However, it must be emphasized that care is needed to ensure that the anterior lingual area of the impression is carefully adapted by the musculature so that the sublingual bar is positioned accurately. The low position is also an advantage in those patients, periodontally affected, who have a reduced alveolar height due to loss of bone.

The cross section employed, with the greatest dimension lying more horizontally than vertically produces greater rigidity and resistance to lateral flexure in function. Figure 10.95 shows a sublingual bar in the mouth.

A lingual bar is contraindicated in the following instances:

1 *Lack of space.* There is sometimes insufficient space between the functional level of the floor of the mouth and the gingival margins to accommodate a sufficiently strong bar. Encroachment on to the floor of the mouth results in either ulceration or an unstable appliance, whereas a lingual bar placed on, or above, the level of the free gingivae prevents the stimulating, cleansing action of the tongue over these tissues, and leads to food impaction on the gingivae. The alternative in these cases is usually a lingual plate.

2 *Instanding teeth.* Bilateral instanding teeth present a complication in the premolar region, although in tapering arches the effect may be noticed more anteriorly. In order to insert a lingual bar in these cases it must be placed at a considerable distance medial to the ridge and consequently it is not well

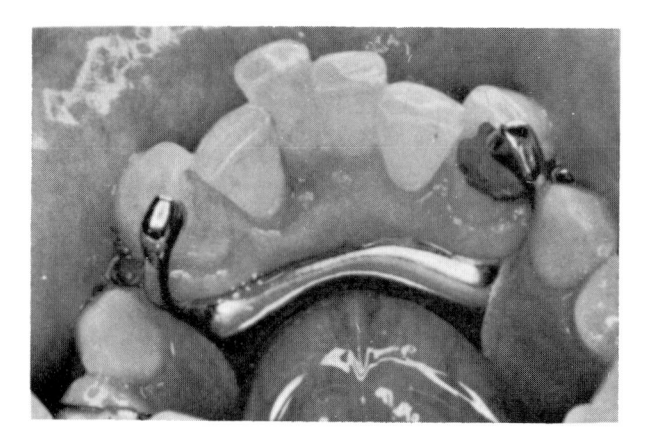

Fig. 10.95. A sublingual bar.

tolerated, particularly in the anterior part of the mouth. Further, such a medially placed bar means a bulky lingual flange to the saddle, which is liable to encroach on the tongue space. The alternative in these cases is a buccal bar.

3 *Anteriorly inclined alveolar process.* Where the anterior alveolar process and teeth have a marked anterior inclination the lingual bar is very prominent and is not well tolerated by the tongue. A lingual plate is often more satisfactory, but a sublingual bar may be applicable.

The lingual plate

The lingual plate contacts the lingual surfaces of the standing teeth and the mucosa covering the lingual aspect of the alveolar process (Fig. 10.96). It is relieved over the gingivae and tissue undercuts.

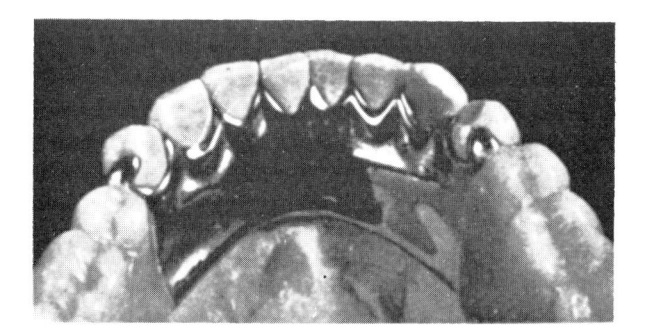

Fig. 10.96. Lingual plate.

Many practitioners construct the lingual plate in acrylic resin for economic reasons but this material is not sufficiently strong or rigid and is too liable to cause an unfavourable reaction in the covered gingivae. Consequently, it is advised that all lingual plates should be made of metal. When cast, preference is given to cobalt chromium on account of the extra rigidity that can be obtained. When a swaged plate is used stainless steel is preferred on economic grounds but it must be of sufficient thickness to be rigid.

The lingual plate is tolerated better than the lingual bar, particularly when the latter is combined with a continuous clasp. It can also be used in those cases where there is only a shallow alveolar process and insufficient space exists between the gingivae and the floor of the mouth for a lingual bar to be inserted. If it is considered that the gingivae should be protected from possible abrasion by hard foods, then a lingual plate is advisable.

A lingual plate is contra-indicated when the gingivae have receded to a

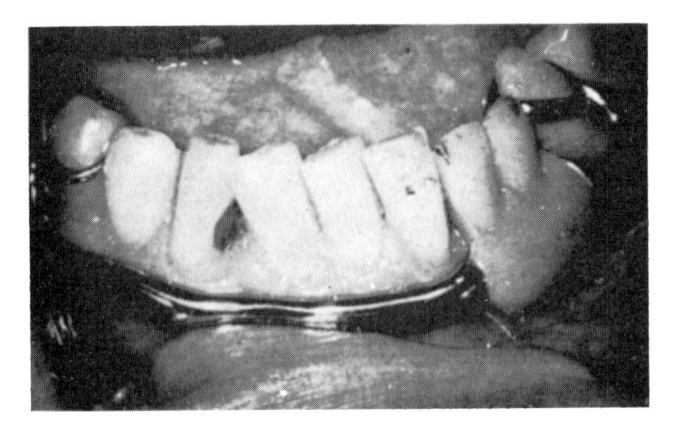

Fig. 10.97. Denture having a labial bar.

marked degree or when gingivectomy has lowered the point of gingival attachment. In either case spaces exist below the interstitial contact points of the teeth and above the gingivae. It is imperative that these spaces should be kept very clean and be readily available for stimulating massage by wood sticks. If a lingual plate is fitted food will inevitably pack into these spaces and cannot be dislodged until the denture has been removed, a procedure which is also necessary before interdental massage can be carried out. In these circumstances a lingual bar is a preferable connector. Figure 10.98 shows a lingual bar connector *in situ*. This denture has been worn continuously for eight years, and the condition of the gingivae is excellent. Whenever a lingual plate is fitted, the patient must be encouraged to practise the highest standards of oral hygiene. Even when a lingual plate is the connector of a denture that is adequately tooth supported, deleterious effects on the underlying gingivae will follow unless oral hygiene is good. With free end saddle dentures lacking as they do complete support, the effects are

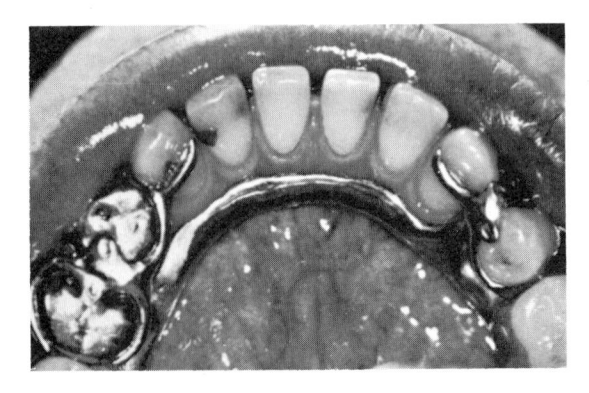

Fig. 10.98. A lingual bar.

likely to be more severe. Nor must it be forgotten that cervical caries is a not uncommon sequelae following the use of a lingual plate.

When a lingual plate connector is used for a Class I lower denture and only the six anterior teeth remain, tooth support for the anterior segment of the denture may be obtained by placing embrasure hooks or incisal rests on two or more of the natural teeth. In such cases, when bone resorption under the saddles has been sufficient to warrant rebasing but this has not been done, the posterior sinkage of the denture will result in a forward movement of the lower border of the lingual plate causing inflammation of the underlying mucosa. Frequent inspection of such dentures is essential, so that rebasing can be undertaken at the appropriate time.

The labial or buccal bar

This bar is situated in the labial or buccal sulcus and lies in relation to, but relieved from, the buccal and labial alveolus (Fig. 10.97). Because of its shape and the complex nature of its design it must be cast. It is always a broader, flatter structure than its lingual counterpart and, because it lies on an arc of greater radius, its section must be greater to give equal rigidity. When long bars are necessary it is an advantage to have them constructed in cobalt chromium alloy as the section required for rigidity is less than if gold is used.

When planning one of these bars the same relationship to mucosal reflection and gingival margins must be observed as was outlined for the lingual bar. Particular attention must be given to freedom of movement for the buccal and labial frenae. The relief over the canine eminence should be increased to two layers of gauge 4 foil as in this region the mucosa is firmly attached to the periosteum with little intervening submucosa and is very liable to traumatic damage.

The labial or buccal bar is most useful in cases of bilateral instanding premolars. It is, of course, possible in some cases to have a labial bar in one area of the denture and a lingual bar in another. Tolerance of labial and buccal bars is usually surprisingly good.

The modified continuous clasp

In certain cases, and particularly when a flap operation or gingivectomy has been carried out in the lower anterior region, little space exists between the floor of the mouth and the gingival margins; thus a lingual bar is contra-indicated. The clinical crown in such cases is long, and it is possible to use a wider type of cobalt chromium continuous clasp as a connector (Fig. 10.99). The advantage of this design over the alternative lingual plate is that the gingivae are not covered and interdental stimulants can be used by the patient with the appliance *in situ*.

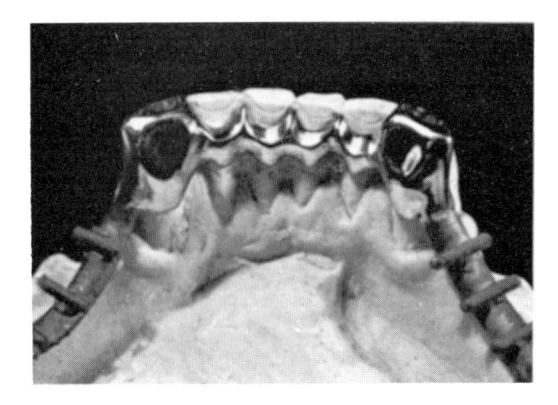

Fig. 10.99. A modified continuous clasp acting as a connector. Tooth support is provided by caps completely covering the incisal edges of the canines.

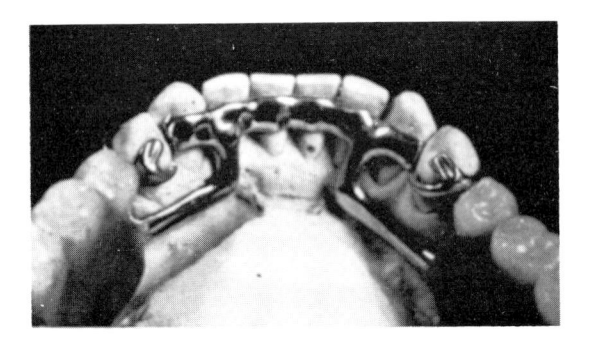

Fig. 10.100. A continuous clasp combined with a lingual bar to form a connector.

If there is some obstruction to a lingual bar such as an abnormal lingual fraenum or bony prominence in the midline, a continuous clasp may be combined with a lingual bar, as shown in Fig. 10.100.

References

ANDERSON J.N. and BATES J.F. (1959) Cobalt-chromium partial dentures—a clinical survey. *Brit. dent. J.* **107,** 57.

ANDERSON J.N. and LAMMIE G.A. (1952) A clinical survey of partial dentures. *Brit. dent. J.* **92,** 59–67.

APPLEGATE O.C. and NISSLE R.O. (1951) Keeping the partial denture in harmony with biological limitations. *J. Amer. dent. Ass.* **43,** 409–19.

APPLEGATE O.C. (1955) The partial denture base. *J. pros. Dent.* **5,** 636–48.

APPLEGATE O.C. (1957) Conditions which may influence the choice of partial or complete denture service. *J. pros. Dent.* **7,** 182–96.

ATKINSON H.F. (1953) Partial denture problems. *Aus. J. Dent.* **57**, 187–90.
AVANT W.E. (1971) Factors that influence retention of removable partial dentures. *J. pros. Dent.* **25**, 265.
BARBENEL J.C. (1971) Design of partial denture components. *J. dent. Res.* **50**, 586.
BATES J.F. (1963) Cast clasps for partial dentures. *Int. dent. J.* **13**, 610.
BATES J.F. (1968) Studies in the retention of cobalt-chromium partial dentures. *Brit. dent. J.* **125**, 97.
BECKETT L.S. (1940) Some fundamentals of partial denture construction. *D. Digest* **49**, 256–61.
BLATTERFEIN L. (1951) Study of partial denture clasping. *J. Amer. dent. Ass.* **43**, 169–85.
BLATTERFEIN L. (1969) The use of the semi precision rest in removable partial dentures. *J. pros. Dent.* **22**, 387.
CHICK A.O. (1953) The correct location of clasps and rests on dentures without stress breakers. *Brit. dent. J.* **95**, 303–9.
CLAYTON J.A. and JASLOW C. (1971) A measurement of clasp forces on teeth. *J. pros. Dent.* **25**, 21.
COHEN M. (1948) Principles of partial denture prosthesis with special reference to the use of the surveyor. *Journal of the dental Association of South Africa* **3**, 450–9.
COLLETT H.A. (1951) Principles of partial denture design. *D. Digest* **57**, 24–9.
CUNNINGHAM D.N. (1970) Indications and contraindications for precision attachments. *D. Clin. N.A.* **14**, 595.
DERRY A. and BERTRAM V. (1970) A clinical survey of removable partial dentures after two years' usage. *Acta Odont. Scand.* **28**, 581.
DE VAN M.M. (1934) The embrasure saddle clasp. *J. Amer. dent. Ass.* **22**, 1352–62.
DE VAN M.M. (1952) The nature of the partial denture foundations; suggestions for its preservation. *J. pros. Dent.* **2**, 210–18.
DE VAN M.M. (1955) Preserving natural teeth through the use of clasps. *J. pros. Dent.* **5**, 208.
FARREL J. (1968) Partial denture tolerance. *Dent. Pract.* **19**, 162.
FIRTELL D.N. (1968) Effect of clasp design upon retention of removable partial dentures. *J. pros. Dent.* **20**, 45.
FRANKS A.S.T. (1961) Influence of occlusal onlays on the electrical output of the masseters. *Brit. dent. J.* **111**, 214.
KENNEDY E. (1942) *Partial denture construction*, 430–43, 510, Dent. Items. Publishing Co. Inc., New York.
LAMMIE G.A., STORER R. and OSBORNE J. (1956) The use of onlays in partial denture construction. *Brit. dent. J.* **100**, 33–42.
MALCOLM J.A. (1943) Occlusal rest in partial denture construction. *D. Digest.* **49**, 256–61.
MATSUMOTO M. and GOTO T. (1970) Lateral force distribution in partial denture design. *J. dent. Res.* **49**, 359.
MATTHEWS E. (1949) Clasp design in partial dentures. *Brit. dent. J.* **85**, 152–8.
J.M. NEY CO. (1949) *The Ney denture book.* Connecticut.
NEVIN R.B. (1955) Periodontal aspects of partial denture prosthesis. *J. pros. Dent.* **5**, 215.
OSBORNE J. and LAMMIE G.A. (1953) Some observations concerning chrome cobalt denture bases. *Brit. dent. J.* **94**, 55–67.
PHILLIPS R.W. and LEONARD L.J. (1956) A study of enamel abrasion as related to partial denture clasps. *J. pros. Dent.* **6**, 657–71.
PREISKEL H.W. (1968) *Precision attachments in dentistry.* Henry Kimpton, London.
ROACH F.E. (1930) Principles and essentials of bar clasp partial dentures. *J. Amer. dent. Ass.* **17**, 124–38.

ROACH F.E. (1934) Mouth survey and design of partial dentures. *J. Amer. dent. Ass.* **21**, 1166–76.

SCHMIDT A.H. (1952) Planning and design of removable partial dentures. *Dent. Pract.* **3**, 3–19.

SCHUYLER C.H. (1942) Factors of partial denture design and construction essential to maintain oral health and function. *J. dent. Soc. St. N.Y.* **8**, 9–17.

SHAFFER F.W. (1970) A method of analysing and surveying for removable partial dentures. *D. Digest*, **76**, 388.

STANDARD S.G. (1951) Problems related to the construction of complete upper and partial lower dentures. *J. Amer. dent. Ass.* **43**, 695–708.

STANSBURY R.R. (1968) An external partial denture attachment. *J. Amer. dent. Ass.* **77**, 88.

STONE E.R. (1936) Tripping action of bar clasps. *J. Amer. dent. Ass.* **23**, 597–617.

TAYLOR R.L. (1948) Partial denture prosthesis—principles of design. *Aus. J. Dent.* **52**, 30–2.

TOMLIN H.R. and OSBORNE J. (1961) Cobalt-chromium partial dentures. *Brit. dent. J.* **110**, 307.

TRYDE G. and BRANTENBERG F. (1965) Den sublinguale barr. *Soertrgh af Tand.* **69**, 873.

WARR J.A. (1959) Friction and partial denture retention. *J. dent. Res.* **38**, 1066.

WARR J.A. (1959) An analysis of clasp design in partial dentures. *Phys. in med. Biol.* **3**, 212.

WILSON J.H. (1949) Partial denture construction—some aspects of diagnosis and design. *Dent. J. Aust.* **21**, 347–363.

11
THE BILATERAL FREE-END SADDLE (KENNEDY CLASS I)

The bilateral free-end saddle denture (Kennedy Class I) is the most common design of partial denture and occurs more often in the mandible than the maxilla. Before considering the design of such a denture it is necessary to understand what happens to it during function, and in particular under the vertical, lateral and antero-posterior loads to which it might be subjected.

Vertical Load

The vertical load that may be exerted on a partial denture can be divided into parafunctional load and functional load, and it has been estimated that the former is at least twice as great as the latter. The functional load can be considered principally as the masticatory load and is applied as the bolus of food is crushed between the upper and lower occlusal surfaces of the teeth before they make contact. It also combines with horizontal loads in the final stages of mastication when the lower teeth move horizontally in contact with their antagonists from a lateral or retruded position into the intercuspal position. In addition an uncomplicated vertical load is likely to be applied intermittently throughout the day in empty swallowing function. The free-end saddle denture by its nature is dependent for its support on two tissues which are completely different. As it can be tooth supported only anteriorly, the posterior edentulous ridge must also bear part of the vertical masticatory load. It is necessary therefore to examine the effect of vertical load on these supporting tissues taking into account the variations in their displacement. A suitable example for consideration is the denture replacing $\overline{765/567}$ with a rigid connector and having three-arm clasps with occlusal rests distally on $\overline{4/4}$, constructed on a cast obtained from a mucostatic impression (Fig. 11.1). In this case the major part of the masticatory load will fall on the saddles. It has been demonstrated that the degree of displacement of the tissues under the saddle of the denture is greater than that of the tooth within its socket, and that this displacement increases towards the retromolar area. When a vertical load is applied to the saddle both the abutment teeth and the soft tissues covering the saddle area are displaced, with the alveolar tissues being displaced to a greater extent than the tooth (Fig. 11.2). The result of this is rotation of the free-end saddle about the abutment tooth or teeth, with the saddle being displaced into the

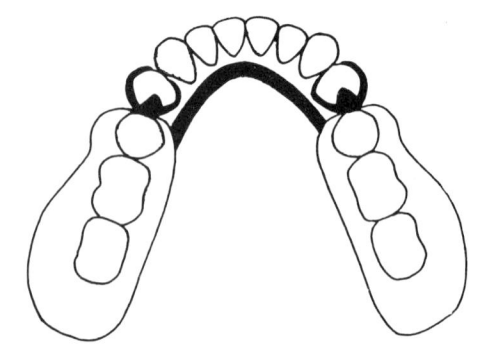

Fig. 11.1. The Class I (Kennedy) partial lower denture being considered.

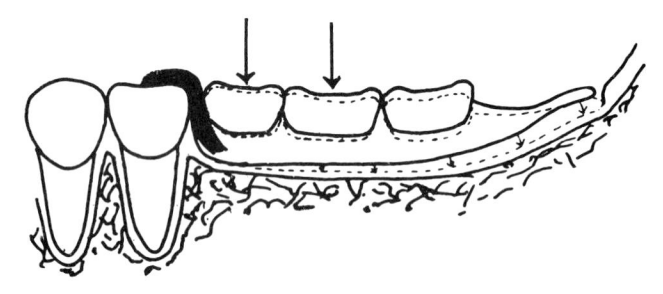

Fig. 11.2. The displacement of the free-end saddle into the soft tissues posteriorly upon vertical loading of the saddle.

soft tissues posteriorly and the clasp arms exerting leverage on the abutment tooth in a distal direction. The occlusal rest present, however, shows virtually no displacement and can be considered as the fulcrum around which this rotatory movement occurs. With a rigid connector present between the saddles the same effect will occur on the opposite side of the arch. Thus in such a design the application of vertical load will cause rotation of the free-end saddles into the tissues overlying the residual ridges, and the line joining the occlusal rests can be considered as the axis of rotation. At the same time as rotation of the saddles into the supporting tissues occurs, so also is there rotation in the opposite direction of the lingual bar connecting the saddles. This is upwards and away from the roots of the lower teeth and their supporting tissues, with the greatest amount of movement being in the midline.

The amount of displacement of both the saddle and the connector is, however, dependent upon the nature and amount of the fibrous submucosa that covers the residual alveolar ridge, and this can be assessed by palpation. The hypothesis that ridge resorption results from the bending inwards of the outer and inner compact plates of bone has been discussed already. Resorption of the intervening cancellous bone is liable to occur when the load placed upon it enters the pathological range, and this can result from either vertical or horizontal forces. It is especially liable to occur when the denture is first worn, and in different degrees. The greater the amount of such resorption the less is the resistance to the deformation of the bony plates and accordingly the greater the loss of ridge contour. Since increased vertical load causes increased bony resorption it is wise to make the saddle cover as large an area as possible in order to reduce the load per unit area and ensure that the residual ridge is subjected to minimal stress. However, even granting maximal saddle coverage, the pressure developed over the bone supporting the free-end saddle is very liable to exceed the tolerance limit especially when the denture is first worn.

If resorption occurs and no attempt is made to restore the fit of the denture by rebasing, further resorption is likely to occur, since the amount of downward displacement under vertical load is increased. An unstable denture with an inaccurate fitting surface will transmit traumatic stress to different parts of the residual ridge crest. This, coupled with the fact that the denture now develops a kinetic energy by virtue of its increasing posterior displacement on vertical loading, accounts for the further ridge destruction that takes place. Much of what has been discussed is dependent upon the magnitude of the applied load, the displaceability of the soft tissues covering the residual ridge, and the health of the alveolar bone and periodontium of the abutment teeth. In addition it must be remembered that the oral mucosa behaves in a visco-elastic manner in its response to load. This response is not only dependent therefore upon the magnitude of the load but also on its duration, rate of application and previous loading history. Apart from the greater displaceability of the saddle tissues under load compared with the periodontal ligament, their rate of recovery is also much slower, extending over several hours. All of these factors will affect directly or indirectly the magnitude and direction of tooth movement.

It has been generally accepted that when the saddle of a Kennedy Class I denture with occlusal rests placed distally on the abutment teeth is loaded vertically, there is a tendency to distal displacement of the abutment tooth. This is not a bodily movement but rather one of tilting due to the arc of rotation of the saddle, which in the gingival area of the abutment tooth is almost parallel to the mucosa, resulting in minimal or no support from the mucosa near the tooth.

This will result in distal bone loss, eventual tooth mobility and of course denture movement, dependent upon the state of the interdental marginal ligament and its regenerative capacity. If however the occlusal rest is placed mesially on the abutment, then the arc of movement of the saddle becomes more perpendicular to the mucosa, and the more mesial fulcrum which is established will increase the support provided by the soft tissues. The direction of force is less likely to cause tissue damage as the abutment tooth tends to move towards the side on which the rest is located and receives additional support from the teeth anterior to it.

It has been shown that bilateral loading of the denture saddles is more favourable to the abutment teeth than unilateral loading and that loads applied to the saddles are transmitted to the abutment teeth primarily through the occlusal rests. Whatever the direction of movement of the abutment tooth, its potential mobility will be dependent upon factors such as the magnitude of the vertical load, the physical characteristics of the overlying mucosa, the angulation of the residual ridge to the horizontal, and above all the periodontal status of the tooth itself.

The effects of clasping are that the more rigid the clasp the greater the leverage on the tooth and the less the load on the alveolar ridge; the more flexible the clasp arms the less leverage on the tooth and more load on the ridge.

This discussion has been concerned, in the main, with the effect of the vertical load on the working side free-end saddle. It must be appreciated, however, that provided a rigid bar connects the saddles a similar state of affairs exists over a large area of bone on the balancing side. This distribution of the load reduces the tendency for the forces to become pathological.

The Lateral Component

Lower free-end saddles may be displaced laterally as a result of the inclined plane action of the cusps of the posterior teeth (Fig. 11.3) and the steeper the cusp inclines the greater will be the load which acts laterally. Lateral loads come into effect during that stage of the masticatory cycle when the opposing teeth, having come into contact in a lateral position, return to the intercuspal position. When that position is reached lateral movement will be resisted by the palatal cusps of the upper teeth. Lateral load may also act on a saddle during those tooth contacts

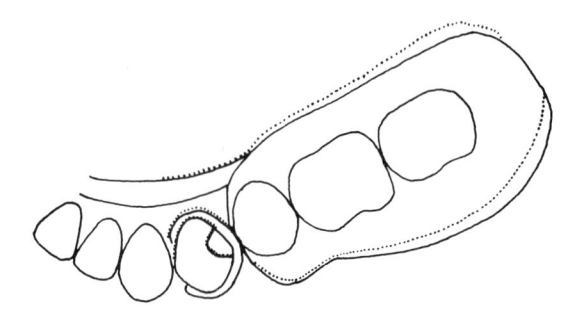

Fig. 11.3. The lateral displacement of the free-end saddle. There is a slight tendency for this to be more marked posteriorly than anteriorly where the clasping provides resistance.

The Bilateral Free-end Saddle (Kennedy Class I) 293

that may take place at times other than during mastication, and, like the vertical forces, will be greater in magnitude.

It has been assumed so far that the denture moves bodily in a lateral direction. This, however, is not quite the whole truth, since there is less resistance to lateral stress at the posterior end of the working side saddle. Anteriorly the buccal clasp arm minimizes movement, but posteriorly the buccal ridge alone resists the lateral displacement. In this it is less effective than the tooth; its efficiency being dependent upon the anatomy of the residual ridge and the condition of the overlying soft tissues. A flat ridge with a marked fibrosis of the submucosa offers comparatively little resistance, but if the ridge is well formed and shows a thinner submucosa, resistance is increased.

The absence of a posterior abutment tooth, therefore, may result in another rotational effect with the clasped abutment tooth as its centre. Fortunately, if there is rigid connection between the two saddles, this rotational torque on the working side is resisted on the balancing side by forward pressure of the saddle against the distal surface of its abutment.

The form of lateral displacement which has been described may have an adverse effect on the residual alveolar ridge, and in this respect the lateral component of load is probably a more major factor in ridge resorption than the vertical component. Providing a rigid connector is used, lateral displacement is resisted by the structures listed in Table 11.1 and Fig. 11.4 with the structures on the balancing side helping to distribute the load over a larger area of bone. If the denture is constructed with some form of flexible connector however, the load applied is borne mainly by the working side tissues.

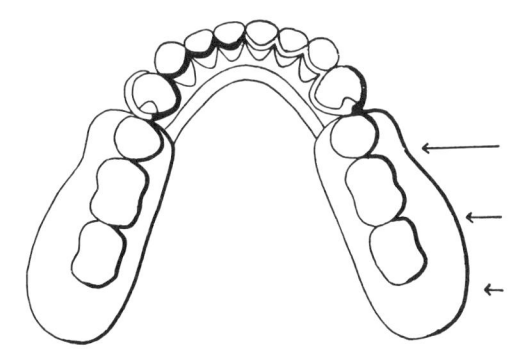

Fig. 11.4. The heavily lined structures communicate lateral stress to the tissues lying beneath them.

If the abutment tooth is held securely by a deep occlusal rest or clasp arms which encompass the tooth on three sides, a rotation tends to be effected about its long axis. The degree to which this takes place depends on the type of clasping. The more rigid the clasp the greater will be the forces acting. Wrought wire or bar

Table 11.1

Stress communicated by:	Resisting structure:
Working side saddle	Buccal ridge plate on working side
Buccal arm of clasp on working side	Abutment tooth on working side
Balancing side saddle	Lingual ridge plate on balancing side
Lingual arm of clasp on balancing side	Abutment tooth on balancing side
Continuous clasp (if included in design)	Teeth on balancing side
Lingual plate (if included in design)	Lingual plate of ridge supporting teeth, and teeth themselves, on balancing side

clasps convey less lateral or rotational force to the abutment tooth than do cast three-arm clasps, but throw more lateral load on the edentulous ridge.

Lateral loads will also be exerted on the denture by the adjacent facial and lingual musculature particularly during swallowing. These loads, which act throughout the day, may total twice the load resulting from masticatory function and their effects can be minimized by using narrow posterior teeth and shaping the flanges so that they do not extend beyond the zone of minimal conflict. In addition, the flanges should be kept thin in order to give a 'streamlined' appearance to the denture.

The Antero-posterior Component

Posterior displacement of the mandible from the intercuspal position takes place only during the first power strokes which are used when a hard or tough bolus is being masticated. Although the magnitude of the load involved is considerable and an anterior displacing load on the lower denture results, it is generally well resisted by the abutment teeth and those anterior in the arch.

Although in masticatory performance a true protrusive movement of the mandible is only used in incision, there is often a protrusive element in grinding. The cusps of the lower teeth, instead of being accommodated in the fossae of the upper teeth, make a contact on the slopes of the upper cusps. This results in an inclined plane action which produces a distal force on the lower denture, the magnitude of which will depend on the musculature and the steepness of the cusp angles. This backward force is in part resisted by the ridge when it slopes upwards into the ascending ramus of the mandible, but the greater part of the resistance comes from the clasped abutment tooth. The arms of the three-arm clasp encompass the tooth almost completely on its buccal and lingual surfaces, and the tips of the arms lie on the mesial half of the crown. Consequently the abutment tooth tends to be pulled in a distal direction. The magnitude of the force applied will be greater if the clasp arms are cast alloy than if they are wrought wire; in the latter case less stress is applied to the tooth but the denture as a whole may be more unstable and there will be more pressure on the ridge posteriorly.

A greater problem arises if the abutment tooth is a canine. Due to the crown morphology of this tooth it is difficult to design a clasp that will encompass the tooth and also be aesthetically acceptable. In such a situation the clasped tooth is unable to offer resistance to the distal displacement of the saddle, which is borne entirely by the residual ridge.

The vertical, lateral, and antero-posterior components of force have been described separately and their effects listed as different entities. In practice however these represent components of a single applied load in three different planes at right angles to each other. Any load applied to the denture therefore can be resolved in the terms of these three components. It is probable that at any one time all these loads will be operative and the stress acting on the abutment tooth or residual alveolar ridge will have the result of combining the effects described.

The Problem of the Free-end Saddle

In the design and construction of any removable partial denture it must be remembered that it is more important to preserve that which remains than to replace meticulously that which is missing. This is generally more difficult in the case of free-end as opposed to bounded saddles, mainly due to the nature of the supporting tissues.

It has been explained already that since the residual alveolar ridge must always bear some of the masticatory load, resorption of that ridge is likely to occur. At the same time the abutment tooth is subjected to load in both antero-posterior and lateral directions which may predispose to premature breakdown of its supporting bony tissues. The approaches to the design of free-end saddle dentures suggested below are based on the appreciation of these two factors.

Treatment of the Free-end Saddle

The suggested methods of restoring the bilateral free-end saddle in this text are based on attempting to control the load delivered to both teeth and residual ridges in order to give the optimum reaction in these tissues. This may be achieved by:
1   Reducing the load.
2   Distributing the load between teeth and residual ridges:
    (i) by varying the connector between clasp and saddle,

a stress breaking,
b combining rigid connection and gingivally approaching clasp,
c combining rigid connection and occlusally approaching clasp,
d the disjunct denture;
(ii) by anterior placement of the occlusal rest:
a the RPI system,
b the balance of force system,
(iii) by mucocompression.
3 Distributing the load widely.
(i) over more than one abutment tooth on each side,
(ii) over the maximal area of edentulous ridge.

1 Reducing the Load

The vertical load on the saddle in mastication may be reduced by decreasing the size of the occlusal table and also by ensuring as wide a coverage of the residual ridge area by the base of the saddle as is compatible with function. This may be affected in antero-posterior and bucco-lingual directions and the following methods are available.

- Using canines and premolars instead of premolars and molars.
- Using narrow teeth or reducing the width of selected teeth by removing the lingual cusp(s).
- Leaving a tooth off a saddle.

This modification has the advantage that it can be used in all cases, and it is surprising that it is so often neglected. It is most necessary when the occlusal load is heavy, the saddle is long, or the bone factor is poor. The load reduction effected in this way is achieved by increasing the efficiency of the denture. In the same way as it requires less effort to cut an object with a knife which is sharp rather than blunt, so the narrow occlusal table allows the patient to penetrate a bolus of food in the same way, with less load being transmitted to the supporting tissues. It should be noted also that a reduction in the masticatory load also reduces the lateral component of force that acts on the saddle during the second stage of mastication, and this is a factor calculated to preserve the ridge form and the supporting tissues of the abutment tooth.

If the reduction in the occlusal table is accomplished by using narrow teeth, then, as discussed previously, there will be a reduction in the degree of lateral force applied by the musculature during function. Omitting the most distal tooth on the saddle will reduce the magnitude of any abutment tooth movement caused by the denture, since it has been shown that the more distally load is applied to a saddle the greater is the magnitude of abutment tooth movement.

2 Distribution of the Load between Teeth and Ridges

(i) By varying the connection between clasp and saddle

(a) *Stress breaking*. The principle of stress breaking in partial denture design is the provision of some degree of movement or flexibility between the clasp unit and the free-end saddle. The stress transmitted by the denture to the tissues is distributed differently therefore and also reduced by the energy absorbed in deformation than if the connection had been rigid. A more descriptive term for this function however might be stress equalization. Any device which allows movement between the saddle unit and the retaining unit is known as a stress breaker.

In general, stress breakers can be divided into two groups:
1 Those having a movable joint between the direct retainer and the saddle.
2 Those having a flexible connection between the direct retainer and the saddle.

The first group is necessary when a precision attachment is used, but can also be used when a clasp is preferred. Many stress breakers of this type have been described in the literature. They vary in their range of movement, some allowing only up-and-down and side-to-side movements, whereas others also permit a vertical hinge action. One of the most satisfactory attachments of this nature is the Dalbo 669 described in the previous chapter.

In the second group where it is decided to incorporate some form of stress breaking this can be provided by constructing a flexible or semi-flexible connector between the direct retainer and tooth supported part of the denture, and the mucosally supported saddle. This is commonly achieved with a distally extended flexible bar connected to the rigid connector, where the degree of flexibility will depend upon its length and cross sectional form. Where a lingual bar connector has been used to join the two saddles it should be distally extended on each side and then recurved along the residual ridge to allow attachment into the matrix resin of the saddle. In such cases it is advisable to design support on the mesial aspect of the abutment teeth, or in the case of a short saddle, on teeth anterior to the abutment teeth (Fig. 11.5).

Alternatively if a lingual plate connector is used a split of an appropriate length can be made at its inferior border. The saddle is attached to the more flexible bar while the clasp units are attached to the rigid part of the framework (Fig. 11.6). The use of such designs allows the mucosa supported saddle a degree of movement which is independent of the rigid tooth supported part of the denture and therefore lessens the stress of the abutment teeth.

Having discussed the methods of stress breaking it remains to consider the principles involved. For this purpose the designs used in Figs 11.5 and 11.6 may

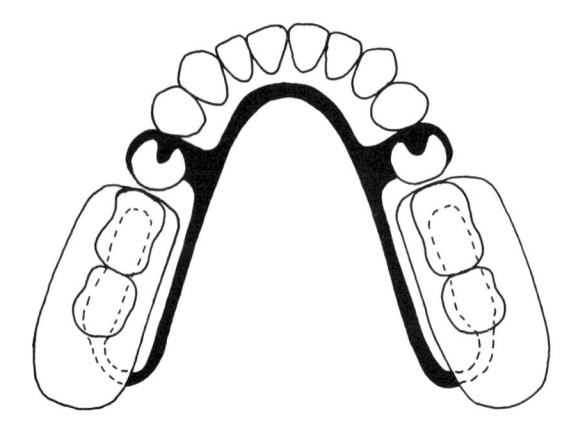

Fig. 11.5. A lingual bar connector with a flexible distal extension. Support is provided on the mesial aspect of the abutment teeth.

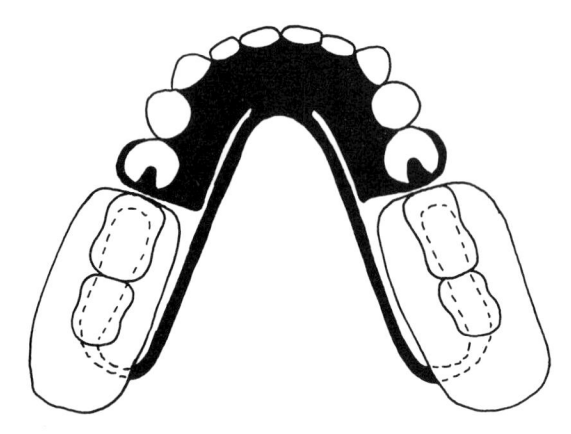

Fig. 11.6. A split lingual plate connector with flexible distally extending bars to the saddle area to allow some independent movement.

be used for discussion. In these situations the distribution of vertical and horizontal load will be as follows.

When a vertical load is applied the saddle is displaced downwards into the soft tissue covering the ridge to a greater extent than where the retainer and occlusal rest have direct connection with the saddle. This means that the ridge bone has to withstand an increased vertical load which is more evenly spread over the whole ridge rather than concentrated at the free end of the saddle. Although not quite accurate it may be assumed that the centre of saddle rotation is at the portion of the connector lying in the midline. This point lies anterior and inferior to the clasped abutment tooth, and, therefore, now causes a downward and slightly forward movement. The premolar receives a reduced vertical force and is more fitted to resist a forward than a backward torque because of the buttressing effect of teeth lying anterior to it.

The net result of the stress-breaking action as far as the vertical component is concerned is a greater assignment of load to the edentulous ridge and less to the abutment tooth. The torque on the abutment is reduced markedly in magnitude and is favourable in direction.

When a lateral component acts on the stress-broken saddle a greatly increased lateral stress is placed on the alveolar bone. Less of the load falls on the abutment teeth, and consequently the magnitude of the damaging lateral torque is reduced. If a continuous clasp or lingual plate is included in the design it is incorporated in the retainer unit and thus plays less part in the distribution of lateral load.

The effectiveness of the action on the posterior component of force depends on the arch form. Where this is square a greater proportion of load falls on the retromolar region whilst the leverage or torque on the abutment tooth is correspondingly less. However where the length of the flexible connector is small, as in a tapering arch form, less backward movement of the saddle occurs and the stresses on the abutment teeth are not so greatly reduced.

Stress breaking has little effect on the anterior component of force acting on the denture saddle during the power strokes; uninterrupted contact between tooth and retainer, and retainer and saddle ensures no saddle movement in an anterior direction and load distribution is accordingly not altered.

It can, therefore, be concluded that the dangerous horizontal torques acting on the abutment teeth are reduced by stress breaking and that, in consequence, their supporting structures are less liable to break down. However, the edentulous ridge is called upon to accept more vertical and horizontal stress and as a result tends to resorb more quickly.

In situations where it is desired to reduce stresses on the abutment teeth as much as possible, such as where the periodontal condition is poor, one must aim for as much flexibility as possible. In other situations, less flexible union may be desired in order to place relatively more stress on the standing teeth and less on the residual ridge. The flexibility of the connector governs the distribution of load between the ridge and the standing teeth, and it can be graded so that greater or less stress is transferred to the standing teeth. This will be dependent upon the length and position of the connector, its cross-sectional shape and dimension, and the physical properties of the material used.

Summing up the principles involved in stress breaking it may be said that, theoretically, decreased stresses are applied to the standing teeth and increased stresses are applied to the edentulous ridge areas. To what extent these theoretical concepts apply in practice will be discussed later.

(b) *Combining rigid connection and gingivally approaching clasping.* When rigid connection between retainers and saddles is used, with gingivally approaching clasps, a condition may exist which is similar in principle to stress breaking. The portion of this type of clasp that is in contact with the abutment tooth is at the end of a bar that is resilient to a degree which depends upon its length and cross section and the alloy used. Now, if the occlusal rest is allowed to move over the occlusal surface of the tooth to a small degree in lateral and antero-posterior directions (and this may occur when saucer-shaped rest seat preparations are used), the action of the clasp bar resembles a stress breaker, since its resilience reduces the horizontal forces on the abutment tooth. The effectiveness of the stress-breaking actions of these clasps may be increased by increasing the resilience of the bar.

(c) *Combining rigid connection and occlusally approaching clasping.* A combination of rigid connection and occlusally approaching clasps is the opposite extreme to stress breaking. In this condition more load is placed on the abutment tooth and less on the ridge. However, the proportion of load falling on tooth and ridge is capable of variation and depends on the type of clasping used. When the arm is resilient, a certain amount of movement of the clasp over the surface of the tooth is permitted. At one extreme a wrought gold wire clasp allows most movement of the clasp over the enamel, whereas a cast cobalt chromium clasp permits least. Thus under vertical and horizontal loading least stress is placed on the tooth when a wrought gold wire clasp is used, whilst the ridge is stressed more heavily. The opposite condition exists with cast cobalt chromium clasps.

It should be emphasized that the extent of these clasp movements is small (otherwise an unstable denture would result), but they may, however, be sufficient to reduce the torques acting on the abutment and keep them within the physiological limit. Once again the indication is for saucer-shaped rest seat preparations; box-shaped preparations have no place in free-end saddle cases unless a stress breaker is used.

The choice between stress breaking and rigid attachment methods. The majority of lower free-end saddle dentures are made with rigid connection between the retainers and the saddles. In view of some of the theoretically desirable features of the stress broken principle it is appropriate to consider the reasons for the overwhelming popularity of the rigid construction.

The stress-breaking principle aims at reducing the loads transmitted to the standing teeth; hence a stress broken design should be particularly applicable to cases in which the standing teeth show periodontal involvement. However, when the condition of the bone surrounding the teeth is poor, the bone of the edentulous areas also is usually poor. Consequently, the increased loads applied in these areas by a stress broken denture result in more rapid resorption than would occur with a rigid design. Although one of the aims of partial denture design should be the preservation of the remaining natural teeth there is much common sense in the observation that teeth that need stress relief should perhaps better be sacrificed. Certainly in the more advanced cases of periodontal involvement a temporizing line of treatment such as the simple 'additive' denture mentioned in Chapter 3 is preferable to a more complex and expensive design.

The economic factor is another reason for the predominance of the rigid design, as designs incorporating flexibility are technically more difficult and time-consuming to construct, and hence are more expensive than the simpler rigid design. However, the more expensive appliance may not necessarily be the best method of rendering an efficient service to the patient. There is merit in simplicity in partial denture design, since a simple design will certainly be better tolerated by the majority of patients.

Another significant disadvantage is that flexible connectors are easily distorted, or even fractured, during use, or by the patient during cleaning. Following such accidents repair is difficult; in fact, a new denture may be required.

If the mucosal tissues covering the ridge areas are highly displaceable and mobile, then there may be an indication for some type of movable or flexible connection between the saddles and the retainer units.

(d) *The disjunct denture.* In the older patient it is not uncommon to find a situation, particularly in the lower jaw, where the few remaining teeth are anterior teeth with considerable gingival recession and a generally poor periodontal condition. The construction of a rigid tooth borne denture or even one incorporating flexible connectors is often contra-indicated due to the state of the periodontal health. A simple tissue supported denture, although possible in some situations is also likely to cause damage to the supporting tissues by virtue of its movement, particularly so where the design of the connector will include coverage of the gingival margins, a situation commonly encountered, as the use of a lingual bar connector is often contra-indicated due to lingual gingival recession.

It has been suggested that such a problem may be overcome by the construction of a two part denture, composed separately of tooth borne and mucosa borne sections each acting independently of each other on its supporting tissues.

The tooth borne part comprises a lingual plate which acts to protect the teeth and the gingivae from the connector of the mucosa borne part, and which also carries retention elements. In addition it is constructed with distally extending buccal bars which are designed to engage a slot in the saddle of the mucosa borne part. These are known as disjunct bars as they are not attached directly and rigidly to the mucosa borne saddle but allow some movement. They are however necessary for its retention.

The mucosa borne section of the denture is the bilateral saddle which replaces the lost teeth, with the connector being a lingual bar from which the

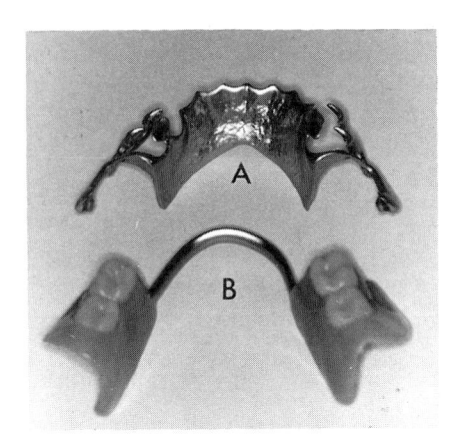

Fig. 11.7. The separate parts of a disjunct denture.
A The tooth borne section with protective lingual plate and disjunct bars.
B The mucosa borne section with its lingual bar connector.

lingual gingival tissues are protected by the lingual plate (Fig. 11.7).

As the two parts of the denture are essentially separate, there is no transfer of the vertical masticatory load from the mucosa borne saddle to the tooth borne section. In addition because of the absence of a rigid connection between the two separate parts there is little transfer of load by means of the disjunct bars. The mucosa borne part can therefore move independently according to the compressibility of the mucosa.

This technique has been suggested as particularly useful in the treatment of the bilateral free-end saddle, where the support contribution of the remaining standing teeth is poor and their periodontal health also might be further compromised by a totally mucosally borne designed denture. The disadvantage of the denture is that it is technically difficult to construct and also that patients occasionally complain of it 'rattling' during function which is of course due to the principles inherent in its design.

(ii) By anterior placement of the occlusal rest

The distribution of load between the abutment teeth and residual ridge can sometimes be altered favourably by anterior placement of the occlusal rest (Fig. 11.8). This has the effect of altering stresses on the saddle from a Class I lever situation where the resistance to the applied load lies on the opposite side of the fulcrum, to a Class II lever where the resistance lies between the applied load and the fulcrum. This permits more even distribution of load and less stress on the abutment teeth. Systems which utilize this principle are the RPI system and the balance of force system.

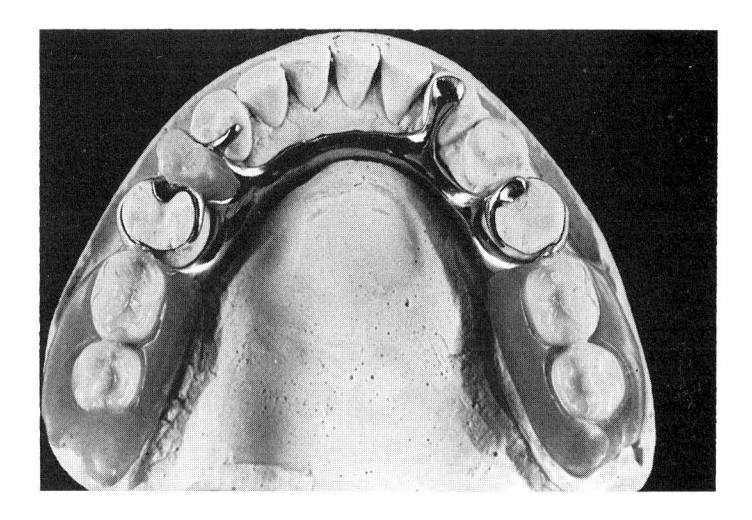

Fig. 11.8. Denture illustrating anterior placement of the occlusal rest.

(a) *The RPI system.* This system of partial denture design involving a clasp unit comprised of a rest, proximal plate and 'I'-bar retainer was developed in an attempt to overcome the problem of providing a rigid partial denture that was dependent upon two different types of support. It is therefore particularly applicable to the free-end saddle prosthesis deriving its support both from the natural teeth and the mucosa of the edentulous saddle areas.

An important consideration of this system is the positioning of the occlusal rest to provide the element of tooth support. If the rest is placed distally on the abutment tooth and load applied to the saddle, it has been demonstrated that the arc of movement of the denture base tends to be mainly perpendicular to the residual ridge in the posterior region. This is less apparent on moving anteriorly, however, until in the region near the abutment tooth the saddle movement is almost parallel to the ridge in an anterior direction. It is clear that in this situation the mucosa adjacent to the tooth can offer little resistance to the applied load, it and the gingival margin being likely to be traumatized by the horizontal movement of the denture against the abutment tooth. This area, where tooth support ends and mucosa support begins, should therefore be protected.

If the occlusal rest is placed mesially on the abutment teeth, it has been shown that the arc of movement of the saddle under applied load will alter and be more perpendicular to the mucosa throughout its length, due to the presence of a mesial rather than a distal fulcrum. This will increase the support provided by the mucosa whilst reducing the anterior movement of the saddle under applied load.

It should also be noted that when the saddle is loaded the abutment teeth will have a tendency to tilt to the side on which the rest is located. If the rest is placed distally then the tooth will tend to tilt distally, where it has little support. If it is placed mesially however, although there will be a tendency to mesial tilting of the abutment tooth, this will be resisted by other teeth in the arch anterior to it. The RPI system therefore incorporates a support unit which engages a rest seat prepared in the mesio-occlusal area of the abutment tooth, and which is connected to the main framework by a minor connector.

In addition to designing for support, stability and retention, potential damage to the gingival tissues distal to the abutment tooth can be lessened if the distal surface of the tooth is covered by a thin plate of cast metal (the proximal plate) which extends on to the soft tissues. This is relieved at the gingival margin where it joins the framework and is highly polished on its fitting surface. It will prevent contact of acrylic resin with the tooth and will be easier to keep clean. Wear and damage will also be limited and the metal will maintain a close adaptation so protecting the tissues from food packing and preventing gingival hypertrophy. In addition the plate should extend lingually on the proximal surface of the tooth in order to provide some reciprocation for the 'I'-bar clasp.

It has been argued that by constructing a conventional occlusally approaching clasp the external contour of the tooth is altered adversely, particularly in relation to natural stimulation of the gingivae and in food shedding. In addition many clasps will exert a leverage effect on the abutment tooth when the saddle is loaded. The use of a gingivally approaching 'I' bar clasp combined with a mesial occlusal rest will minimize interference with tooth contour and will also avoid stress on the tooth (Fig. 11.9). The bar should cross the gingival margin at right angles, being relieved from the soft tissues at the greatest mesiodistal prominence

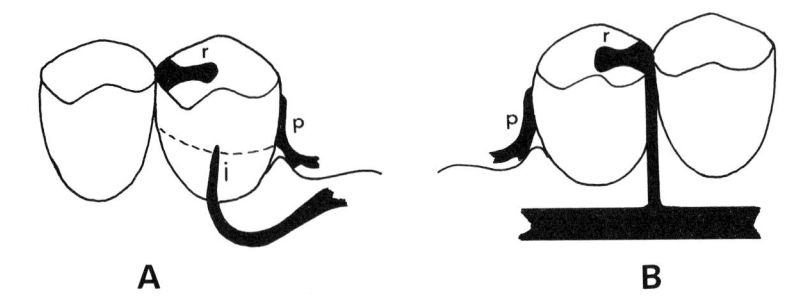

Fig. 11.9. Buccal (A) and lingual (B) views of the RPI system showing the rest (r), proximal plate (p), and I-bar clasp (i). Note the position of the minor connector on the lingual aspect.

on the buccal surface of the tooth tapering slightly towards its tip. If its tip is placed towards the mesial portion of the tooth it also serves to bring the proximal plate into tight contact with the distal surface. As the denture is depressed on to its basal seat the clasp will move forwards and downwards and out of contact with the tooth so removing any possibility of leverage.

The entire system (Fig. 11.9) is composed therefore of a mesial occlusal rest, a proximal plate and a gingivally approaching 'I' bar clasp arm (RPI). The mesial rest is linked to a minor connector which also provides some reciprocation and is placed in the mesio-lingual embrasure but free of the adjacent tooth anterior to it. With applied load to the saddle, the rest acts as a fulcrum point, ensuring mesial rather than distal loading of the abutment tooth. The proximal plate usually requires the preparation of a guide plane, which should extend from the junction of the occlusal and middle thirds of the proximal surface of the tooth on to the mucosal tissues. Under load it will be depressed tissuewards further into the undercut area without exerting torque or leverage on the abutment tooth. The 'I'-bar crosses the gingival margin at right angles and contacts the tooth in its gingival third and at the greatest mesiodistal prominence of the tooth, its precise position of contact being immediately below and above the survey line. Besides being retentive, it will move mesio-gingivally away from the tooth under applied load. As the 'I'-bar and proximal plate are free of the abutment tooth during saddle loading they will therefore reduce stress on the tooth.

The RPI system will result in a denture where there will be enhanced mucosal support due to perpendicular loading, reinforcement against mesial tilting of the abutment tooth, adequate retention with minimal effect on natural tooth contour, no adverse stress on the abutment tooth during masticatory loading, and protection of the transitional region between the tooth and the mucosal area of the edentulous saddle. It is therefore particularly suitable for the free-end saddle situation, although contra-indicated in cases where there is gingival recession and abnormally tilted teeth.

(b) *Balance of force system.* The balance of force system, can be considered as a further refinement of the RPI system being based on the mechanical principles of a Class II lever. As the magnitude of masticatory loads on the abutment teeth are much greater than those of the forces of displacement, and as the tooth is less able to withstand this, the design has been developed to ensure that loads during masticatory performance are directed vertically along the long axis of the tooth so avoiding torque and leverage. As the design evolved through an analysis of the force acting on the abutment tooth by the clasp arm it is essentially a principle of clasp design.

In the construction of such a denture tooth preparation is essential. A rest seat must be provided on the part of the occlusal surface of the abutment tooth that is distant from the saddle. This will act as the fulcrum point and ensure vertical loading on the tooth during function. In free-end saddle dentures this would be a mesially placed support unit. In addition to rest seat preparation an interproximal access area of about 1 mm must be created between the abutment tooth and the anterior tooth adjacent. It is in this area that reciprocation for the clasp arm will be positioned together with the minor connector.

The clasp unit is designed so that the retentive tip of the clasp arm is positioned on the interproximal surface of the abutment tooth adjacent to the edentulous saddle. It should lie below the maximum convexity of this surface engaging a degree of undercut according to the physical properties of the material. The reciprocation for the retentive force of the clasp arm in resisting displacement is provided by a vertical plate in the prepared access area on the mesial surface of the abutment tooth. The mesial rest, vertical reciprocation plate and clasp arm are joined by a minor connector running lingually on the abutment tooth above its maximum convexity. The vertical plate is joined to the major connector.

The unit should be so designed that the flexible tip of the clasp arm, the occlusal rest and the contact surface of the vertical reciprocating plate are in line with the crest of the edentulous ridge. Retention is therefore achieved mesio-distally as opposed to bucco-lingually and the design ensures that the greatest loads on the tooth are applied mesio-distally where it is well supported. Such a system of clasp design is shown diagrammatically in Fig. 11.10.

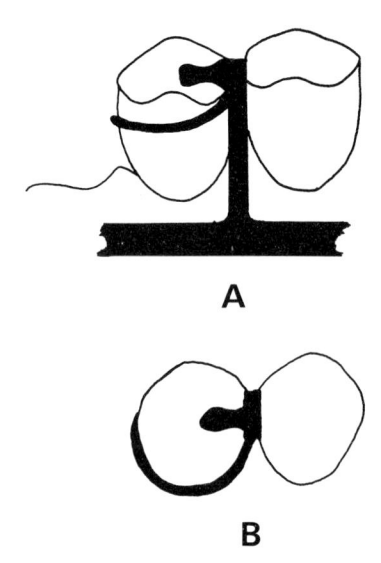

Fig. 11.10. Lingual (A) and occlusal (B) views of the clasp design used in the balance of force system. Note the interproximal access area with its minor connector and reciprocation plate, the proximally positioned clasp arm and the mesially placed occlusal rest.

When masticatory load is applied to the distal extension saddle its downward movement towards the underlying tissue is accompanied by a similar movement of the retentive tip of the clasp arm. This allows the clasp to disengage the tooth as it moves into an area of increased undercut, thus eliminating horizontal tooth loading. The mesial occlusal rest will direct loads vertically along the long axis of the tooth whence it is better able to withstand them.

If a displacing force is applied to the denture, the saddle and clasp tip once again move in the same direction occlusally. The clasp tip will now engage the proximal surface of the tooth below its maximum convexity thus providing resistance to further displacement. Reciprocation during this action is provided by the vertical interproximal plate on the opposite side of the tooth.

This system of denture construction demonstrates stability during masticatory function and retention against displacement whilst attempting to minimize damage to the abutment teeth. If greater retention is desired specific spring loaded denture attachments have been designed for use with this technique. In the United Kingdom and the United States of America dentures using the balance of force system are constructed under license and known as Equipoise™ designs.

(iii) By mucocompression

The third method of distributing the load suitably between abutment teeth and the edentulous ridge is by compressing the mucosa covering the ridge.

It is necessary at this stage to differentiate between mucostasis and mucocompression. A cast poured from a mucostatic impression represents the tissues as they are at rest. Such impressions are taken with materials of very low viscosity, when only a small amount of pressure is required for them to flow into every detail of the teeth and mucosal surfaces. In consequence, there is little or no displacement of the mucosa. Examples of such mucostatic impression materials are the low viscosity alginates.

On the other hand, a cast poured from a mucocompressive impression reproduces the tissues as they are under load. A mucocompressive impression is taken with a material which has a high viscosity. Consequently, more pressure is required and part of this force is directed through the more rigid material to the underlying mucosa which is displaced. However, the amount of displacement is not uniform throughout the mucosa, the tissues overlying the retromolar areas being displaced to a greater degree than those lying more anteriorly. There is also a tendency for the displacement to be maximal on the crest of the ridge as a result of the increased pressure which acts in this area.

Impression compound or zinc oxide paste in a close fitting tray may be used for a mucocompressive technique, either to take the working impression or in a rebasing method. The techniques are discussed later. The more viscous the paste used for taking the impression the more nearly will maximum displacement be approached. However, such a state is not ideal. The terms mucostatic and mucocompressive are only relative and do not refer to two fixed states. It is more accurate to regard impression techniques as effecting varying degrees of tissue displacement, the so-called mucostatic techniques showing minimal displacement, and the mucocompressive methods causing varying degrees of greater displacement.

The degree of tissue displacement achieved depends upon the viscosity of the material and its thickness. Alginates provide the least displacement and impression compound and zinc oxide pastes the most. Silicones and other elastomers are intermediate in their mucocompressive abilities.

Having established that different impression materials give varying degrees of mucosal displacement it is in order to consider the effects on the lower free-end saddle in particular. The saddle base fitted accurately against the mucosa from which tissue fluid has already been displaced, sinks less under the masticatory load than if fitted against an undisturbed mucosa. Therefore, the greater the amount of displacement the less is the magnitude of the torque and load on the abutment, when a vertical load is placed on the saddle.

It will be evident, too, that the amount of displacement affects the distribution of load between abutment and ridge bone. The greater the displacement the more evenly is the stress distributed between the abutment and the edentulous ridge.

It can be assumed that reduction of leverage and torque action and uniform loading of the edentulous ridge are desirable features to be gained by maximal displacement. However, the mucosa cannot be continuously subjected to such heavy pressure since this will result in decreased blood supply to, and drainage from, the soft tissues. Coupled with the fact that the tissue fluid is also reduced, this may result in a trophic disturbance. There is an inadequate supply of chemicals essential to the vitality of the cells and metabolites collect. These would eventually cause necrosis of the parts concerned, but long before this stage is reached pain is induced necessitating the removal of the denture. This pain is also caused by direct pressure on the nerve endings in the submucosa.

The natural tendency of the displaced tissue is to recoil in a visco-elastic manner. In assuming that the saddle is maintained in the closest approximation with the displaced mucosa, the presence of some force to hold it in this position is also assumed. This force can only come from rigid clasping of the abutment tooth and results in a continuous force acting on the abutment. The fact that its magnitude is small is offset by its continuous nature.

It is thus seen that the use of rigid connection and clasping together with maximum displacement leads to an unacceptable situation in respect of potential damage to the abutment and covering mucosa. If maximum displacement is to be used, arrangement must be made to allow some recoil of the mucosal tissues. This can be achieved either by very light clasping, generally wrought gold wires of thin gauge, or by a stress breaker giving flexible connection between the saddles and retainer units.

The writers never use the method of maximum displacement coupled with light clasping directly attached to the saddles for the following reasons:

- The retention of such a denture is inadequate because of the light clasping and poor adhesion, the latter being due to the uneven thickness of saliva film between the mucosa and the fitting surface of the denture after recoil of the tissues.
- Lateral stresses are resisted largely by the edentulous ridge, which is, therefore, liable to resorb.

At the other extreme, with mucostasis, even when cast clasps are directly attached to the saddles, no forces act either on the ridge or abutment when the saddle is not under load. In the resting state, too, adhesion is maximal. Mucostatic impression techniques are simple, and provided manufacturer's instructions are carried out, good results are obtainable even by those whose experience is limited.

With such a technique and where rigid clasping directly attached to the saddle is used, maximal leverage and torque is placed on the abutment teeth, which are, therefore, predisposed to periodontal breakdown. The amount of downward movement of the saddle posteriorly can be marked where the tissues are easily displaceable and results in the patient having a sense of insecurity when using the denture. With this type of impression, too, the bone is not evenly stressed, the areas underlying thinner and firmer mucosa receiving an increased share of the load.

There is, however, a condition intermediate between maximum displacement and mucostasis, that has considerable advantages. If a small amount of displacement is effected under a free-end saddle, the amount of tissuewards movement which can be produced when vertical pressure is applied is reduced considerably. This has the effect of reducing leverage and torque in the abutment tooth if the clasp is attached directly to the saddle. It would appear that when only a small amount of tissue fluid is displaced and the pressure exerted against the blood vessels is not marked there is no trophic disturbance, and the complication of pain is not clinically evident. Thus a compromise between stasis and maximum displacement seems to give a result with the advantages of each present to some degree.

It is realized that the preceding discussion of mucocompression and mucostasis is very theoretical. In practice it is difficult to secure the correct amount of tissue displacement for any particular case, but the techniques that may be employed for this purpose will be discussed later.

3 Wide Distribution of Load

The third general way of preserving the teeth and ridges in an optimal state of health is by distributing the load widely.

(i) Wide distribution of load over the teeth

The vertical load cannot readily be distributed over more than one tooth on each side of the arch because of the rotation which takes place about an axis through the two most posteriorly placed occlusal rests on each side when the saddles are loaded vertically. Some degree of distribution does, however, take place in the method illustrated (Fig. 11.11).

When clinical circumstances permit, the procedure is to move the occlusal rest anteriorly so that it lies not on the tooth that immediately bounds the saddle, but on the occlusal surface of the tooth that lies immediately anterior. If a rest is placed on this tooth some of the vertical load is placed upon it and its marginal ridge becomes the fulcrum point. If two flexible arms now arise from this and encompass the buccal and lingual surfaces of the posterior tooth, and if these arms lie above the survey lines then some of the vertical load is dispersed. Part is dissipated in opening the clasp arms and part is directed down the long axis of the tooth. The retaining clasp is on the rested tooth, which accepts vertical load through the occlusal rest. Lateral load is distributed to the two teeth by the clasp arms.

(ii) Wide distribution of load over the ridge

The saddles of the denture should always cover the largest possible area, so that the pressure falling on any unit area of the edentulous ridge is reduced under vertical and horizontal loading. Whilst full coverage over the retromolar area and the buttress bone both buccally and lingually is desirable for load distribution it may not always be acceptable to the patient. In addition distal coverage may lead to denture displacement due to action of the lower fibres of the temporalis. It is not uncommon to have to undertake reduction of such extensions to produce a denture that corresponds more to the dimensions of the natural teeth and mucosa which has been lost.

Pain

The deleterious effects of stress on the abutment teeth and alveolar ridge have been discussed in order to emphasize the long-term importance of tissue preservation. However, from the viewpoint of the patient, pain when the denture is

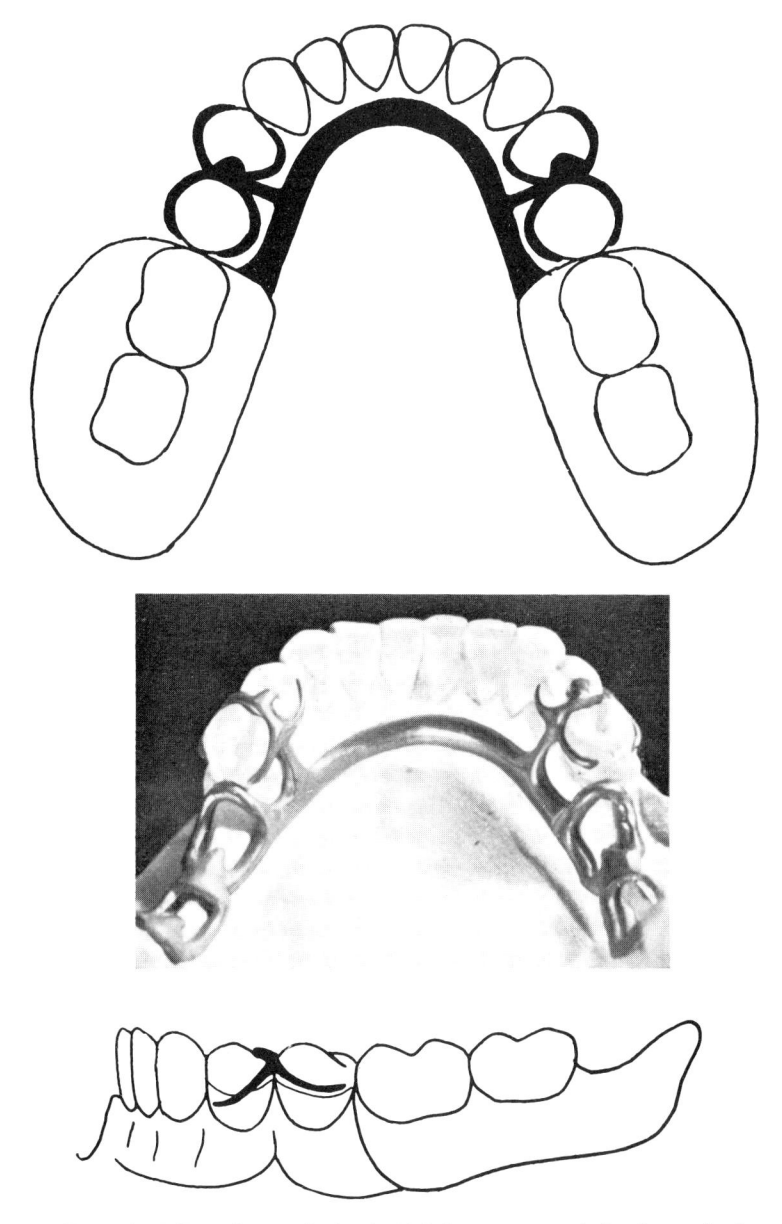

The Bilateral Free-end Saddle (Kennedy Class I) 311

Fig. 11.11. Distributing the load widely by a compound clasping method.

worn may be a more immediate complication. It is often so severe as to necessitate removal of the denture and many bilateral free-end saddle lower dentures are never worn again after a short period when pain was marked and continuous.

Pain may be experienced when the alveolar ridge is covered by a thin atrophic mucosa and submucosa. Generally pain is located posteriorly and lingually over the alveolar ridge where the thickness of soft tissue is minimal. The area involved is usually the mylo-hyoid ridge but is sometimes the more superior edge of the lingual plate of cortical bone. These areas are first traumatized in the power strokes of mastication when the pain is most marked; later, however, the pain becomes continuous. When a patient with such a condition is eating he directs his whole conscious attention to the act; it is a 'main act' and in no sense automatic as it is normally. Moreover it is apparent both from visual observation and electro-myographic records that a testing contraction precedes the comminuting contraction to ensure that the traumatic effect is bearable.

Two methods of treatment may be used for this painful condition. The first is the surgical removal of the bony prominences. However there are many contra-indications to surgery and it is always better to avoid surgical interference if possible. The prosthetic approach is the use of a resilient lining on the fitting surface of the saddles. The principle used is that the resilient layer, being no longer present in the atrophied tissues, is replaced over the fitting surface of the denture saddle. This layer absorbs energy in its compression when load is applied to the saddle and it also serves to distribute the load over all the bone-bearing area rather than concentrate it over the sharp bony ridges.

It is inevitable that some small degree of downward saddle displacement is introduced when saddles with soft linings are brought into occlusion with an intervening bolus of food. This is to some extent counteracted by the use of a paste impression effecting some displacement; its amount is however limited by the atrophic nature of the covering tissues. The approach of choice is to limit the downward saddle rotation by using the minimal thickness of soft material that will be effective in reducing the pain, increasing its thickness locally where sharp ridges of bone are noted. The method should only be used with a design which allows an intermediate amount of independent saddle movement in relation to the ridge.

Two technical points require emphasis with regard to this method. The bond strength of some of the silicone soft lining materials to acrylic resin is not as strong as is desirable. To overcome any tendency for the soft layer to be pulled away from the underlying resin the periphery of the saddle should always be formed of hard resin; a boxed-in effect is therefore secured. The abrasive resistance of these materials is lower than that of a hard resin; cleaning should therefore be limited to rinsing under running water and no brushing should be carried out on this surface.

Pain associated with an abutment tooth is a complication that may occur after a bilateral free-end saddle lower denture has been worn for a period of time. It usually results from a load in excess of the physiological limit being applied to the tooth by the relative clasp arm or by the occlusal rest.

When the gingivae are covered by any component of a partial denture, they are liable to become inflamed. This is particularly true of the gingivae on the distal and lingual aspects of the abutment teeth of free-end saddle lower dentures. It is a reaction which follows the slight loss of fit of the saddles which in turn produces slight movement of the anterior end of the saddle against the abutment gingivae. The prevention of such a situation developing is dependent upon adequate and frequent rebasing of the saddles.

The Necessity for the Regular Inspection of the Free-end Saddle Denture

The regular inspection of all bilateral free-end saddle partial dentures is important for two reasons. First, it is necessary to check the position of clasp arms and verify that they have neither been displaced in such a way as to lie out of contact with the enamel, nor are exerting a continuous force, instead of lying in passive contact with the tooth. The necessity for this inspection is more marked with long arm, gingivally approaching types of clasp than with the occlusally approaching variety. If the denture is stress broken by a flexible connector then its position must be examined regularly. The danger of displacement is greater with the more resilient wrought wire than with the cast connector. Precision attachments must be checked for wear and for the tension of springs when these are present.

Second, it is important to assess whether rebasing of the saddles is necessary. The results of failure to rebase free-end saddle dentures constitute a menacing complication. The end result of negligence in this direction has too often been attributed to an inherent weakness in the principle of construction, whether that be stress breaking or rigid connection. The tendency for saddle movement to occur under vertical and horizontal loading is due to displacement of the soft tissues covering the ridge. Normally the degree of displacement is small but it is increased when, after ridge resorption, a space exists between the fitting surface of the saddle and the ridge. Consequently, the leverage and torque acting on the abutment and its surrounding gingivae become magnified and can enter the pathological range. The energy released on to the ridge is also increased by the more kinetic nature of the force applied by the saddle. Timely and efficient rebasing of the saddles is essential to preserve the ridge, the abutment teeth and the gingivae in a healthy state.

Rebasing should not be deferred until the patient complains of either ridge soreness or failing ability to manage the denture. A slight rotational movement about the occlusal rests as elicited by light pressure on the saddles, is the indication when no stress breaker has been used. The sensation is not visual but tactile and is developed as a result of experience. When a stress breaker has been used the decision is more difficult. After an assessment has been made of the displaceability of the ridge tissues by palpation, the stability of the free-end saddle to vertical pressure is tested. Once again only experience can teach the amount of movement that is indicative of the need for rebasing. The need for regular inspection of saddles which have a resilient lining is even more necessary than with those made of acrylic resin. The danger of the ridge resorbing remains the same but there is the additional hazard that the lining may be abraded thereby increasing the discrepancy between saddle and ridge forms.

Modifications of the Bilateral Free-end Saddle Lower Denture

The bilateral free-end saddle lower is seen more frequently than its modifications. However, two modifications occur often enough to warrant special consideration.

The first is where an anterior saddle is present in addition to the two free-end saddles. A variable number of anterior teeth may be missing and molar replacements will be required posteriorly. The anterior saddle displays some of the difficulties encountered with a free-end saddle. Although the saddle is, strictly speaking, bounded, the abutments both lie posterior to the saddle. In other words, the anterior extremity of the saddle cannot, under masticatory stress, be supported by teeth and consequently is partly mucosa borne. During incision this saddle is displaced downwards at its anterior extremity, and a rotation of the denture takes place about its rested abutments. The stress on the abutment teeth, if these are clasped, depends on the saddle length and shape as well as on the displaceability of the mucosa overlying the ridge. How far the mesio-incisal point lies in front of the fulcrum line through the rested abutments depends on the length and shape of the edentulous arch (Fig. 11.12). The greater the distance, the greater is the stress acting on the clasped abutments, and the greater the danger to the teeth. The longer the saddle and the more tapering its form, the

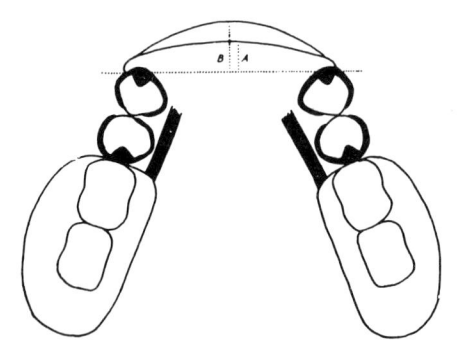

Fig. 11.12. The effect of the arch shape on the relationship of the mesio-incisal point to the fulcrum axis.

greater is this distance, while the shorter the saddle and the more square its form, the less is this distance. Since, in practice, such saddles are usually short, square in form and overlie a relatively firm mucosa, the danger to the abutments during incision is not so marked as when load is placed upon the posterior free-end saddles. This applies equally when lateral stresses are considered.

In such cases a rigid construction is advisable. By clasping the four abutment teeth, vertical and horizontal forces are resisted by two teeth on each side, thus facilitating wide distribution of load.

It is necessary to consider a variation of this modification where bilaterally only the two natural premolars remain. A design used in such cases is shown in Fig. 11.13 where lingual bars and continuous clasps have been used, the purpose of the latter being to distribute lateral load. They may be replaced by cast lingual plates when indicated. The clasps are constructed in wrought wire, but where the ridges are well formed and covered by a firm mucosa they may be constructed in cast alloy. A complication exists when the premolars on both sides are instanding. When the lingual inclination is severe, buccal bars may replace the lingual bars, back action clasps arising from common struts attached thereto (Fig. 11.14).

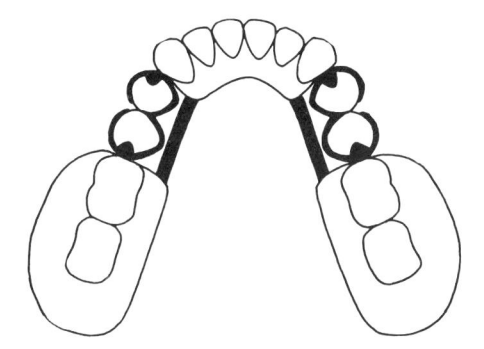

Fig. 11.13. A design used in a Kennedy Class I, modification 1, partial lower. The clasping is of gold and the lingual bar of wrought stainless steel wire.

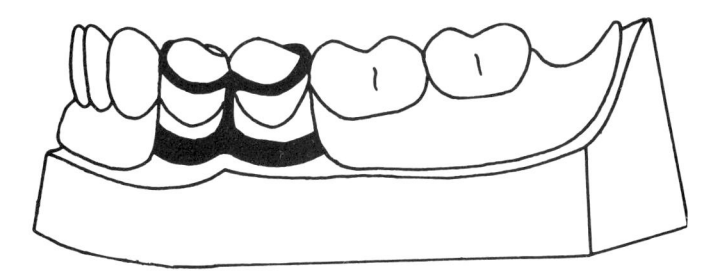

Fig. 11.14. The use of reverse back action clasps and a buccal bar in a Class I, modification 1, partial lower denture, where the teeth are lingually inclined.

The final variation of this modification is where only two canines remain. As stated earlier the retention of these teeth in order to stabilize the lower denture is a desirable form of treatment, even if it is certain that it is only a temporary measure. In such circumstances a simple acrylic resin mucosa supported denture can be constructed. If the canines require extraction at a later date it is simple to convert this into an immediate complete lower denture. If the supporting structures of the teeth are satisfactory and the root canals negotiable, endodontic treatment can be undertaken and the coronal portion of the tooth removed. A simple overdenture can then be constructed. Where retention is a problem intraradicular attachments or magnetic retention units can be incorporated into such an appliance.

The second variety of modified bilateral free-end saddle denture which requires consideration is where an otherwise long free-end saddle is interrupted by a single standing tooth. A typical instance is where a second premolar remains as the only tooth posterior to the standing canine. It may sometimes be advisable to extract a single standing tooth to avoid a single tooth saddle, but if the supporting tissues are healthy it should usually be retained for the following reasons:

- It reduces the length of the free-end saddle, thereby reducing the moment of the leverage or torque acting on the abutment tooth under vertical and lateral load.
- Some of the masticatory load falls directly on a natural tooth.
- Since clasping and resting are permitted on two abutment teeth wider distribution of load is possible.

A typical design for such a case is illustrated in Fig. 11.15.

In the less common situation when a molar is a single standing tooth, it will often be sensible to dispense with the small free-end saddle posterior to the tooth. In the case illustrated (Fig. 11.16) no natural tooth in the upper jaw opposed the left lower molar region.

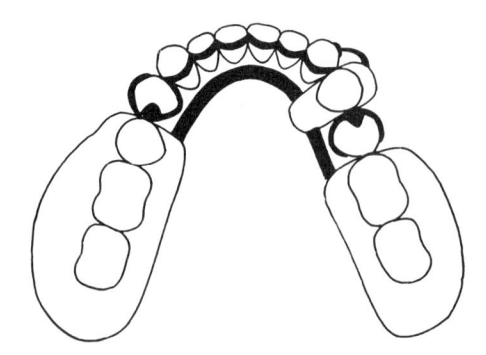

Fig. 11.15. A design often used for a Class I, modification 1, partial lower denture with an interrupted long saddle. The clasping is in wrought wire.

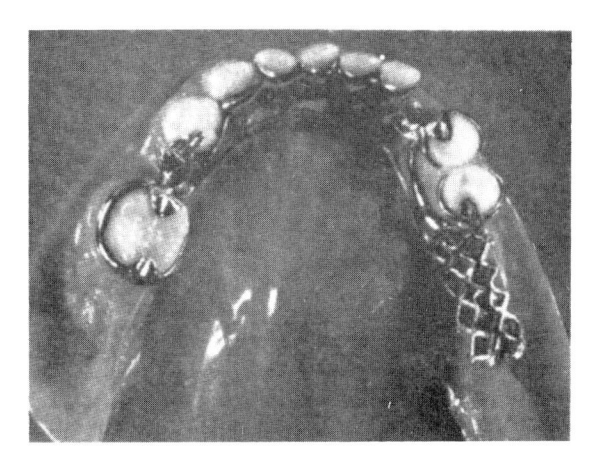

Fig. 11.16. A short edentulous area distal to a single standing molar not replaced by a denture saddle.

The Bilateral Free-end Saddle Upper Denture

The basic problems encountered with bilateral free-end saddle upper dentures are similar to those found with lowers. However, these cases do not occur so frequently in the upper as in the lower jaw.

As in the lower jaw, when the teeth come into occlusion the saddles sink posteriorly more than anteriorly; however, this tendency is less marked in the upper for two reasons. First, the submucosa covering the upper tuberosity generally has a denser fibrous structure than that of the retromolar area in the mandible. Second, additional area is provided by palatal coverage and this reduces the pressure, and consequently the displacement under the masticatory load. Thus, under equivalent conditions the stress applied to a clasped abutment tooth in the upper is less than in the lower.

Under vertical load, before the teeth have come into occlusion and are still separated by a bolus of food, there will be no tendency for antero-posterior displacement of the denture provided the occlusal plane lies approximately parallel to the edentulous ridge. In the rare cases where this is not so, the denture may be forced anteriorly or posteriorly. For example, if the plane is low posteriorly then the denture will be displaced in that direction. Factors which also affect antero-posterior movement are the shape of the palate and the prominence of the tuberosities. Obviously posterior displacement is not likely if there is a prominent tuberosity.

Due to the inclined plane action of the teeth during movement in occlusion from a lateral to the tooth position, there is a lateral movement of the saddle. Its direction is, however, opposite to that in the lower. Similar structures resist the displacement, with the important addition of any rigid component of the denture which covers the palate on the side where mastication is taking place. Resistance to lateral movement is shared over a greater area of bone and hence the lateral load falling on the supporting structures of the clasped abutment tooth is less than it may be in the lower jaw. In moving from protrusion to the tooth position, with the teeth in occlusion, the inclined plane action of the cusps tends to cause an anterior movement of the upper denture. This may be effectively resisted by the anterior teeth, a favourable condition when compared with the lower, where the movement is backward and unresisted by standing teeth. When the opposing cuspal inclines approximate at the end of a power stroke the saddles are displaced posteriorly. Resistance to this movement comes from clasped premolar or canine teeth which should be encompassed sufficiently by the clasps to assure stability of the appliance. For this purpose circumferential clasps are better than those of the bar type.

The upper jaw presents a more favourable condition for denture support than the lower jaw in view of its different bony architecture. The maxillary bone has a thinner cortical plate than the lower jaw but shows a spongiosum with more closely related trabeculae. It is considered that when stress is applied by a saddle the physiological limit of the bone in the upper is higher than in the lower.

Against these favourable factors is the disadvantage that retention presents a greater problem than in the lower. This is sometimes insurmountable and consideration may have to be given to more sophisticated treatment such as the use of intracoronal attachments or implant therapy, or even in some cases extraction followed by a complete denture. In the upper the weight of the appliance acts as a displacing rather than a retaining force as it does in the lower. This is particularly so when the denture is made of metal and is consequently heavier. The retention of this class of denture can only be effected through the combination of direct and indirect methods.

The use of direct retention is not always a simple matter. The aesthetic wishes of the patient must be considered and patients often refuse to wear a denture which shows any clasping. This creates a problem not necessarily confined to canines but extending back in some cases to the second premolar. The use of bar clasps lying in the closest admissible relationships to the gingival margin can often solve this difficulty provided some component such as an embrasure hook placed more anteriorly is also used to prevent posterior displacement of the denture.

Indirect retention is more necessary with the upper than with the lower Class I denture. To the displacing forces acting on the saddle, whether they act through a sticky bolus of food or through muscular action at the periphery, must be added the weight of the denture. Indirect retention is obtainable in these cases by the following methods:
- continuous clasp

- Cummer arms
- anterior extension of the palatal bar
- anterior palatal bar
- extension of any palatal plate to cover the rugae.

It will be appreciated that these possibilities offer varying chances of success. The most efficient indirect retention will be achieved by a component placed as far anteriorly as possible and resting preferably on tooth structure rather than on the rugae area of the hard palate; however, in some instances this tissue may be very resistant to displacement. Two factors which may modify the type of indirect retention, or even nullify its use, are lack of tolerance and a deep anterior vertical overlap. The latter complication often prevents the use of a continuous clasp.

Every precaution should be taken to ensure that the denture as a whole fits accurately. However, it is not possible to use soft tissue displacement throughout the peripheral length of the denture and consequently the positive retention that may be developed in a full denture cannot be employed. Some adhesive force should be developed as an additional aid to retention and the denture must be kept as light as possible, and its centre of gravity kept as far anteriorly as possible so that the weight lying posterior to the clasped teeth will be reduced. This contra-indicates broad posterior palatal coverage and the use of posterior palatal bars, and indicates thin anterior palatal plates.

The same general principles that governed the lower, apply to the upper in respect of occlusal table size, selection of impression method, necessity for early rebasing, and wide distribution of load. Where premolars are the abutment teeth, bar or wrought wire clasps buccally, together with rigid cast palatal arms lying above the survey line are the methods selected to permit a slight movement of the clasp arms over the surface of the teeth.

Modifications of the Bilateral Free-end Saddle Upper Denture

As in the equivalent lower, two modifications occur frequently. In the first a single standing tooth, very often an upper second premolar, converts what would otherwise be a long free-end saddle into a more readily manageable shorter saddle. Again, the retention of such a tooth, if it is healthy, is to be commended. These cases are treated by a rigid design and the gingival margin of the single standing tooth is covered by a relieved palatal plate.

The second common modification is where one, or more, of the anterior natural teeth are missing. In general, the design used in these cases follows the principles laid down for an unmodified bilateral free-end denture and the additional tooth or teeth is carried on the palatal plate or on a continuous clasp.

Another modification is a case displaying a series of single tooth saddles separated by single standing teeth. There is often evidence for extracting some or all of these teeth, but treatment must be decided upon individual factors, not least among these being the patient's opinion as to whether they wish to retain the teeth or not. If no teeth are to be removed a horse-shoe-shaped metal base covering the hard palate is often the treatment of choice. Clinically it has been found that the tissue reaction, and in particular the gingival health, under such dentures, remains excellent, provided the patient maintains good oral hygiene. Dentures of this type should be adequately tooth supported and the retention augmented by suitable clasping. Whilst metal is to be preferred for this type of denture on the grounds of strength and oral health, acrylic resin can also be used, but care should be taken to protect the gingival margins.

If, for some reason, adequate tooth support cannot be provided, then the denture will have to be of the mucosa-borne variety. This type of design must result ultimately in some gingival damage, but owing to the resistance of the hard palate the effect is likely to be less serious and much longer delayed in the upper jaw than in the lower.

The Swing Lock Denture

The term swing lock describes a specific design of partial denture which can be used in any situation in the mouth, but is particularly useful where there has been loss of a considerable number of teeth. As such it is perhaps most appropriate to include it within the chapter on the bilateral free-end saddle, although it is possible to use it in other situations.

The appliance is designed with a rigid lingual or palatal plate connector to which is attached, by means of a hinge, a labial or buccal bar. This bar is placed in the sulcus and has struts of 'fingers' extending to contact the labial or buccal surfaces of the natural teeth below the survey line, so providing retention. The depth of undercut engaged is relatively unimportant as, due to the nature of the design, the retentive struts do not pass over the maximum convexity of the tooth on insertion. Occasionally for aesthetic reason the struts are replaced by an acrylic veneer (Fig. 11.17).

The labial bar or acrylic veneer is designed to pivot on its hinge in the manner of a gate. The denture is inserted with the 'gate' open and when it is closed it is fastened to the main framework by means of a latch or lock positioned on the opposite side of the arch from the hinge. The framework and bar is constructed in cast cobalt chromium alloy, with the hinge and lock attachments provided as preformed plastic patterns which are invested and cast in metal in the normal fashion.

The principle behind this type of denture is that it allows wide distribution of stress during function to all remaining teeth and residual ridges rather than to just a few abutments. When the appliance is inserted and locked into position the

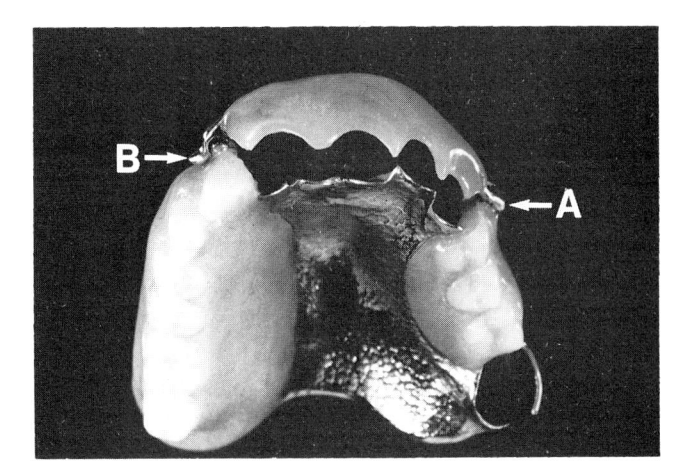

Fig. 11.17. An upper swinglock partial denture with a labial acrylic veneer. The veneer pivots open at its hinge (A) to allow the denture to be inserted. Once the denture is in position the veneer is closed and locked (B).

enclosed natural teeth are held rigidly in a fixed position. This has a splinting or stabilizing action on these teeth which may have often a poor periodontal condition, or be particularly unsuitable for isolated loading due to their anatomical form. The splinting therefore spreads the applied load allowing it to be shared, and also resists tipping and rotation of the appliance. Additional occlusal support may be achieved by the use of rests, and retention is gained from the labial struts or acrylic veneer.

The principles involved in the construction of a swing lock denture are the same as for any partial denture. It should be noted however that in order to be effective the lock and hinge units on opposite sides of the cast must be placed at the same height. Due to its rigidity and methods of load distribution, stress broken designs are deemed unnecessary, although it has been suggested that an altered cast technique should be used in its construction. If rests are used, these should be placed on the mesial aspect of the most distal abutment for reasons discussed earlier. The retentive element of the denture must be positive which means that the labial struts must contact the surface of the teeth when the denture is inserted. If they do not, rotation and movement of the appliance may occur. In this respect it may be necessary to adjust them from time to time to maintain a constant relationship with the reciprocating element of the denture.

This denture is therefore suitable for use in compromised clinical situations, and is particularly useful where only a few teeth remain and load distribution may be a problem due to mobility or inadequate periodontal support. It can also be used where it is difficult to develop sufficient denture retention by means of a conventional design, where unfavourable undercuts exist, and where the necks of the teeth are exposed resulting in unfavourable aesthetics. Its use is contraindicated where a poor standard of oral hygiene exists, or where there is a lack of sulcus depth for positioning of the hinged bar. In this respect some 6–8 mm of sulcus depth is required together with 2–4 mm of attached gingivae.

The use of the swing-lock denture is, to some extent, still somewhat controversial. Although not suitable, nor even required, for every case it is a useful addition to the clinical armamentarium.

References

APPLEGATE O.C. and NISSLE R.O. (1951) Keeping the partial denture in harmony with biological limitations. *J. Amer. dent. Ass.* **43**, 409–19.
BASKER R.M., HARRISON A. and RALPH J.P. (1983) Overdentures in general dental practice. 2: Indications for overdentures: patient selection. *Brit. dent. J.* **154**, 321.
BECKER C.M. and BOLENDER C.L. (1981) Designing swinglock partial dentures. *J. pros. Dent.* **46**, 126.
BECKETT L.S. (1940) Some fundamentals of partial denture construction. *Aus. J. Dent.* **44**, 365–7.
BERG T. (1984) I-bar; myth and countermyth. *D. Clin. N. A.* **28**, 371.
BOLENDER C.L. and BECKER C.M. (1981) Swinglock removable partial dentures; where and when. *J. pros. Dent.* **45**, 4.
BRILL N. (1955) Adaptation and the hybrid-prosthesis. *J. pros. Dent.* **5**, 811.
CECCONI B.T., ASGAR K. and DOOTZ E. (1971) The effect of partial denture clasp design on abutment tooth movement. *J. pros. Dent.* **25**, 44.
CECCONI B.T., ASGAR K. and DOOTZ E. (1971) Removable partial denture abutment tooth movement as affected by inclination of residual ridges and type of loading. *J. pros. Dent.* **25**, 375.
CECCONI B.T., ASGAR K. and DOOTZ E. (1972) Clasp assembly modifications and their effect on abutment tooth movement. *J. pros. Dent.* **27**, 160.
CHRISTIDOU L., OSBORNE J. and CHAMBERLAIN J.B. (1973) An investigation into the effects of partial denture design on the mobility of abutment teeth. *Brit. dent. J.* **135**, 9.
CLARKE D.A. and MURPHY W.M. (1973) The swinglock partial removable denture. *Dent. Tech.* **26**, 77.
DE VAN M.M. (1952) The nature of the partial denture foundations; suggestions for its preservation. *J. pros. Dent.* **2**, 210–18.
DOLDER E.J. (1961) The bar joint mandibular denture. *J. pros. Dent.* **11**, 689.
FRECHETTE A.R. (1951) Partial denture planning with special reference to stress distribution. *J. pros. Dent.* **1**, 700–7.
GEISSLER P.R. and WATT D.M. (1965) Disjunct dentures for patients with teeth of poor prognosis. *Dent. Pract.* **15**, 421.
GILLINGS B.R.D. (1981) Magnetic retention for complete and partial overdentures. Part I. *J. pros. Dent.* **45**, 484.
GOODMAN J.J. and GOODMAN H.W. (1963) Balance of force in precision free-end restorations. *J. pros. Dent.* **13**, 302.
GOODMAN J.J. and GOODMAN H. (1968) The C and L attachment—a functional retentive device. *Ann. Dent.* **27**, 49.

JONES R.R. (1952) The lower partial denture. *J. pros. Dent.* **2**, 219–29.
KRATOCHVIL F.J. (1963) Influence of occlusal rest position and clasp design on movement of abutment teeth. *J. pros. Dent.* **13**, 114.
KROL A.J. (1973) Clasp design for extension-base removable partial dentures. *J. pros. Dent.* **29**, 408.
KROL A.J. (1973) RPI (Rest, Proximal Plate, I-Bar) clasp retainer and its modifications. *D. Clin. N. A.* **17**, 631.
KYDD W.L., DUTTON D.A. and SMITH D.W. (1964) Lateral forces exerted on abutment teeth by partial dentures. *J. Amer. dent. Ass.* **68**, 859.
KYDD W.L., DALY C.H. and WHEELER J.B. (1971) The thickness measurements of masticatory mucosa *in vivo. Int. dent. J.* **21**, 430.
LAIRD W.R.E, SMITH G.A. and GRANT A.A. (1981) The use of magnetic forces in prosthetic dentistry. *J. Dent.* **9**, 328.
LAMMIE G.A. and STORER R. (1958) A preliminary report on resilient denture plastics. *J. pros. Dent.* **8**, 411–24.
LANE R.P. (1947) Practical stress breaking in partial dentures. *Dent. J. Aust.* **19**, 314–22.
LOOS A. (1950) Bio-physiological principles in the construction of partial dentures. *Brit. dent. J.* **88**, 61–8.
MACGREGOR A.R., MILLER T.P.G. and FARAH J.W. (1978) Stress analysis of partial dentures. *J. Dent.* **6**, 125.
PARFITT G.J. (1960) Measurement of the physiological mobility of individual teeth in an axial direction. *J. dent. Res.* **39**, 608.
PREISKEL H.W. (1969) *Precision attachments in dentistry.* 3rd Ed. Henry Kimpton Ltd, London.
SCHULTE F.D. and SMITH D.E. (1980) Clinical evaluation of swinglock removable partial dentures. *J. pros. Dent.* **44**, 595.
SHOHET H. (1969) Relative magnitude of stress on abutment teeth with different retainers. *J. pros. Dent.* **21**, 267.
SMITH G.A., LAIRD W.R.E. and GRANT A.A. (1983) Magnetic retention units for over-dentures. *J. Oral Rehab.* **10**, 481.
STEFEL V.L. (1951) Fundamental principles involved in partial denture design. *J. Amer. dent. Ass.* **41**, 534–44.
STEFEL V.L. (1963) Clasp partial dentures. *J. Amer. dent. Ass.* **66**, 803.
TAYLOR R.L. (1948) Partial denture prosthesis—principles of design. *Aust. J. Dent.* **52**, 30–2.
WATT D.M. (1958) A preliminary investigation of the support of partial dentures and its relation to vertical loads. *Dent. Pract.* **9**, 2.
WATT D.M. and MACGREGOR A.R. (1985) *Designing partial dentures.* John Wright & Sons Ltd, Bristol.
WILLS D.J. and MANDERSON R.D. (1977) Biochemical aspects of the support of partial dentures. *J. Dent.* **5**, 310.
WILSON J.H. (1949) Partial denture construction, some aspects of diagnosis and design. *Dent. J. Aust.* **21**, 347–63.
WRIGHT W.H. (1951) Partial denture prosthesis; a preventive oral health service. *J. Amer. dent. Ass.* **43**, 163–8.

12

THE UNILATERAL FREE-END SADDLE DENTURE
(KENNEDY CLASS II)

The main problem with the unilateral free-end saddle (Kennedy Class II) denture is the same as with the bilateral free-end saddle denture. As a free-end saddle it must accept part of the vertical and lateral loads, and there are the same relative differences in displaceability at each end of the saddle area.

The fact that a similar saddle is not present on the other side of the mouth may complicate the problem of retention. In bilateral situations the presence of a saddle on the other side increases the retention by adhesion, by the retentive action of the tongue and buccinator muscles on the polished surfaces, and by the additional weight. In order that the retention of the unilateral free-end saddle denture may be equal to that of the bilateral, additional retention must be provided on the side where the arch is complete. It is obtained by clasping more than one tooth on this side, and by using the more rigid types of clasp.

As far as design is concerned unmodified unilateral free-end saddle dentures divide into two groups, depending on the nature and length of the edentulous ridge and the condition of the abutment.

The first group can be dealt with by combining relatively rigid clasping of the abutment tooth with rigid connection between the saddle and this retainer. There are two indications for this type of design.

First, the very short saddle is such an indication, where the majority of mastication occurs on the side where all the natural teeth are standing. Even longer saddles may only receive a balancing load during the final stage of mastication. Consequently, rigid clasping, together with rigid connection between clasp and saddle, can be considered practical with a longer saddle in a unilateral case than in a bilateral. Given a sound periodontal situation the design shown in Fig. 12.1 will usually be satisfactory.

The second indication is where the ridge is prominent and the mucosa is of normal thickness. Hence there is little saddle displacement on loading. These conditions are not uncommon and are most frequent in young adults. The extractions have often been caused by caries which has affected the teeth on one side, teeth which have been supported in well developed bone with no periodontal disease. The bone factor therefore, is very favourable, and as a result

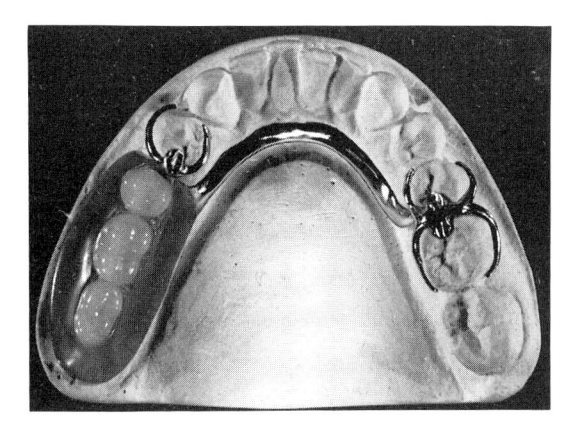

Fig. 12.1. A typical unilateral free-end saddle lower denture with rigid clasping and a rigid connector between clasp and saddle.

rigid clasping and rigid connection of saddle and retainer can be safely recommended.

The second group are the less common cases where the condition of the abutment, the length of the saddle, and the displaceability of the mucosa, contra-indicate the above approach. Since, to give adequate retention, rigid clasping is necessary on the side where the arch is intact, there is no possibility of the lingual bar, or other connector, being rotated upwards as the saddle is displaced into compressible tissue under vertical loading. Therefore, a wrought wire clasp, which would allow some rotation of the appliance about the abutment tooth, has not the same application with unilateral free-end saddle dentures since rotation of the appliance as a whole cannot take place.

Thus, the treatment of choice where it is considered unwise to use the rigid type of appliance, is to connect the saddle and retainer unit by a flexible or semi-flexible connector. Two alternative designs may be considered.

The first is more applicable with shorter saddles as it involves anterior placement of the occlusal rest, generally on the first pre-molar on the side where the saddle is required. This tooth is clasped and joined to the clasping system of the opposite side by a lingual bar of sufficient thickness to give rigidity. The saddle is joined to this retainer unit by a semi-flexible bar whose slight resilience allows some movement in relation to the rigid retainer unit (Fig. 12.2). In this case the thinner section lingual bar attached to the saddle allows some stress-breaking action.

The second design is a split casting modifying a lingual plate. A split of appropriate length is made at the inferior border of the plate and to the lower more flexible bar thus created, the saddle is joined, while the clasp on the same

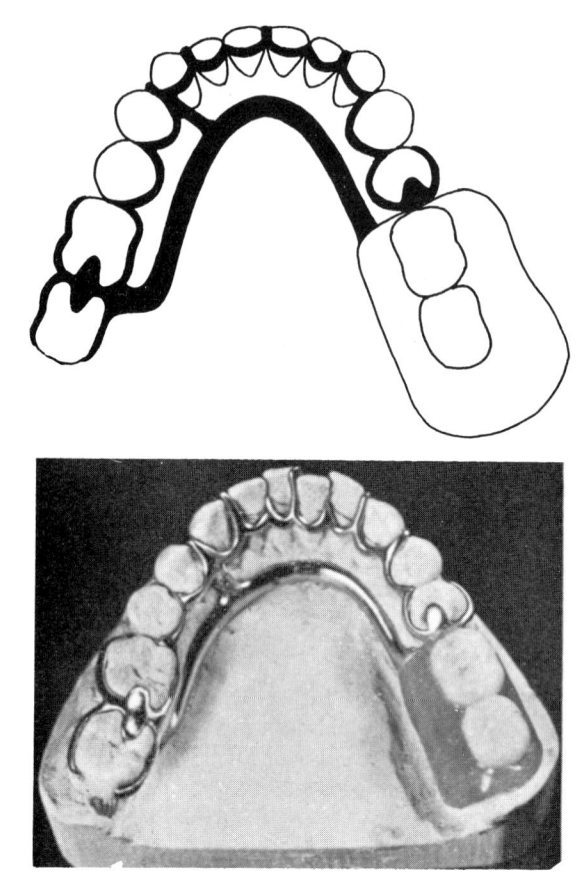

Fig. 12.2. A unilateral free-end saddle lower denture with the occlusal rest and clasp placed anteriorly. A semi-flexible lingual bar provides the posterior saddle connection.

side is attached to the rigid more superior part of the plate (Fig. 12.3). The lower bar must be more flexible in the vertical than the horizontal plane in order that the appliance has a lateral rigidity to distribute horizontal forces widely. This can be achieved by making its section wider than it is deep. If gold is used a very narrow slit can be achieved by incorporating a fine stainless steel strip in the wax pattern in the position where the break is required. Basically the design has the disadvantage that the slit opens slightly in function and theoretically is liable to trap either the tongue or food particles. In practice this does not seem to constitute a serious drawback if the saddle is short and the slit is accordingly situated posteriorly. With a long saddle, however, the slit is anteriorly placed and in this position may be intolerable to some patients. The slit can be cleaned easily by the patient using dental floss.

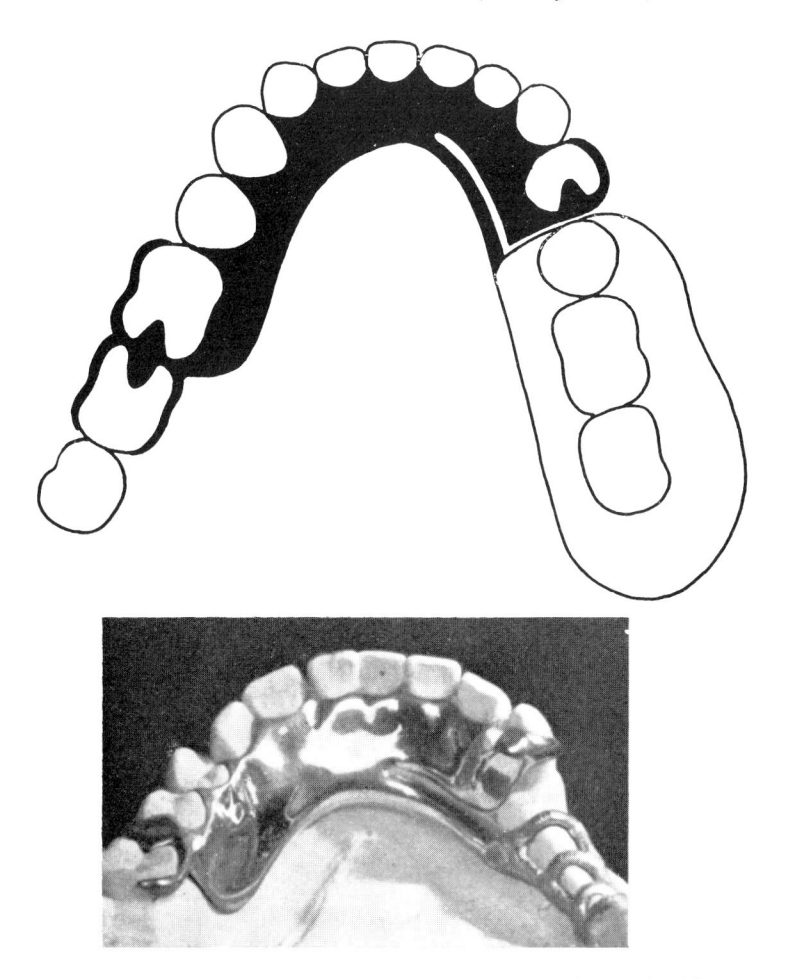

Fig. 12.3. A split casting used in the replacement of a long free-end saddle.

Modifications of the unilateral free-end saddle are encountered commonly in the lower jaw with a bounded saddle usually in the posterior region on the opposite side.

The denture shown in Fig. 12.4 is typical of the type of replacement required in these cases. Retention on the side of the bounded saddle is dependent upon the ability of the single molar tooth to withstand the loads applied. When rigid construction is employed, frequent inspection of the appliance is essential so that resorption under the free-end saddle may be compensated by rebasing. If this is not done, a damaging torque will be applied to the single standing molar leading at best to increased tilting and at worst to loosening and eventual loss.

If the periodontal condition of such a single standing tooth is doubtful, it may

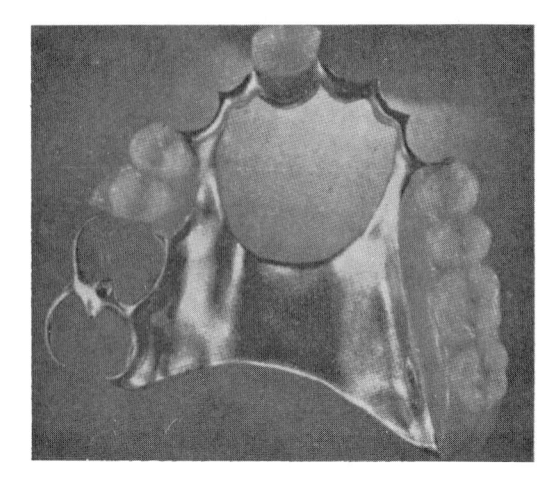

Fig. 12.4. A typical modification of a single free-end saddle denture.

be possible to design the denture incorporating a flexible connector to the distal extension saddle as already described. In addition less stress will be applied to the tooth if wrought wire instead of cast metal is used for clasp construction. In the upper jaw unmodified unilateral free-end saddle dentures are not common, but those with modifications are encountered frequently. Unmodified situations, when they do occur, are almost always due to the loss of teeth due to caries, and hence a well-formed ridge is present. Rigid constructions are almost always used, and clasping is normally necessary on the abutment tooth and on appropriate teeth on the opposite side of the arch. However, if for any reason complete palatal coverage with a plate is used, clasping may be unnecessary.

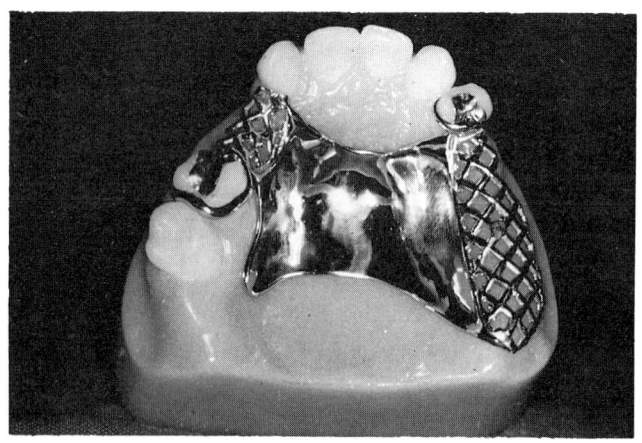

Fig. 12.5. A suggested design for a unilateral free-end saddle upper denture where a single standing premolar is present. The positioning and use of clasp arms are, however, dependent on the morphology of the crowns of the abutment teeth.

As with bilateral free-end saddles the single standing premolar may be a complication. The type of design illustrated in Fig. 12.5 is often effective, however, where palatal coverage is associated with adequate tooth support.

13
THE BOUNDED-SADDLE DENTURE (KENNEDY CLASS III)

The bounded-saddle denture (Kennedy Class III) is not required as frequently as its modifications. Unilateral edentulous spaces of varying length are, however, commonly seen and they often present a problem in treatment planning.

It has been suggested that bounded saddles should be sub-divided into three groups according to the clinical presentation and consequently the type of treatment indicated. It is appropriate, therefore, to discuss these groups separately.

Group A

Cases are designated Group A when the saddles are short, the abutment teeth are healthy and there has been the minimum of bone loss around their roots. In such cases fixed bridges will normally be the restorations of choice, but a well-designed and constructed unilateral removable partial denture can be satisfactory in the unmodified case.

In cases when aesthetics is not involved, it is often difficult to decide whether or not a restoration should be made. There are those who contend that the loss of any single tooth demands a replacement if the masticatory mechanism is to be preserved in its healthiest state. It is said that only in this way can the integrity of the dental arch be maintained, tilting and overeruption of teeth avoided, and the incidence of premature occlusal contacts consequently reduced. Thus it is claimed that one of the big factors causing occlusal derangement is treated preventively, and that the incidence of periodontal disease and joint disturbances will be reduced significantly. It is not always practical, nor even desirable, however, to make a replacement for every extracted tooth. So often poor oral hygiene, the complication of erupting teeth and a susceptibility to caries, make it impracticable to do anything other than leave the condition as it exists and carry out frequent examinations of the patient. In this respect it is important to balance the beneficial effects of restoring the edentulous space against the deleterious effects on the remaining dentition which may result from the wearing of a partial denture.

Group B

These are the cases in which one or more of the abutment teeth cannot, by themselves, assume the support and bracing of the denture, particularly the lateral loads that may be applied. The reasons for this may be that the saddle is long, that the root shape or length of the abutment tooth or teeth is poor, that occlusal loading will be excessive, or that there has been bone resorption around the abutment teeth. In these circumstances, a bilateral denture will be required and never a unilateral denture or a fixed bridge. Whenever possible it may be desirable to obtain support from teeth adjacent to the weaker abutment teeth, either by splinting the abutment tooth to them or by multiple clasping or resting.

Group C

These are cases in which the saddle is exceptionally long and one of the abutments is unable to provide any support for the denture. A typical example of such a situation is when the posterior abutment is a second or third molar and the anterior abutment is a short-rooted lateral incisor. In these cases the anterior saddle extension has to be mucosa borne.

The Unilateral Denture

The essential feature of this type of denture is that it covers the tissues of one side of the mouth only (Fig. 13.1). Such an appliance however may be unstable and permit only a limited distribution of load. As such dentures are invariably tooth supported, the resistance to vertical load is nevertheless favourable particularly if the abutment teeth have large root areas.

Ideally, when the teeth come together in working occlusion the buccal inclines of both buccal and lingual cusps of the lower teeth contact the lingual inclines of the corresponding cusps of the uppers (Fig. 13.2). This ideal occlusal pattern is rarely seen, and it is frequently found that primary contact is made only by the buccal cusps.

In patients who employ any degree of lateral jaw movement during mastication the construction of a unilateral denture in which there is only single cusp contact during lateral occlusion will result in instability. This is particularly so if the line of application of the vertical component of load acts externally to a line through the buccal extremities of the occlusal rests at either end of the saddle (Fig. 13.3). In such a situation the line of action of the load will not be within the limits of the stable quadrilateral base formed by the lines joining the buccal and

Chapter 13

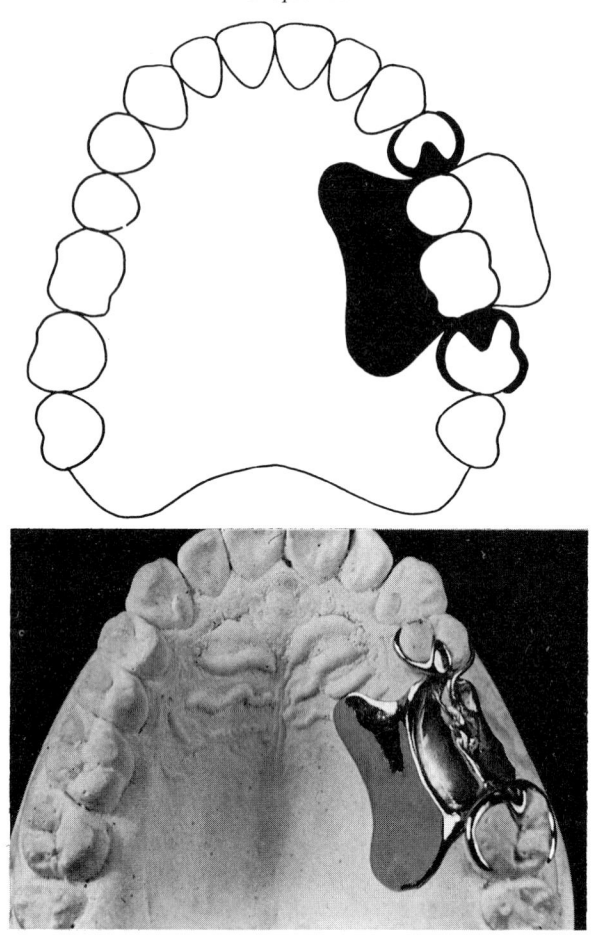

Fig. 13.1. The unilateral partial denture.

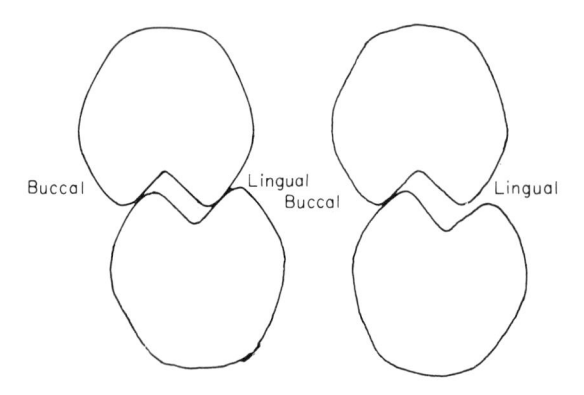

Fig. 13.2. Two possible tooth relationships in lateral excursion.

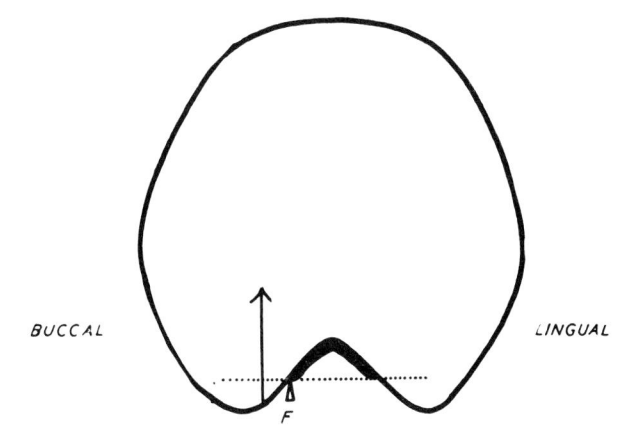

The Bounded-Saddle Denture (Kennedy Class III) 333

Fig. 13.3. The line of action of the vertical component of force lying buccally to the occlusal rest, resulting in an unstable appliance.

lingual margins of the rests (Fig. 13.4). The load will therefore act over more displaceable tissue and the denture will tend to rotate and sink into this tissue. In addition, because of the inclined plane action the lateral component of the applied load will tend to displace the appliance buccally. It must be conceded however that the degree of movement that takes place is small and is governed by the bracing effect of the lingual clasp arms and occlusal rests, the amount of palatal tissue covered, and the inclination of the palatal vault. In this respect a palate with more vertical sides will resist lateral displacement of the denture more effectively. If this tendency for the saddle to be displaced laterally is considerable, a space will develop between the fitting surface of the buccal plate of the appliance and its underlying ridge. This further decreases the stability of the appliance since more sinking under the vertical force can now take place. This vertical force does in fact effect a rotation of the saddle about an axis joining the buccal corners of the two occlusal rests where they pass over the marginal ridges of the abutments.

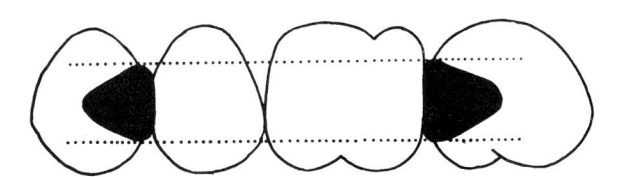

Fig. 13.4. The steady quadrilateral base formed by the lines joining the buccal and lingual margins of the rests, inside which the line of action of the vertical force should fall to give a stable appliance.

The following measures may be undertaken in order to limit this tendency to instability in the unilateral partial denture.

1 *Provision of lingual and buccal cusp contacts.* When the patient uses any degree of lateral movement in mastication or empty movements it is necessary to arrange for simultaneous contact of lingual and buccal cusps during working occlusion. In this way vertical components of load will act on both lingual and buccal cusps. This will ensure that the area of combined load application is most likely to fall within the width of the occlusal rests, even though the buccal component may act externally to a line joining the buccal edges of the occlusal rests (Fig. 13.5).

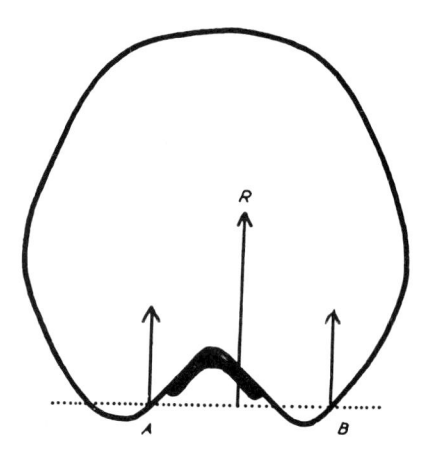

Fig. 13.5. The stabilizing effect of a lingual cusp contact when the buccal contact lies outside the maximum width of the occlusal rests. The resultant of the two forces acts within the lines joining the margins of the rests.

In order to achieve this stability it is necessary to restrict the prescription of a unilateral denture to patients who either have minimal horizontal movements during mastication or who have an occlusal arrangement approaching the ideal, with low cusp angles in the natural teeth. In some cases a less than ideal occlusion may be improved by judicious grinding and reshaping of cusps, although this is not always acceptable to the patient. In order to develop the optimum occlusal relationship for such a case it is useful to employ a fully adjustable articulator, although final adjustments to the occlusion will require to be made with the denture in the mouth.

2 *Use of wide occlusal rests.* The width of the occlusal rests, particularly in a buccal direction, should be maximal. This keeps the axis of rotation as far buccally as possible and helps to ensure that the vertical component of force acts

lingually or palatally to this axis. It is necessary to bear this in mind when preparing rest seats in the abutment teeth.

In those cases where the rests on the abutments cannot for any reason be buccally extended the possibility of employing an auxiliary occlusal rest buccally placed on a more posterior molar must be considered. This measure has the effect of moving the axis of rotation buccally.

3 *Provision of adequate bracing.* Bracing of the unilateral denture, against buccal movement must be substantial. This can be achieved simply by extending the denture on to the more vertical part of the hard palate (Fig. 13.1). Further bracing should be provided by clasp arms on the abutment teeth and it may be necessary also to clasp contiguous teeth to allow wider distribution of lateral load. It is an advantage to use a deep and square rest seat preparation for supplementary bracing.

The periodontal condition of the abutment and contiguous teeth requires to be assessed accurately by clinical and radiographic examination. These teeth are required to accept a substantially increased lateral load and the operator must be certain that their reaction will be physiological. This type of appliance is consequently most often suitable for the young adult in very good oral and general health. Similar reasoning may preclude the possibility of using a unilateral appliance where one of the abutments is a third molar if, as is often the case, its roots are short.

4 *Provision of adequate retention.* As we have already seen, a unilateral denture is not only subject to vertical displacement from its basal seat but also to buccal displacement through its tendency to buccal rotation about an axis through the buccal margins of the occlusal rests. It is therefore necessary to provide retention against such displacement and this may be achieved by clasping. In a bilateral denture the clasps on the opposite side of the jaw provide the retention, but in a unilateral appliance only the palatal clasp arms can be effective. It is, therefore, essential that the palatal clasp arms engage tooth undercut. When conically shaped teeth do not allow this, a unilateral clasp retained denture is contraindicated.

When the contours of the teeth are suitable for clasps, palatal bracing and retention are both required, hence the cast circumferential clasp is the only possibility. From the bracing point of view cobalt chromium is the alloy of choice and its use on molars is to be commended. However, it is often preferable to combine this with cast gold clasping on premolars as the shorter cobalt chromium clasp arm does not display adequate resilience for retention.

To secure retention against vertical displacement it is wise to augment the retention gained from the palatal clasp arms by retentive clasp arms on the buccal surface of the abutments. Thus the teeth must show suitable convexity on both buccal and lingual surfaces. It will be appreciated, therefore, that neither canines nor third molars are normally suitable as abutments for unilateral dentures.

Where there are contra-indications to a bilateral denture and a conventional unilateral denture cannot be constructed due to adverse coronal morphology of the abutment teeth, use can be made of intra or extra-coronal attachments. If use is made of such appliances it is even more important to ensure that the applied vertical load falls within the quadrilateral area formed by the lines joining the buccal and lingual margins of the attachments since more lateral stress will be applied to the abutment teeth. For further information on the use of preformed attachments the reader is advised to consult an appropriate text.

When the lower unilateral denture is considered it will be noted that the lateral component of load acts towards the lingual rather than the buccal and consequently tends to stabilize the denture in function. In spite of this few dentures of this type are required for the lower jaw. This is due to the reduced incidence of the short bounded saddle in the lower jaw, to the generally more unfavourable shape of the teeth as regards undercut areas, and to the more delicate nature of the lingual mucosa.

The Sectional Denture

In order to overcome the problems presented by proximal undercuts in relation to unilateral partial dentures the provision of a sectional or two-part denture has been suggested. A typical situation where such a denture may be employed is shown in Fig. 13.6 where undercuts are present in the mesial aspect of the distal abutment tooth and the distal aspect of the mesial abutment tooth. A conventional partial denture would require that either or both of these undercuts should be masked out and a careful path of insertion selected. This however can sometimes result in a denture with poor retention and stability, unacceptable aesthetic properties and a tendency for food impaction to occur.

A sectional partial denture is designed to engage and utilize opposing proximal undercuts on mesial and distal abutment teeth, which will result in

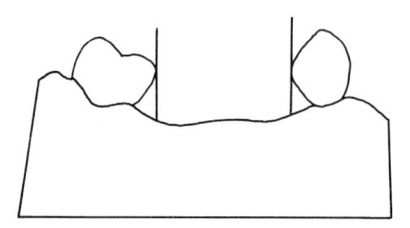

Fig. 13.6. A typical situation where the tooth loss might be restored to advantage by using a sectional denture to engage both mesial and distal proximal undercut areas.

The Bounded-Saddle Denture (Kennedy Class III) 337

positive retention in both a vertical and lateral direction often without recourse to conventional clasping. Each part of the denture will therefore have its individual path of insertion and once in position the parts will be maintained in position by means of a locking bolt (Fig. 13.7) so forming a rigid unit. Such a denture will completely restore the edentulous space with no unsightly or unhygienic gaps thus improving aesthetics and lessening food impaction.

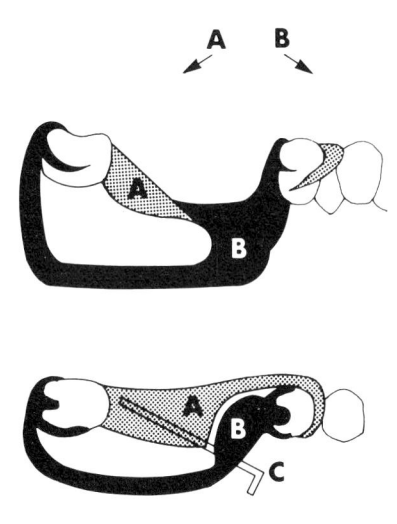

Fig. 13.7. Diagrammatic illustration of a sectional denture. Portion A is inserted first from in front and then portion B from behind. Locking bolt C secures the two portions together.

The technical construction of such an appliance is naturally more complex than a conventional denture. The master cast is required to be surveyed relative to the paths of insertion of each part with a posterior tilt used for the part engaging the undercut relative to the posterior abutment and an anterior tilt for the part engaging the undercut relative to the anterior abutment. The posterior section also has an anterior guiding arm and support approaching the anterior tooth lingually to its mesial aspect. The anterior surface of the posterior section, which is closely approximated to the mesial surface of the posterior abutment tooth should be inclined parallel to the distal surface of the anterior abutment in order to define its path of insertion. It will also be provided with a locating channel which will be engaged by the locking bolt (Fig. 13.8) The anterior part will contact the distal surface of the anterior abutment and also the anterior surface of the posterior section. This part will carry the locking bolt in its sleeve, within an acrylic matrix secured to the casting. (Fig. 13.9).

Such a denture is always constructed in cast metal, usually cobalt chromium alloy. It is inserted by the patient placing its separate parts in position and then locking them in place, with its removal being the same operation in reverse.

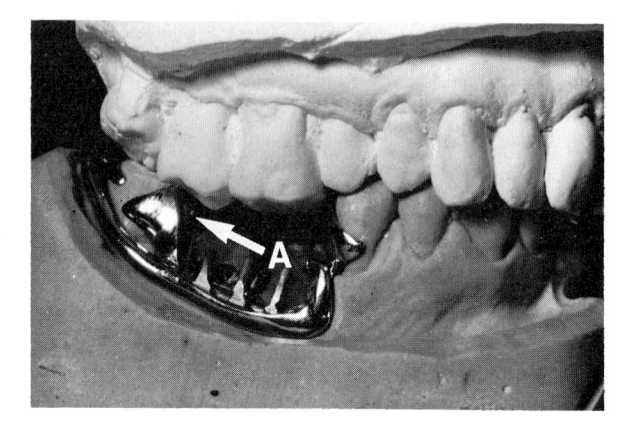

Fig. 13.8. The posterior part of a sectional denture with the locating channel (A) for the locking bolt.

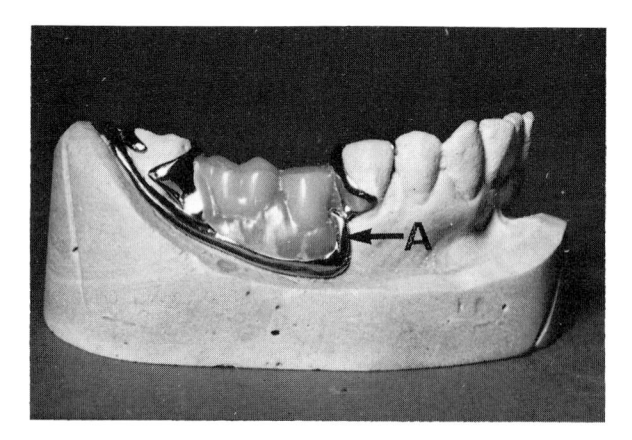

Fig. 13.9. The assembled sectional denture with the handle of the locking bolt (A) recessed into the matrix acrylic.

The Bilateral Denture

Although this requires a certain degree of manual dexterity it is usually learned quickly, and due to the close fit into approximal areas around abutment teeth such dentures are extremely stable and comfortable in function.

The Bilateral Denture

The bilateral denture has the advantages of increased stability and wider load distribution. It is, therefore, preferred in those cases where either the crown shape, root size, or periodontal condition of one or more of the abutments are not considered suitable for the support of a unilateral denture. If a removable rather than a fixed appliance is to be made, then a bilateral denture is normally preferable. Moreover, with a large rather than a small appliance the possibility of swallowing or inhaling is reduced.

The treatment of choice is a cast denture (Fig. 13.10) having clasps at either end of the saddle and on the opposite side of the jaw. This last retainer unit may be a compound clasp, joined to the saddle by a palatal or lingual bar. A continuous clasp may be included in the design, its purpose being mainly distribution of lateral load. In the upper, when a metal denture is contra-indicated on economic grounds, an acrylic plate may be used provided that there is adequate clearance of the gingival margins of the unclasped natural teeth (Fig. 13.11).

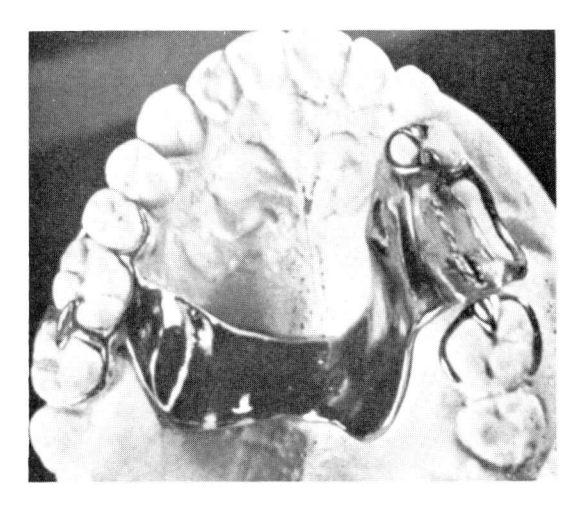

Fig. 13.10. A bilateral skeleton denture employed in an unmodified Class III case with a short saddle.

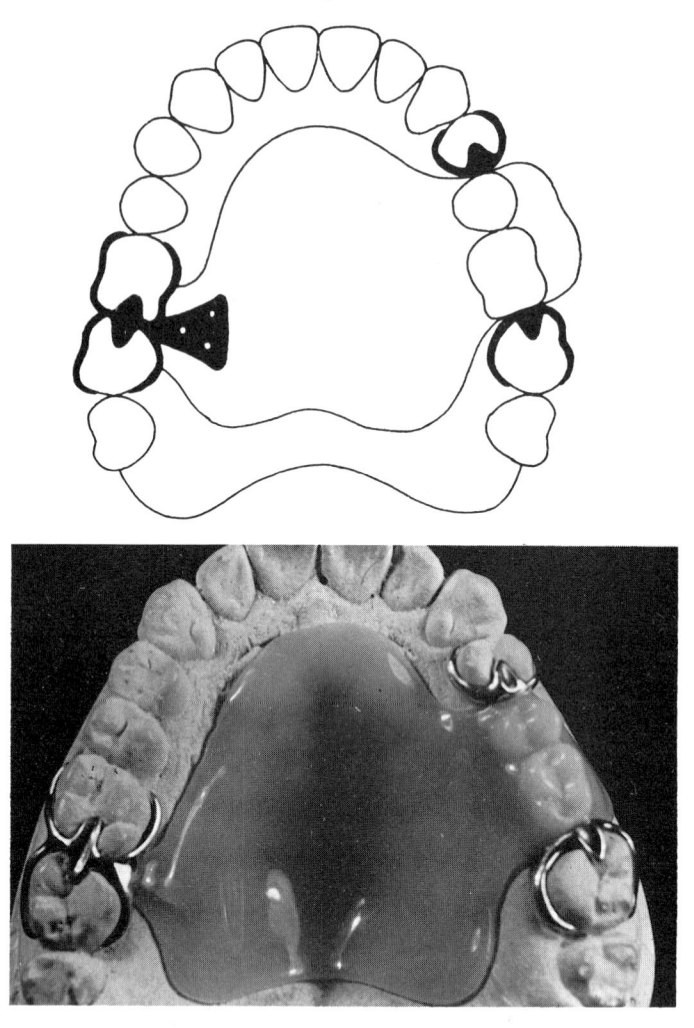

Fig. 13.11. A design suitable for an acrylic resin plate.

The Long Posterior Saddle

It is more common for the long saddle to present as a Kennedy Class III with modification(s) (Fig. 13.12). In such instances it is not uncommon to find the abutment teeth affected by periodontal disease and unable to accept any additional loads that might be imposed by supporting a fairly large tooth borne partial denture. In such a situation we must accept the fact that the denture must be mucosa supported. Maximum coverage of the mucosal tissues including the palate should be provided, compatible with avoidance of damage, so that the bone

The Bounded-Saddle Denture (Kennedy Class III)

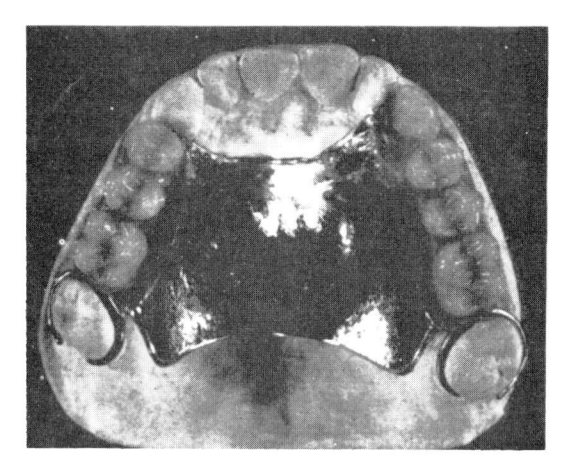

Fig. 13.12. A suitable design for an upper bilateral denture for a patient with some periodontal involvement.

of the residual alveolar ridge and the hard palate will bear the maximum load. Such a design will provide a reasonable amount of retention by adhesion, but this should be supplemented by wrought wire clasps on appropriate teeth (Fig. 13.12) and a correctly developed peripheral form to the saddles. The denture base may be constructed in cast cobalt chromium alloy or in acrylic resin with swaged stainless steel indicated in some situations.

When a long saddle is present and the standing teeth are supported firmly in healthy bone, then a tooth-borne design may be satisfactory. However, in the case illustrated (Fig. 13.13) the anterior abutment teeth are canines, and hence some

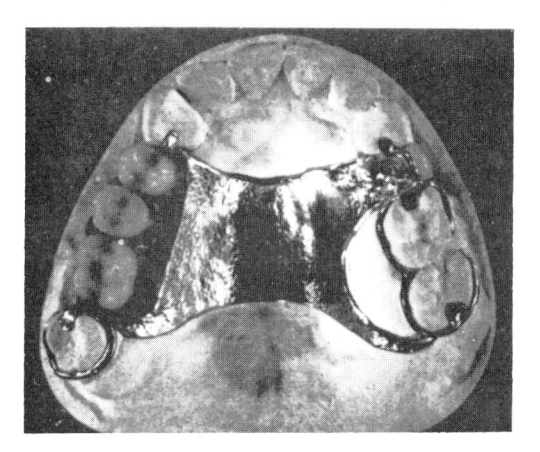

Fig. 13.13. Anterior tooth support provided by rests fitting into rest seats in three-quarter crowns on the canines.

provision should be made for the reception of rests. These can either be cut into the enamel, in which case they should be carefully polished and treated with a fluoride containing compound, or alternatively built up on the enamel surface using an adhesive restorative material.

Modifications of the Bounded Saddle

Modified bounded saddle cases are common, particularly in the maxilla. Where the saddles are short and the support of the abutment teeth is good, a cast metal tooth-supported partial denture with suitable bar connectors is an appropriate choice of treatment. In the lower the additional saddle may be connected by means of a lingual bar or lingual plate. Where plate connectors are used a third or additional saddle can easily be carried on the extension of the plate. As a general principle it is preferable to cover the gingival margin of a single tooth which lies between two saddles (Fig. 13.14a), the denture base material making contact with either the cingulum in the case of an anterior tooth, or the enamel immediately above the survey line on a posterior tooth. The danger of creating a food trap is marked when an attempt is made to keep the metal clear of the gingival margin of a single tooth. Where more than one standing tooth is present the connecting bar can be brought well away with every assurance that the gingiva will remain healthy (Fig. 13.14b).

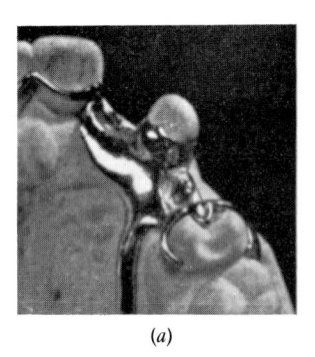

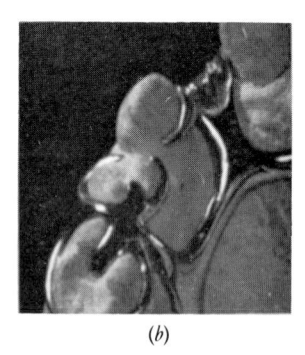

(a) (b)

Fig. 13.14. (a) Casting covering a single standing tooth.
(b) Clearing the gingival margin when there is more than one contiguous standing tooth.

In an upper denture with a large number of modifications a design using connecting bars becomes impracticable because of the large number of single standing teeth necessitating gingival coverage and the complexity of the resultant design. In such cases a palatal plate covering the hard palate and all the gingival margins is the treatment of choice. Such a plate may be made in acrylic resin or cobalt chromium. Where there is a hard bony area in the centre of the palate the central part of the plate may be omitted if cobalt chromium is used, but should be relieved if acrylic is employed. The condition of the gingivae under acrylic resin is always best when these have been relieved on the cast. As well as ensuring that the tissues are not abraded, this imparts a highly finished surface to that part of the acrylic fitting surface in proximity to the gingival margins. Even with this precaution a better result can be expected from highly polished cobalt chromium in this region. Adequate tooth support should be provided whenever possible although sinking of a purely mucosa borne plate will be slow due to the broad palatal coverage.

Great care must be taken that space does not exist at any point between the free margins of these plates and the enamel of the standing teeth immediately above the survey line. This demands accurate impressions and careful surveying. It is always desirable to eliminate tooth and tissue undercuts with wax, duplicate the cast, set up and process on the duplicate, and fit back finally on the master cast. A denture made in this way, even when many modifications exist, should be able to be inserted into the mouth without any grinding of the denture margins.

The Every Denture

In situations where two or more bounded saddles in the upper jaw require restoration, and where the long term prognosis for the remaining teeth is doubtful it is possible to achieve a satisfactory result with a totally mucosa borne denture of the design described by Every. This design aims to use broad palatal coverage alone to resist the vertical load. Lateral load is resisted by the palatal tissues and the standing teeth of the posterior segment of the arch with antero-posterior load being resisted by the hard palate and the standing anterior teeth.

One of the principles of this type of denture is to achieve a point contact between the artificial teeth and the adjacent abutment teeth. By this means the horizontal component of the vertical load is distributed mesio-distally along the arch. The arch morphology is better adapted to withstand mesio-distal than bucco-lingual stresses, as a load tending to move a tooth in the direction of its contact, that is in the mesio-distal direction, has an opposing force with components from the membrane surrounding the root together with the adjacent tooth with which it is in contact. It is important that a contact point is developed rather than an area, which will tend to produce a lateral or bucco-lingual component of applied load. Satisfactory contact points can only be achieved if the contacting proximal surfaces are convex and are placed slightly buccal to the axial midline than is usual in the natural dentition. The artificial tooth should maintain a tight contact at or just above the survey line and in this respect the use of porcelain teeth is preferable to acrylic teeth in order to reduce subsequent wear which would destroy the contacts. In addition to those already described, a further contact is developed with the distal surface of the most posterior tooth on each side of the arch, usually by means of a wire attached to the acrylic base. This is designed to prevent distal movement of this tooth so ensuring that the more anterior contacts between artificial and natural teeth are preserved.

Lingually to the contact point the denture is constructed with a wide embrasure area between the natural teeth and the saddle. This allows natural stimulation of the gingivae, and by the provision of a sluiceway prevents food impaction so minimizing caries and periodontal disease. Stagnation areas are also reduced by ensuring that the denture base is kept clear of the gingival margins of the natural teeth, and at no point, either buccally, palatally or inter-proximally should the acrylic cross gingival tissue, particularly in relation to the abutment teeth. Although maximum palatal coverage is indicated so that the tissue can react more favourably to vertical and lateral loading, the margins of the palatal plate are kept at least 3 mm clear of the gingival margins (Fig. 13.15).

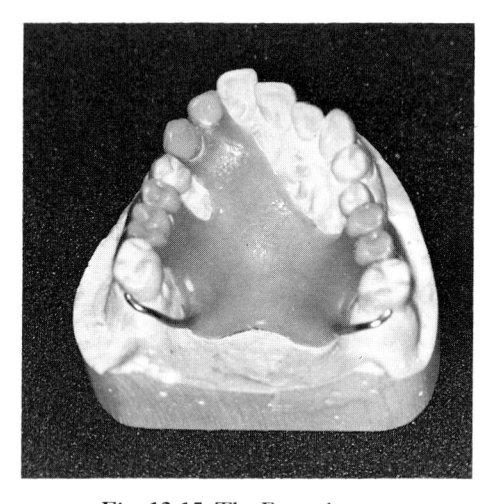

Fig. 13.15. The Every denture.

Retention of the denture is by adhesion, and is achieved by optimum coverage of the denture bearing tissues with full extension of the denture periphery into the depth and width of the functional sulcus. Full use should be made of peripheral damming both anteriorly and posteriorly. Further factors which aid retention are careful shaping of the polished surfaces to harness muscle control and the establishment of a free sliding occlusion to minimize displacement due to lateral or uneven loading applied to the artificial teeth.

This type of denture can only be used in the upper jaw with its broad palatal coverage and is not effective in the distal-extension saddle situation. Being constructed in acrylic it lacks strength and has the disadvantage of flexibility although this can sometimes be overcome by constructing a cast cobalt chromium base. The design however has much to commend it.

The Claspless Denture

The majority of bounded saddle dentures with modifications are retained in position by the use of clasps. Clasping is however not always acceptable to the patient, partly because clasps may be a source of discomfort, but more particularly in the anterior region from an aesthetic point of view, if they are visible during laughing and speaking. In such a situation it is possible to construct a denture which is retained satisfactorily using direct retention, but which does not have the aesthetic disadvantage of clasps, or even intra-coronal attachments with their necessary destruction of dental tissue for their placement, together with the associated expense. The construction of such a denture is dependent upon the use of a spring loaded nipple incorporated in the appliance, which will engage an undercut present on the proximal surface of an abutment tooth adjacent to the saddle area. A diagrammatic example of such a retentive aid is shown in Fig. 13.16. Several commercial examples of this type of attachment are available, but perhaps the most common is the ZA-Anchor system (Metrodent Ltd, Huddersfield, England). This system embodies a spring loaded metal or nylon nipple housed in an externally threaded casing which may be screwed into position in the resin matrix of the finished denture, the screw pathway having been determined by the use of a threaded processing dummy which is discarded.

The principle of operation of such an appliance is very simple. As the patient inserts the denture with the attachment in position, the nipple comes in contact with the maximum convexity of the tooth. It is then depressed against the spring and retracts into its housing, so allowing the denture to be seated. Once in

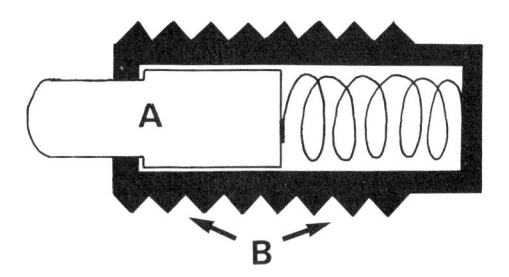

Fig. 13.16. A diagrammatic representation of a longitudinal section through a ZA Anchor, with its spring loaded nipple (A) and externally threaded casing (B).

position however, the recoil of the spring allows the nipple to engage the proximal undercut present on the abutment tooth. This it should do passively. Subsequently during wearing the resistance of the spring to compression prevents the nipple being depressed and moving back over the maximum convexity of the tooth, thus ensuring retention until the denture is forcibly removed by the wearer. The design of the attachment incorporates a collar which limits the amount of projection of the nipple from the housing, although the appliance can be set to achieve any desired fit. Such attachments are usually small enough to be included in a single tooth saddle. It is however necessary to have an adequate thickness of resin around them in order to avoid breakage during function. For most effective retention they should be positioned in relation to the undercut, and parallel to the residual ridge. Once in position adjustments may be made if required, using special tools provided.

It is considered that the use of an attachment with a metal nipple may cause some abrasion of the tooth substance or a synthetic restorative material. This is avoided if nylon is used, although nylon will wear more readily than metal and require more frequent adjustment. Ultimately the whole unit will require replacement but this can be done easily without remaking the denture.

References

APPLEGATE O.C. (1960) An evaluation of the support for the removable partial denture. *J. pros. Dent.* **10**, 112.
APPLEGATE O.C. (1960) The rationale of partial denture choice. *J. pros. Dent.* **10**, 891.
BATES J.F. (1970) *Partial denture construction*, pp. 128. John Wright & Sons, Bristol.
CRADDOCK F.W. (1951) *Prosthetic dentistry*, 2nd edition, 274–76. Kimpton, London.
DYER M.R.Y. (1972) The 'Every' type acrylic partial denture. *Dent. Pract.* **22**, 339.
EVERY R.G. (1949) The elimination of destructive forces in replacing teeth with partial dentures. *N.Z. dent. J.* **45**, 207–14.
EVERY R.G. (1949) A new design for removable partial dentures. *Dent. Pract.* **14**, 284.
HOBKIRK J.A. and STRAHAN J.D. (1979) The influence on the gingival tissues of prostheses incorporating gingival relief areas. *J. dent.* **7**, 15.
LANE R.P. (1947) Practical stress breaking in partial dentures. *Dent. J. Aust.* **19**, 314–22.
LEE J.H. (1964) A new design for removable partial dentures. *Dent. Pract.* **14**, 284.
LEE J.H. (1963) Sectional partial metal dentures incorporating an internal locking bolt. *J. pros. Dent.* **13**, 1067.
L'ESTRANGE P. and PULLEN-WARNER E. (1969) Sectional dentures—a simplified method of attachment. *Dent. Pract.* **19**, 379.
MALCOLM J.A. (1943) The occlusal rest in partial denture construction. *D. Digest.* **49**, 256–61.
WRIGHT S.M. (1984) Use of spring-loaded attachments for retention of removable partial dentures. *J. pros. Dent.* **51**, 605.

14

THE ANTERIOR BOUNDED SADDLE (KENNEDY CLASS IV)

By definition an anterior bounded saddle (Kennedy Class IV) partial denture is that type in which a single saddle lies entirely anterior to the abutments. This class has no modifications, but the length of the saddle may vary from a single tooth to include posterior teeth in both sides of the jaw. Such dentures may be required for either upper or lower jaws, but are commonest in the upper.

Loss of one or more upper anterior teeth may occur in childhood and adolescence on account of trauma, and a large number of anterior saddle restorations are made for children, generally boys, who have met with some accident while playing games. It is also not uncommon to find congenital absence of a single upper tooth or even a pair of teeth, particularly with upper lateral incisors. Although this can often be treated orthodontically, sometimes the space is so large that prosthetic replacement is required. The more extensive situations are usually not encountered until adult life and their incidence is not high.

The lower anterior saddle denture is rarely necessary before adult life since the lower incisors, being less prominent than the uppers, generally escape damage from trauma, and are less liable to caries. By far the most frequent is the one that replaces the four incisors lost through periodontal disease.

The treatment in the upper jaw depends largely upon the age of the patient. There is little doubt that the best ultimate treatment in many instances, particularly when only one or two teeth have been lost, is by bridgework. Generally this can only be a second line of treatment, and in a young person a denture is usually required in the first instance for one of the following reasons:

- The roots of the abutments may be incompletely formed.
- A space retainer may be required immediately as eruption of other teeth may be in progress.
- Expensive forms of treatment are often better delayed until danger of further trauma has been reduced in later years.
- To allow alveolar resorption to take place.

The Treatment of Children

As indicated, the treatment of children is related generally to traumatic loss of teeth or absence of development of one or more incisors. As treatment of the

348   *Chapter 14*

relatively young child is essentially a temporary or holding operation until he is older, it is most appropriate to consider a simple design of denture. Ideally this should be replaced by a more permanent appliance when the condition of the mouth has stabilized at the cessation of growth. In spite of this however, some of the denture designs utilized for young patients are necessary also in adult life where more sophisticated techniques are contra-indicated.

When providing a denture in the developing dentition it is particularly important that apart from restoring appearance and function, the appliance should not cause damage to the natural teeth or their supporting structures. It is

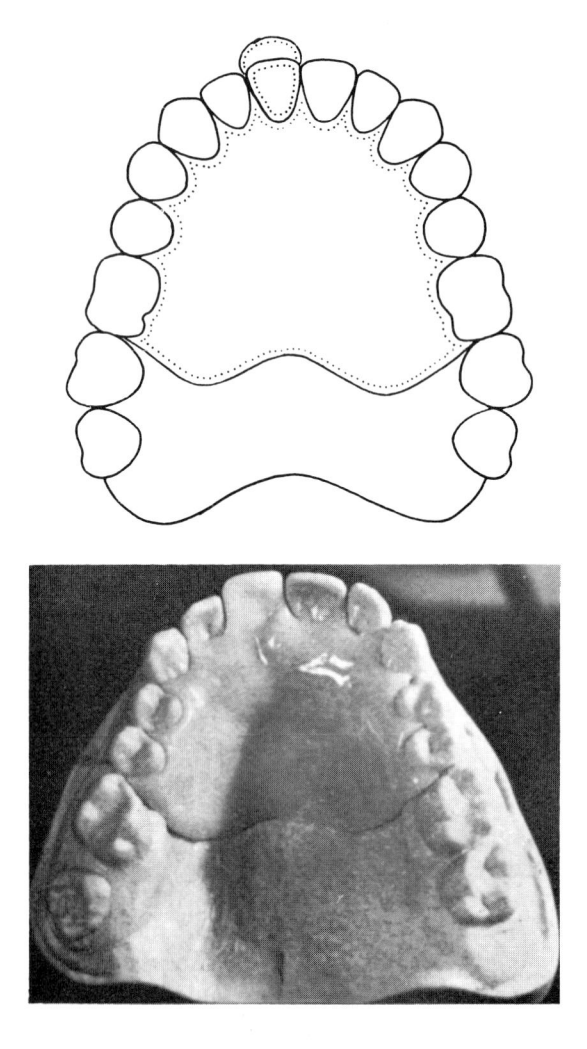

Fig. 14.1. The mucosa borne acrylic resin denture covering the gingivae.

unfortunate that simplicity of a denture often equates with abrogation of responsibility in relation to acceptable principles of design and construction. A design seen all too commonly in children is the mucosa borne acrylic resin covering a large area of the palate and the gingival margins of the natural teeth (Fig. 14.1). In many cases the master cast has not been surveyed, undercuts have not been masked out, and the periphery of the denture finishes below the maximum convexity of the tooth. The necessary removal of acrylic resin to allow insertion of the denture results in an appliance where the contact between tooth and denture base is lost at the periphery. This will encourage food packing with resultant mechanical trauma to the gingival margin. The degree to which either of these conditions may progress will depend, amongst other factors, on the adaptation and support of the rest of the denture together with the oral hygiene of the patient.

One possible design which may be utilized in this situation is the so-called spoon denture which can be constructed in either acrylic resin or cast metal. This will cover a large area of the hard palate, but the periphery is kept clear of the gingival margins by some 3–4 mm (Fig. 14.2). If desired, tooth support can be provided in the cingulum areas of the abutment teeth. Since obliteration of palatal undercuts is unnecessary the technical and chairside time required is small, and because the gingival margins are left uncovered and no extensive contact is made with the standing teeth, gingivitis and caries are not caused.

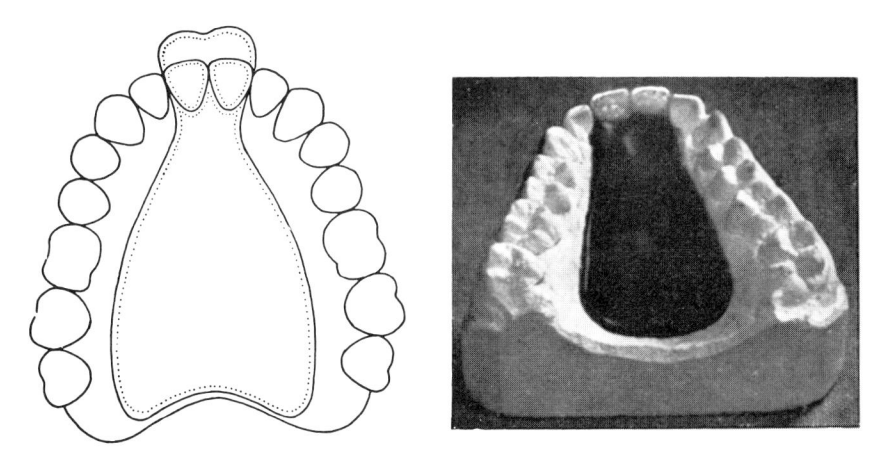

Fig. 14.2. The spoon denture.

The disadvantage of the spoon denture is its relatively poor retention. This depends on adhesion and the action of the dorsum of the tongue. Since adhesion is directly proportional to the area covered, extension of the base to the junction of the soft and hard palates is essential. This posterior extension also helps the action of the tongue since its upwards pressure against the posterior part of the base helps to stabilize the denture against vertical displacement.

The spoon denture tends to be displaced during incision. When only one or two teeth are carried on the denture incision can generally be made by the remaining standing teeth and embarrassment avoided. If more teeth are missing it is only under the most favourable conditions that a spoon denture can be advised. In general, children very quickly accommodate to such a denture, but with adults less success is achieved. Due to the poor retention of this denture and its displacement during function it is advisable to use radio-opaque resin in its construction, in case of traumatic displacement into the oesophagus or trachea.

In estimating the possible success of a spoon denture the following points should be noted:

1   *The nature of the mucosa.* The best retention is obtained where a normal amount of firm fibrous tissue is present in the submucosa. When the palatal bone is covered by a very thin mucosa, and this is quite frequently the case in children, the retention of the spoon denture may not be adequate.

2   *The form of the hard palate.* A large palate is more favourable as adhesion is greater. A palate that has steep sides is better than one that is flat, as it offers more resistance to lateral movement of the appliance and thus gives it added stability. Where the palate has a marked vault it may be necessary to produce a bifid design.

3   *The use of an anterior flange.* The presence of an anterior flange stabilizes the appliance against posterior displacement and helps to resist downwards vertical displacement of the posterior portion. Whenever possible a flange should be used, but aesthetics must often have prior consideration.

4   *The closeness of the occlusion.* This complication is considered below in more detail.

5   *The degree of vertical overlap.* In cases where more than one tooth has been lost, a deep overlap may mean increased stress applied to the denture during incision. This will particularly apply if the related horizontal overlap is small.

When it is considered that a spoon denture would not have adequate retention or stability, two modifications may be considered. In the first, extensions of the palatal plate are brought into contact with the first permanent molar teeth which are clasped with Adams cribs constructed in 0.7 mm stainless steel wire. These provide retention by point contact in the buccal embrasures, while the buccal arm extending between these areas lies clear of the buccal surface of the teeth (Fig. 14.3). Point contact on the less readily cleansed buccal surface is calculated to reduce the risk of caries, and gingivitis of the palatal

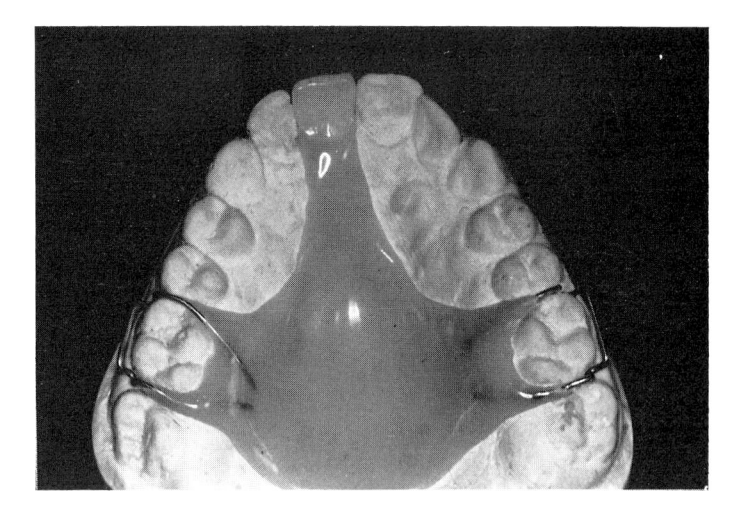

Fig. 14.3. Spoon denture modified by use of Adams cribs.

gingiva is minimized by finishing the acrylic resin occlusally to the survey line together with the resting effect of the occlusal arms of the Adams' cribs. This design may be used where it is possible to accommodate the thin wire between the opposing arches without interfering with the occlusion. Whereas in adults the writers do not hesitate to grind enamel to accommodate a clasp arm, they deprecate this procedure in children where the risk of caries is high.

A further modification of the spoon denture is the production of a cast cobalt chromium base with clasps engaging the buccal undercuts of the molar teeth. (Fig. 14.4). Although this design is useful in the adult mouth it is less effective in children where there is often insufficient buccal undercut for the retentive part of the clasp arm to engage. If a cast base is desired for a child this can often be achieved by combining an anterior cast portion with a posterior extension in acrylic resin which can carry the Adams cribs necessary for retention.

The complication of a close occlusion

It is sometimes found that insufficient space exists between the incisal edges of the lower incisors and the hard palate for the inclusion of an acrylic base of adequate thickness. In such cases a metal base is essential and can be constructed to the designs already mentioned and according to the requirements of the patient. Due to the limited space it is sometimes difficult however to attach the teeth effectively to the base using acrylic resin and a conventional cast meshwork, and metal backings may have to be provided as an integral part of the casting.

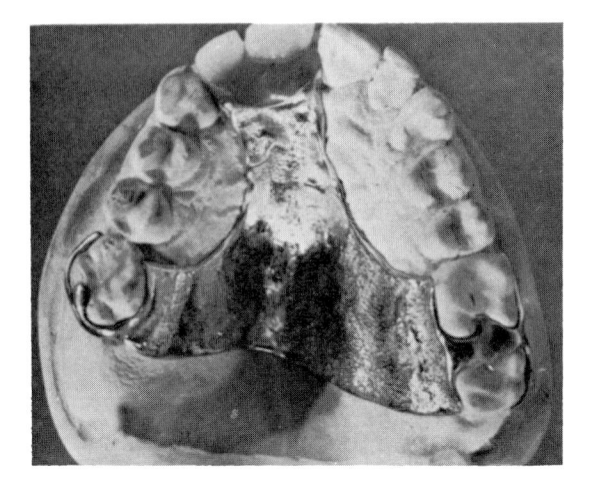

Fig. 14.4. T-shaped cobalt chromium denture.

Other Anterior Saddle Designs

When a stable oral situation has been reached alternative methods of treatment may be considered. In many instances a fixed bridge will be the best type of restoration, but it may be contra-indicated for the following reasons:
- Ridge resorption may necessitate the addition of an anterior flange.
- The condition of the abutments may not be suitable for bridge support.
- Personal factors may contra-indicate extensive abutment preparation.
- The length or curve of the edentulous span may put too great a strain on the abutments.

If, for any of these reasons, a bridge cannot be made then treatment must be the provision of a removable partial denture. When the saddle is short a metal denture cast in cobalt chromium is a most satisfactory replacement (Fig. 14.5). The retention of this type of appliance during incision should be considered.

When a vertical force is applied to the saddle towards the ridge, a displacing rotation tends to take place, having as its axis a line between the cingula of the abutment teeth on which the saddle is supported. The moment of this force depends on how far in front of this axis the artificial teeth are placed, while its effective magnitude depends on the nature of the mucosa covering the ridge; the more compressible is this tissue, the less is the direct resistance it offers to the displacement. The displacing rotation is resisted largely by the clasping placed posterior to the rotatory axis. On a principle of moments, the more posteriorly the clasping is placed the greater is the retention of the appliance.

The general design of such a denture is in the form of two palatal bar

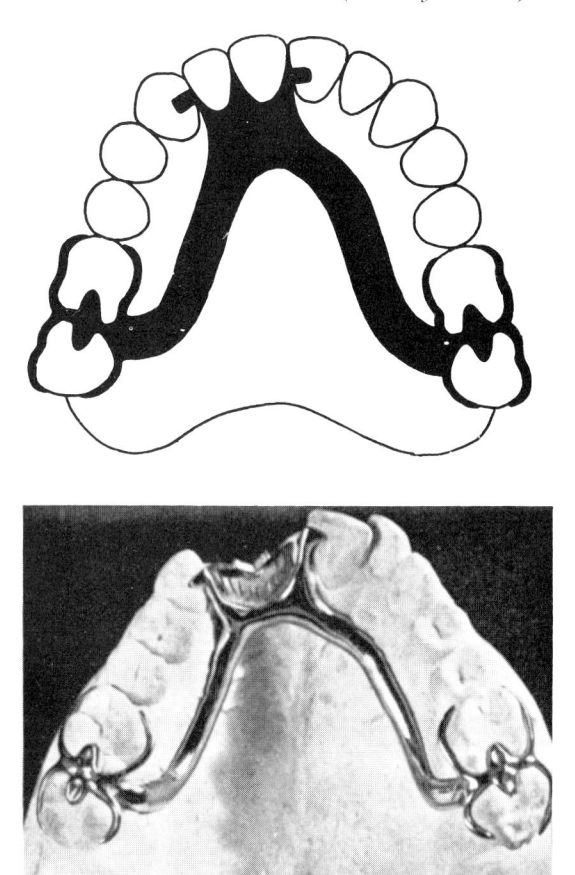

Fig. 14.5. Skeleton denture with posterior clasping.

connectors arising from the saddle and placed on the lateral walls of the plate equidistant between the gingival margins and the midline. To their distal ends are attached the clasps, usually two on each side (Fig. 14.5). If the bars are cast in cobalt chromium alloy there is usually no need for a posterior palatal connecting bar. Rest seats are always prepared in the abutment teeth if they are central incisors or canines. Before rests are placed on lateral incisors their condition should be assessed both clinically and radiographically. If there is any doubt the rest should be placed on the more distal canine to avoid loading the lateral incisor excessively.

A complication which sometimes arises with this type of denture is vertical displacement of the saddle as a result of the weight of the appliance. One method of overcoming this is to engage a soft tissue undercut with the labial flange of the denture. If this is not possible and the denture is heavy, occlusal rests bilaterally

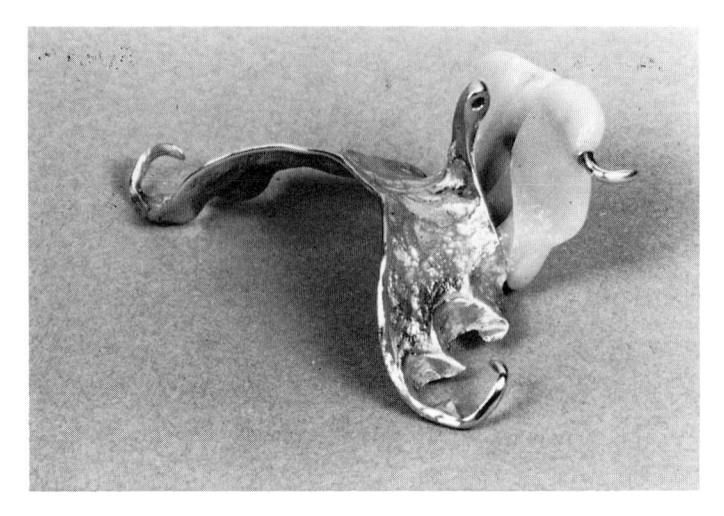

Fig. 14.6. A hinged sectional denture with a locking bolt (courtesy of Mr G.A. Smith).

on the distal aspect of the most posterior molars, together with more anteriorly placed clasping may overcome the problem, by providing a degree of indirect retention.

Exceptionally long, anterior bounded saddles, when perhaps even the premolars require replacement on one or both sides, occur only in adults. Usually the periodontal condition of the remaining teeth is good and varying degrees of displaceability are found in the mucosa that covers the ridge.

This type of denture presents a similar problem to that found in bilateral free-end dentures. The saddle, although bounded by teeth at each end, has the feature of the free-end saddle in that its part most remote from the teeth is mucosa supported. The solution to the problem, however, is not so difficult as with the free-end saddle. In the first place, the whole of the hard palate may be covered anterior to a line between the abutments of each side and consequently sinking of the denture is well resisted and retention is assisted by adhesion. Furthermore, the clasping possibilites are generally better since the teeth which remain include the multi-rooted molars, and the danger of applying a damaging stress to these teeth is less than to premolars. Multiple clasping is often employed, which not only acts as a splint to the remaining teeth but also distributes any torque or leverage action. With such dentures good retention is necessary as with the premolars used in the mastication of sticky foods displacement of the saddle away from its basal seat is likely. Indirect retention can be obtained by posterior extension over the hard palate whilst posterior resting is also possible. A denture showing the above features is shown in Fig. 14.7.

As with free-end saddles frequent inspection and rebasing are necessary since only a slight degree of rotation about the occlusal rests will open up a space

The Anterior Bounded Saddle (Kennedy Class IV) 355

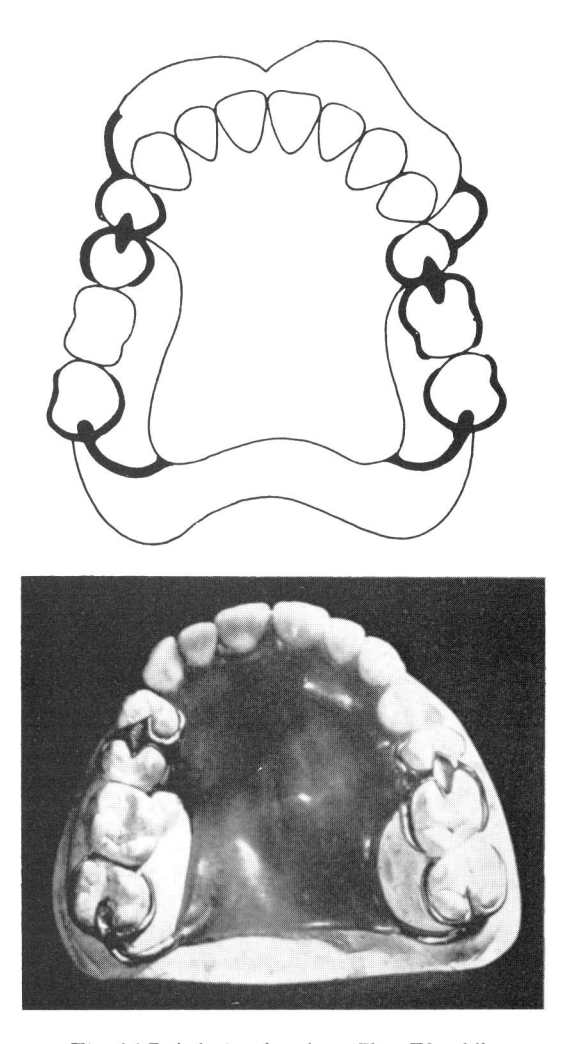

Fig. 14.7. A design for a long Class IV saddle.

between the posterior periphery of the denture base and the hard palate, into which food will find its way.

An alternative form of treatment when the saddle is short is the sectional denture. In principle such a denture follows the system described earlier for unilateral bounded saddles in the posterior region of the mouth. One section is cast in metal and is inserted from the palatal aspect of the ridge which enables the proximal undercuts of the abutment teeth to be engaged. The labial section which carries the teeth and the labial flange is inserted from below in an upwards and backwards path. It is frictionally retained to the first section by means of split post matrices attached to the cast portion, which will engage a stainless steel tube matrix in the labial section. A design can also be used which incorporates a hinge between the two parts, with the anterior flange and teeth being rotated into place and held in position by a locking bolt (Fig. 14.6). In cases of large proximal undercuts on the natural anterior teeth an improved appearance may be achieved with this type of denture but retention and stability are sometimes less than adequate. Retention may be improved by use of intracoronal attachments for the first section.

The Anterior Bounded Saddle Lower Denture

This denture is usually required in adults who have lost the four lower anterior teeth through periodontal disease or rarely caries. Occasionally it may also be seen in teenagers who have succumbed to juvenile periodontitis. In this situation a cast metal denture is the treatment of choice. The design consists of bilateral lingual bars extending posteriorly from the saddle, terminating in clasps; continuous clasping may or may not be present (Fig. 14.8). The saddle must be adequately tooth supported anteriorly, and this can be accomplished by using rests on the mesial aspect of the occlusal surfaces of the premolars. The use of the

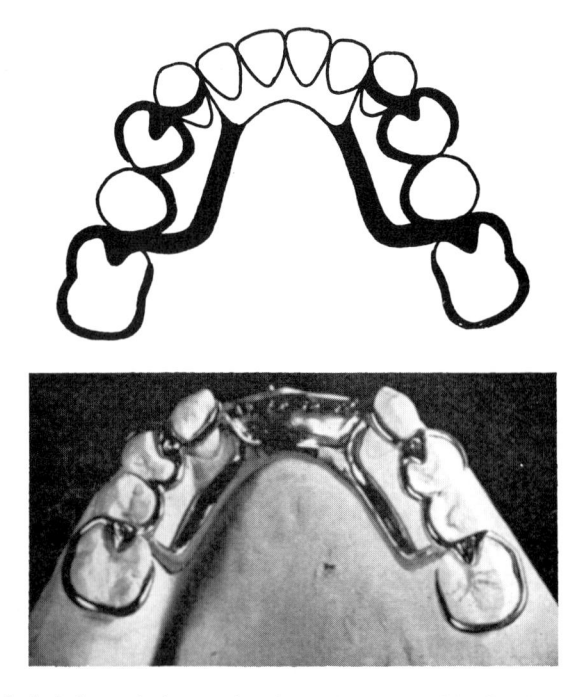

Fig. 14.8. A skeleton design used in the replacement of the four lower incisors.

canines for support has the advantage of bringing the axis of rotation forward so that the posterior clasping is consequently more effectively but will necessitate extensive preparation of the teeth to provide effective seats for the rests on the cingula or else the use of incisal edge rests with their obvious aesthetic disadvantages.

Composite Bonded Bridges

In many instances the permanent replacement of a single lost anterior tooth by a removable partial denture is not entirely satisfactory. This is often due to the size of the appliance in respect of tissue coverage, and its inherent instability and poor retention, together with the possible adverse effects which it may have on the remaining dentition. The possibility of restoring the loss by means of a fixed bridge may also be rejected where this entails removal of healthy tooth substance, and also on economic considerations.

Most of these objections can be overcome by the use of an etched cast ceramometal restoration which can be bonded to minimally prepared and etched enamel surfaces. Although not a partial denture in the strictest sense, it nevertheless should be considered in the restoration of a one- or two-tooth anterior bounded saddle.

The earliest of these appliances was in the form of a perforated retainer with a pontic attached, which had been prepared on a master cast. A composite resin was applied to the etched enamel on the lingual or palatal surfaces of the abutment teeth and the retainer placed in position. Retention of the bridge to the teeth relied upon the resin escaping through the perforations and being adapted around the retainer before polymerization. This system however produced only limited retention of the resin to the framework, and with its low abrasion resistance and tendency to allow leakage of the oral fluids it had limited success.

Retention of the framework however was improved by subjecting its fitting surface to an electrolytic etching process. This improved the resin bond by establishing mechanical retention between the micropores of the etched alloy surface and the composite resin in a manner similar to its attachment to an etched enamel surface.

This technique therefore can be used to provide a fixed partial denture of a limited span, most commonly in the anterior region, but also occasionally in the posterior region of the mouth. In deciding to provide such a restoration due consideration must be given to the health of the supporting tissues of the abutment teeth, and to select an adequate number of abutments to allow load distribution. Teeth with inadequate support, large carious lesions, extensive restorations, and evidence of severe attrition are not suitable for use as abutments.

Tooth preparation for this prosthesis should be minimal. Enamel may be reduced to free the occlusal if necessary, but it must be stressed that it is preferable that the attachment is placed on a non-functional surface. This will reduce the possibility of mechanical displacement. A definitive path of insertion should be created which should be vertical with small grooves or slots prepared on the proximal surfaces of the abutment teeth to improve retention, and lessen the chance of lingual or palatal displacement. Additional resistance to displacement in this direction can be achieved by incorporating a slightly curved guiding surface on the labio-proximal surface of the teeth adjacent to the space so giving a 'wrap around' effect. Defining a cingulum rest area will also provide additional vertical support. The whole area of the preparation should be kept clear of the gingival margin by at least 1 mm.

Once tooth preparation is complete an impression is recorded using either polysulphide or silicone impression material. An impression of the opposing arch is also necessary together with an interocclusal registration. The cast should be poured in stone and a duplicate made in refractory material on which the casting will be produced. The resultant casting is produced in non-precious alloy upon which the ceramic pontic can be bonded. The casting should be about 0.5 mm thick for rigidity but should taper to a knife edge at its margins. Once the pontic has been built the casting is subjected to electrolytic etching on its fitting surface, the other areas being protected by wax. Following etching it must be kept free of any contamination. An example of such a restoration is shown in Figs 14.9 and 14.10.

At insertion the tooth surface is prepared in the normal manner for an acid etched restoration. A bonding agent is used on the enamel and the luting composite applied to the casting. The restoration is seated firmly in position and maintained until the resin has polymerized.

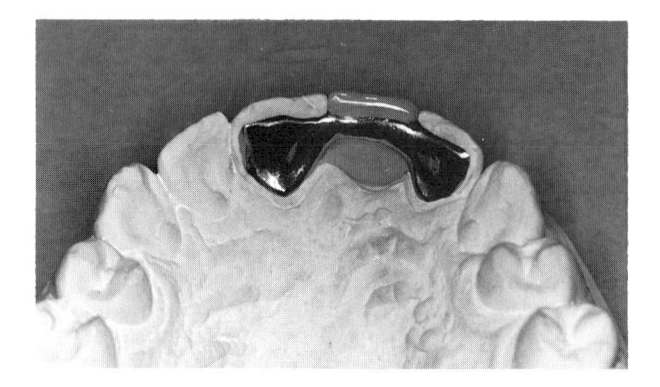

Fig. 14.9. A composite bonded bridge to replace an upper central incisor tooth.

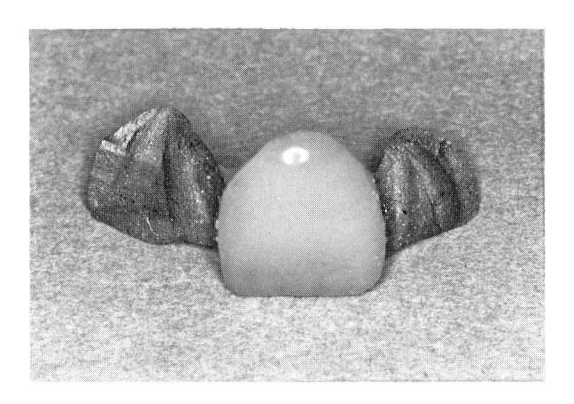

Fig. 14.10. The ceramometal restoration showing the etched metal fitting surface.

The advantages of this technique are that a saddle of limited span can be restored economically without loss of healthy tooth substance or the wearing of a large partial denture. For aesthetic reasons it is not suitable where there is obvious soft tissue loss, but otherwise offers an alternative to the conventional partial denture.

References

ANDERSON J.N. and LAMMIE G.A. (1952) A clinical survey of partial dentures. *Brit. dent. J.* **92**, 59–67.
BARRACK G. (1984) Recent advances in etched cast retorations. *J. pros. Dent.* **52**, 619.
BENINGTON I.C. (1972) The problem of replacement of the upper lateral incisor in the young patient. *Dent. Pract.* **22**, 405.
BRAVER G.M. (1981) The desirability of using radiopaque plastics in dentistry: a status report. *J. Amer. dent. Ass.* **102**, 347.
DIMMER A. (1970) A method of treating the anterior bounded saddle. *Dent. Pract.* **20**, 271.
FISH S.F. (1970) Partial dentures 5. Design. *Brit. dent. J.* **128**, 446.
HOOLE A.J. (1939) The replacement of a single upper anterior tooth. *Proc. Congress Aust. dent. Ass.* 499–513.
HOWE D.F. and DENEHY G.E. (1977) Anterior fixed partial dentures utilizing the acid-etch technique and a cast metal framework. *J. pros. dent.* **37**, 28.
LAIRD W.R.E (1969) Child dental health: the role of the prosthetist. *Dent. Pract.* **19**, 341.
LEE J.H. (1964) A new design for removable partial dentures. *Dent. Pract.* **14**, 284.
L'ESTRANGE P.R. and PULLEN-WARNER E. (1969) Sectional dentures—a simplified method of attachment. *Dent. Pract.* **19**, 379.
L'ESTRANGE P.R. and PULLEN-WARNER E. (1969) Sectional dentures—aids to removal and adjustment. *Dent. Pract.* **20**, 135.

LIVADITIS G.J. and THOMPSON V.P. (1982) Etched castings: an improved retentive for resin bonded retainers. *J. pros. Dent.* **47**, 52.

OSBORNE J. and LAMMIE G.A. (1953) Some observations concerning chrome-cobalt denture bases. *Brit. dent. J.* **94**, 55–67.

ROCHETTE A.L. (1973) Attachment of a splint to enamel of lower anterior teeth. *J. pros. Dent.* **30**, 418.

STILEMAN R.D.W. (1951) Spoon dentures. *Brit. dent. J.* **91**, 294–97.

15
IMPRESSION TAKING

Preliminary Impressions

In the first stage of partial denture construction it is necessary to obtain casts from a preliminary impression of the teeth and denture related tissues. These casts are poured in dental stone, surveyed and may be mounted on a movable articulator with the aid of an interocclusal registration if appropriate. This will allow the clinician to produce a tentative design. In the light of this, further decisions can be made on the need for tooth modification to develop guide planes and undercut areas. Alterations in occlusal morphology to accommodate support elements or to reduce cuspal interference on mandibular excursion may also be required. Preliminary impressions must therefore be accurate, as unless the occlusion and tooth form can be observed with exactness, decisions cannot be made in respect of rest seat preparations or grinding which must be carried out prior to taking the master impression.

Preliminary impressions are normally recorded in alginate material using stock trays which are available in a variety of sizes and materials. Such trays, however, do not usually fit the mouth well. Before attempting to take an impression, therefore, it is important to ensure that there is adequate coverage of all the tooth surfaces and related soft tissue areas together with sufficient clearance of the tissues by the tray flanges. This is done by placing the tray in the mouth and examining its coverage both laterally and antero-posteriorly, together with its peripheral extension. Generally it will be necessary to modify the adaptation and extension of the stock tray, particularly in the maxillary tuberosity region, the disto-lingual sulcus, and the vault of the palate. This can be done most effectively by adding impression compound to the tray in the deficient areas and then inserting it into the mouth in order to mould the compound while it is still plastic (Fig. 15.1). On removal the compound is chilled, and the modified tray can be used to record the preliminary impression in alignate material after an adhesive has been applied both to the compound and to any non-perforated areas of the tray. Whilst such an impression is not necessarily accurate in respect of its peripheral extension it avoids areas of unsupported alginate which would be liable to manipulative distortion, and ensures good reproduction of tooth surfaces, so enabling decisions to be made regarding tooth preparation. In this respect the use of impression compound on its own for recording preliminary

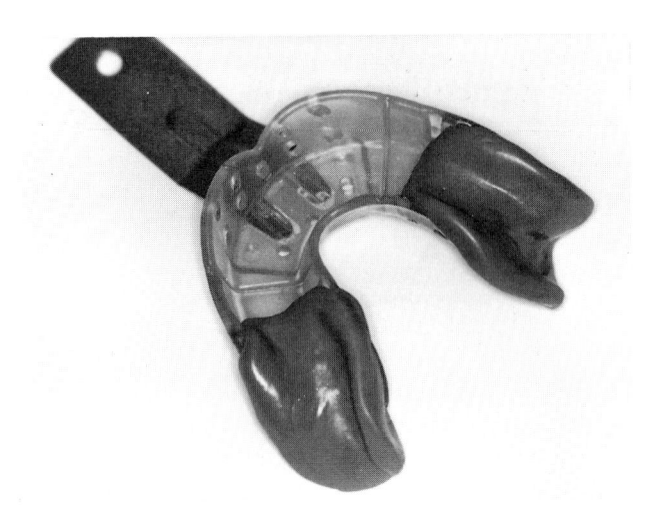

Fig. 15.1. Lower stock tray modified by addition of compound.

impressions for the partially dentulous mouth is contra-indicated, as it is unable to record with any degree of accuracy the form of the standing teeth thus precluding surveying the cast and producing a design.

Master impressions

Master impressions are only recorded after a decision has been made on the design of the partial denture. Any desired tooth or tissue preparation including routine restorative work, scaling, oral hygiene instruction and tissue conditioning should have been completed, and the tissues should be clinically and radiographically healthy. In particular, impressions should not be recorded immediately following subgingival scaling and the initial phase of oral hygiene instruction, in order to allow gingival tissues time for resolution, or following occlusal adjustment where some tooth movement might be anticipated.

The master impression should always be recorded in an individual tray which has been designed and constructed on the preliminary cast. Such trays should allow adequate space for an even substantial thickness of impression material between their fitting surface and the denture bearing tissues. In addition the periphery should not extend beyond the junction of the reflected and attached mucosa (the mucogingival line) which would lead to displacement of the tissue of the sulci during border moulding. Care must be taken also to ensure that the rigid tray does not extend into any undercut area which may make its insertion and seating difficult. Individual trays must be capable of supporting the impression material adequately in order to limit distortion. In this respect they must be strong and inflexible, and acrylic resin is therefore the material of choice rather than a thermoplastic material which is insufficiently rigid. The most popular material for recording master impressions is undoubtedly alginate (irreversible hydrocolloid). Although reversible hydrocolloids can also be used, the technique requires special equipment and is somewhat time consuming. More recently the elastomeric materials such as the polysulphides, silicones and polyethers have gained in popularity, particularly where a cast alloy framework is to be constructed, due to their dimensional stability.

Alginate Impressions

Alginate impression material is supplied as a powder, which when spatulated with the correct amount of water, produces a fluid, which changes in a few minutes to an elastic gel. Typically an alginate impression powder would contain a mixture of sodium or potassium alginate, calcium sulphate dihydrate, trisodium phosphate, modifiers and fillers such as diatomaceous earth, together with flavouring and colouring agents.

Sodium alginate is a colloidal substance prepared from various species of seaweed. It is the salt of alginic acid and a natural polymer. Sodium alginate dissolves in water to produce a viscous sol. However the calcium salt of alginic acid is insoluble and its colloidal structure can hold considerable quantities of water. It is therefore known as a hydrocolloid gel. If sodium alginate and calcium sulphate are mixed together in the presence of water, then the jelly-like calcium alginate is immediately formed by a double decomposition reaction. In the case of impression materials, however, a working time of at least two minutes is required and a retarding agent is necessary. This is tri-sodium phosphate which competes preferentially for calcium ions, so making them unavailable for reaction with the sodium alginate. The time taken to sequester the calcium ions depends on the amount of trisodium phosphate present. Once this has been used up, the calcium ions immediately precipitate the calcium alginate gel.

The modifiers, which include magnesium oxide and carbonate, and sodium fluoride and fluosilicate, produce good setting and a good surface. The filler gives body to the material.

To obtain optimum results with alginates, two issues must be attended to; the first is the proportion of powder to water, which should be as recommended by the manufacturer, whilst the second concerns thorough spatulation of the powder and water which can be achieved by using a flexible bowl and a curved rigid spatula.

Alginates are usually supplied as a bulk powder, which necessitates proportioning. However, some manufacturers supply pre-measured sachets, in which case only the water has to be proportioned. The popularity of alginates is due to the fact that they are easy to use and inexpensive; they also show reasonable elastic recovery.

Dimensional accuracy

When used correctly and according to the manufacturer's instructions, alignates can be relied upon to provide impressions which give accurate reproduction of surface detail and undercut areas. Faults may arise, however, from time to time and may be recognized as either surface or dimensional inaccuracies.

The commonest surface inaccuracy is the 'blow hole' or void. Small voids are usually due to the presence of air bubbles which have become entrapped in the alginate mix, while larger ones are caused by air being trapped between the surfaces of the impression material and the tissues. A second surface fault arises as a result of an adhesive film present on either the mucosa or the teeth. A viscous gelatinous film of mucus, which in some patients arises from the palatal glands situated on the posterior part of the hard palate, may be sufficiently thick to cause a surface inaccuracy, the impression showing characteristic punctate deficiencies and a surface covered with adherent ropy mucus. It is generally found that a small part of this mucous film is present before the impression is taken and that the presence of the impression material, although undoubtedly acting as a stimulus to secretion, does not account for a great increase in its thickness. A film of tenacious mucus or one of materia alba may be present on the teeth and prevent the close adaptation of the impression material to the enamel surface. Fortunately, all these surface inaccuracies can be eliminated by attention to details of technique, which will be considered later.

The second error is dimensional inaccuracy and its prevention is a more difficult problem, although much can be done by careful attention to technique. Dimensional changes may be caused by stress acting on the material either during or following its gelation.

Stresses that act during the set of the impression material may be induced as a result of either the calcium alginate expanding during its formation, or as a result of forces developed by the operator in his manipulation of the impression tray. The expansion of the gel is resisted by the tray and the mouth tissues and this results in the development of strains in the areas where the expansion has been restricted. The later release of these strains, after removal from the mouth, may lead to distortion. The other cause of strain is continuous pressure applied by the operator after the tray has been correctly seated and after gelation has occurred in the layer of alginate in close proximity to the warm tissues, but while the material next to the impression tray is still plastic. Such pressure may be applied with the mistaken idea that soft tissue displacement can be affected at this stage, or it may be developed accidentally as a result of closure of the mandible on to the operator's fingers. In either case, pressure is communicated through the rigid tray to the setting gel which, in consequence, is compressively stressed. A further cause of strain inducement is movement of the tray during gelation which is likely to produce permanent deformation. Whilst a careful operator is not likely to allow gross movement to occur, a small degree of movement may take place, if, during gelation, the operator changes his finger hold on the tray. In particular, a change of finger position is likely to allow a lower tray to move slightly upwards and this may produce a small error in the incisal edges of the anterior teeth. When placing the fingers on the tray in the first instance, a comfortable position should be selected so that it should not be necessary to change it until the impression is ready to be removed.

Distortion of the set impression material may occur either during or after its removal from the mouth. There can be little doubt that permanent deformation of the gel often occurs during removal of the impression from the mouth. This is particularly so if the impression is removed slowly from undercut areas rather than rapidly which allows elastic recoil. Stress applied at this stage may be beyond the elastic limit without causing visible damage to the impression or may be in excess of the proportional limit when tears in the material may be evident. Although it has been suggested that tears in alginate material can be repaired by the use of a cyanoacrylate adhesive it is the opinion of the authors that any impression in which a tear is apparent should be discarded as some distortion of the gel is almost certain to have occurred. One disadvantage of alginate materials is, however, that these tears need not necessarily be apparent on the surface of the impression. Consequently, a technique of removal is necessary which stresses the impression material minimally.

Permanent deformation is essentially dependent upon the stress applied to the material and the time during which this stress is applied. The degree of strain is governed by the overall shape of the jaw concerned and will be increased considerably by the presence of teeth with large undercuts. However, the time during which the stress is applied is, to a large extent, within the control of the clinician. Hence it is essential to remove the alginate impression as quickly as possible. In cases of severe undercuts it may not be possible to secure an undistorted alginate impression and a material with superior elastic properties such as silicone should be used.

During the setting reaction of alginates, the pH value of the fluid mass changes. Because of this, some manufacturers include acid/base indicators in their formations so that a colour change of the setting mass indicates that a certain point has been reached, usually the point at which the tray should be loaded or inserted into the mouth. These materials are usually referred to as chromatic alginates.

After removal from the mouth the alginate may be distorted either as a result of its losing or gaining water, or during pouring of casts. When the alginate gel is placed in water or an aqueous solution it absorbs water and consequently swells. This is known as imbibition. When the 'set' gel is allowed to stand in an atmosphere not saturated with vapour it loses water and consequently shrinks.

During pouring of casts, pressure may be exerted on the elastic gel causing its deformation. Distortion at this stage is maximum in those areas where the thickness of the impression is greatest or where the periphery of the impression is unsupported by the tray.

Technique

The patient

The patient must be seated comfortably in the dental chair with the head in line with the trunk and the occlusal plane horizontal. The chair should be at such a height that the operator is able to have complete control of the patient. Clothing should be protected by a plastic bib or napkin.

Prior to recording the impression the patient should be instructed to rinse their mouth with a warm solution of sodium bicarbonate. As this is a solvent for mucus it effectively removes any surface film from the palatal area and from the natural teeth. As well as improving dimensional accuracy therefore, it reduces the likelihood of retching by removing irritant mucus strands which track down on to the sensitive soft palate. This mouthwash also has a cleansing effect on the teeth, but this may be augmented by rubbing all surfaces of these with a dry napkin immediately prior to loading the tray. Some patients have such large interdental undercuts between their standing teeth that it is impossible to remove an impression without distortion of tearing. Packing such spaces with soft carding wax prior to impression taking is often necessary.

When recording the impression it is preferable to take the lower impression first. This lessens the possibility of retching and consequently inspires confidence. In addition less saliva is likely to pool in the floor of the mouth at this stage which can compromise the surface of the material.

Individual trays

The advantages of using individual trays for alginate impressions may be summarized as follows:

1   The peripheral extension of the impression can be recorded accurately. A tray which is over-extended will produce distortion of the tissues at the reflection of the sulcus and result in a denture periphery which is overextended. An under-extended tray does not give support to the set alginate and the unsupported gel is liable to be stressed either during, or subsequent to, removal from the mouth. This may produce deformation not only in the unsupported alginate but also in material which although supported is in immediate proximity to the periphery. It is advocated, therefore, that when using alginate, the tray is extended even in areas where the impression is not essential to denture construction.

Impression Taking 367

One possible exception to full peripheral extension is where a deep undercut exists in an area that is not required in the construction of the denture. Such an area is often present labially in the lower incisor region. In removing alginate from such a site it is necessarily strained and liable to distortion and the possibility of cutting the tray short should be considered (Fig. 15.2).

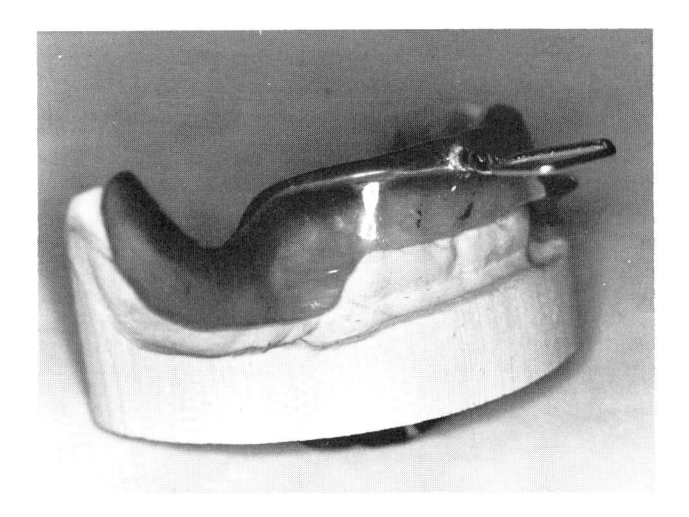

Fig. 15.2. Lower tray cut away labially in the incisor region.

2 It is possible to have a uniform thickness of material throughout the impression which again contributes to dimensional accuracy. Large, thick and therefore relatively unsupported bulks of alginate in the palatal vault, for example, are easily distorted during cast pouring, whilst varying thickness of material from one area to another may lead to inaccuracies in the reproduction of tooth and tissue undercuts.

3 There is less discomfort to the patient when taking the impression owing to the smaller tray and reduced mass of material. It is also much easier to control the flow of alginate on to the soft palate if an individual tray is used.

4 There is considerable economy of impression material.

Individual trays for alginate impressions should normally be constructed in autopolymerizing acrylic resin with a clearance of two thicknesses of base plate wax between the fitting surface of the tray and the preliminary cast. This ensures a tray of adequate strength and rigidity which can still be modified easily at the chairside if appropriate. The tray handle should be positioned centrally so that it is free from lip interference. In order that the alginate will adhere to the tray, it should be coated with a proprietary adhesive designed for this purpose. In this respect it is important that the adhesive be carried on to the labial, buccal and lingual surfaces of the tray to ensure adhesion of the peripheral roll of the material when it is formed by border moulding. Adhesive solutions are particularly efficient when the bond is stressed in tension. However where there are marked undercuts buccally and labially it may be necessary to include perforations in the tray to provide additional bonding against shear stress. An example of the type of tray preferred is shown in Fig. 15.3.

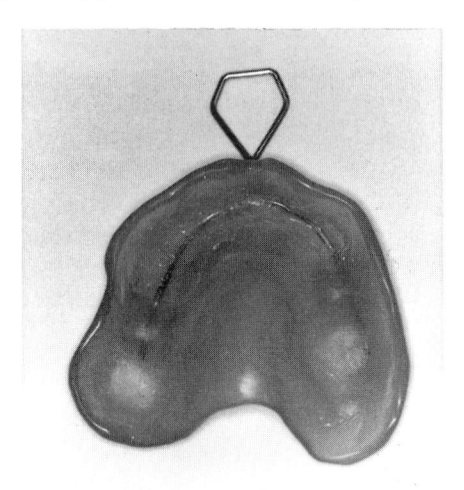

Fig. 15.3. Individual tray for alginate impression.

Prior to taking the impression the individual tray is tried in the mouth to assess its extension. In order to ensure that the border of the impression will be accurate it is important that the periphery of the tray does not extend beyond the mucogingival line. This can often be achieved by ensuring that on the preliminary cast the periphery is finished approximately 2 mm short of the depth of the functional sulcus (Fig. 15.4). The posterior extension of the upper tray should not be extended beyond the vibrating line and it is often an advantage to adapt either low fusing impression compound or an autopolymerizing acrylic border moulding material to the tissues in this area in order to control the escape of impression material on to the sensitive tissues of the soft palate and the dorsum of the tongue.

In addition this will ensure adequate consolidation of the fluid alginate over the posterior palatal tissues. It is sometimes useful to define accurately the buccal and labial peripheries of the tray also, by addition of impression compound or a border moulding material and allowing the patient to mould it by muscular movements of the lips and cheeks. If this is done, care should be taken that the resultant rigid material does not extend into undercut areas so making the tray difficult to insert.

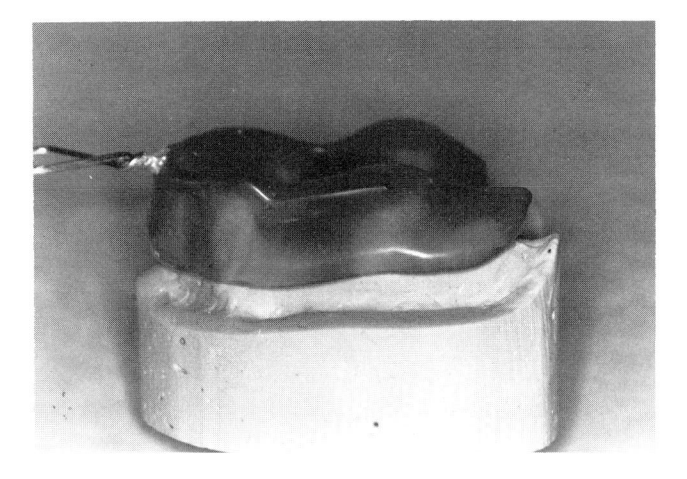

Fig. 15.4. Reduction of tray periphery.

The lower tray should be checked particularly for its lingual peripheral relationship to the floor of the mouth and lingual fraenum. Restricted movement of the tongue should be possible without gross movement of the tray. When the standing teeth are lingually inclined, adequate space should be allowed for impression material in this area otherwise tearing of the alginate material may occur. In such cases the partial denture may be designed with a labial bar connector and if this is anticipated the periphery of the tray must be adjusted so that the depth and width of the functional sulcus may be recorded accurately.

When recording the impression, care must be taken to avoid placing excessive load on the tray. This may be evident as the tray showing through the completed impression, particularly in the edentulous areas. This is inaccurate and will result in an areas of pressure in the finished denture, and can be avoided by placing stops of low fusing impression compound or any other suitable material. These stops should be placed in the tray whilst mouldable and the tray inserted into the mouth when the material will be moulded into the appropriate anatomical form (Fig. 15.5). When the tray is filled with impression material the stops will help to prevent the tray contacting the mucosa and will also aid in its spatial location.

Mixing

It cannot be too strongly emphasized that the manufacturer's instructions regarding proportioning the powder and water, checking the water temperature, and the mixing time should be followed accurately. These factors control the physical properties displayed by the material when it is inserted into the mouth and, together with the time the impression is held in the mouth, determine the nature of the final gel.

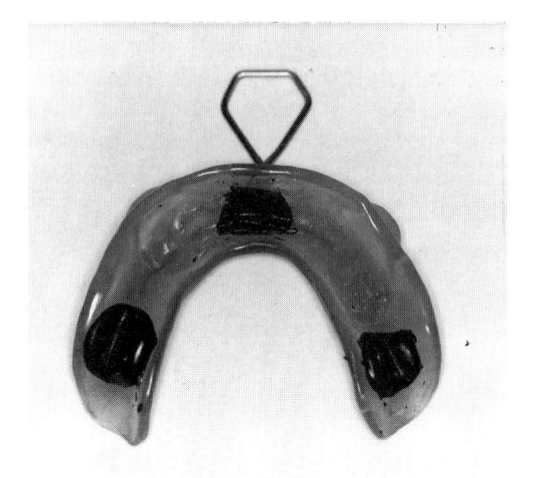

Fig. 15.5. Compound stops.

Different brands of alginate have different viscosities when mixed and whichever is preferred is a matter of personal choice. It must be understood, however, that if a high viscosity material is used then greater seating pressure is required to achieve sufficient flow. In addition there is a greater liability to entrap air and cause blow holes although this can be minimized by careful attention to technique.

Problems in accuracy may arise when measuring the proportions of powder and water. The amount of water presents little problem being measured volumetrically in a small cylinder provided by the manufacturer. Similarly if the powder is presented in individual package form for each impression there is no possibility of error. The majority of alginates are supplied, however, as loose powder, and it is not always particularly satisfactory to use the volumetric measure. The mass of powder so obtained is dependent upon its degree of consolidation in the measure and differences of up to 45% in weight can be demonstrated with supposedly similar volumes of the same material. Clearly variations such as this will produce mixes of differing viscosities, setting times and ultimate properties. In this respect it is suggested that the alginate container should be shaken vigorously to ensure dispersion of all the ingredients, following which a scoop of the loosened powder is tapped lightly against the side of the container and levelled off with the blade of a spatula. In this manner some standardization of mixes and their properties should be achieved.

As the gelation time of alginates is accelerated by an increase in temperature, particular attention should be paid to the manufacturer's instructions in respect of the mixing water. The use of water at a temperature in excess of that recommended, although reducing the time that the impression may be in the mouth, is likely to produce a mix which is not sufficiently plastic. This may result in additional pressure being required to seat the impression with excessive stress production within the gelling alginate. Both of these factors may result in distortion of the material on removal from the mouth.

The time and method of mixing have a marked effect on the condition of the material when it is placed in the patient's mouth. The time should be controlled by a watch with a second hand. The working times advocated by the manufacturers presume *thorough* and *vigorous* mixing and a combination of these factors ensures a smooth, homogeneous mix in which the chemical reactions have proceeded to the desired amount. Mixing should be carried out with a rigid curved mixer in preference to a flexible spatula. Initially the mixing should be slow and controlled so that the alginate powder is thoroughly wetted and none is lost from the mixing bowl. This period is followed by energetic spatulation when the material is worked against the *side* of the bowl.

Clinical technique

Once the impression material has been mixed for the required time and to the desired consistency it is loaded on to the modified individual tray. The correct volume of impression material is that equal to the two layers of wax used in the construction of the tray, but in practice some excess over this quantity is necessary. However, any great excess of material causes either an exudation over the buccal or posterior margins of the tray, thereby predisposing to retching, or an increased impression thickness. The impression material should be adapted during loading so that it approximates to the form of the arch and palatal vault. Less air is likely to be entrapped if the loading is done quickly with one or two lots of material on the mixing spatula.

The impression is then positioned in the mouth. In the case of the upper the tray may be located accurately by placing the anterior part of the tray in position whilst retracting the upper lip with the free hand to allow good visibility. The posterior part of the tray can then be raised into position using a slight 'puddling' motion, in order to improve the flow of the material into the undercut areas. The patient should partially close his mouth to allow appropriate border moulding to be carried out. This technique however has a disadvantage in that it drives impression material over the posterior border of the tray on to the soft palate and the dorsum of the tongue which may stimulate the retching reflex. In patients who are predisposed to retching the posterior border should be placed initially and then the anterior area rotated into position. Such a technique however may cause some difficulty in seating of the tray, and occasionally deficiencies may occur in the vault of the palate caused by the entrapment of air.

On insertion of the loaded lower tray some difficulty may be experienced if the patient has natural anterior teeth present in both jaws. In this case the mouth should be opened widely, and once the tray is located over the teeth, the mouth should be partially closed in order to relax the buccal and labial musculature and to allow seating of the impression. When seating the impression the buccal and labial tissues should be displaced outwards with the fingers to allow the impression material to flow over the periphery of the tray and avoid trapping of air or a fold of tissue. Border moulding should be then carried out buccally and labially by the operator and lingually by the patient. In this respect the patient should be instructed to protrude the tongue towards the handle of the tray and to maintain it in that position until final gelation has occurred. This will serve to mould the periphery of the impression in the disto-lingual region and to raise the floor of the mouth to its likely maximum extent during function. An impression so moulded will result in a denture which is not easily displaced by the surrounding musculature during normal functional movements.

This procedure of positioning and seating the impression should be carried out as rapidly as the skill of the operator permits in order to allow the maximum period of undisturbed gelation. When the tray has been correctly seated it must be supported without movement for the time advised by the manufacturer. The pressure applied at this stage should be sufficient only to support the tray in position, as any excessive pressure will not only cause displacement of the soft tissues but will also result in straining of the gel and subsequent distortion.

If the alginate has been mixed properly, the tray loaded correctly, and the appropriate clinical techniques followed then a satisfactory impression will be obtained. Departure from the techniques described is likely to result in an impression which will not be adequate for denture construction.

The period during which the impression remains in the mouth is critical. If it is short gelation may not be complete, while if the recommended time is exceeded the patient is subjected to unnecessary discomfort. Accordingly this period should be carefully timed according to the instructions of the manufacturer.

The method of removal, as well as the stage at which it is done, is important. In order to obtain an impression with the least amount of distortion or breakage, it is imperative that the hydrocolloid materials be removed from the teeth suddenly, by what almost amounts to an impact force or jerk. Removal should, therefore, be sudden and rapid.

Removal should be attempted in one downwards or upwards path, according to whether the impression is upper or lower and should normally be in the long axis of the teeth. Manipulation of the handle of the tray upwards and downwards has the effect of alternatively compressing and stretching the material anteriorly and posteriorly, which will result in deformation within the impression which may be permanent (Fig. 15.6).

If the tray is withdrawn vertically without any rotation, particularly in cases where the soft palate lies more nearly horizontal and when excess alginate posteriorly is minimal, a space is immediately created between the palate and material which allows the ingress of air so facilitating the removal of the impression rapidly and with minimal distortion.

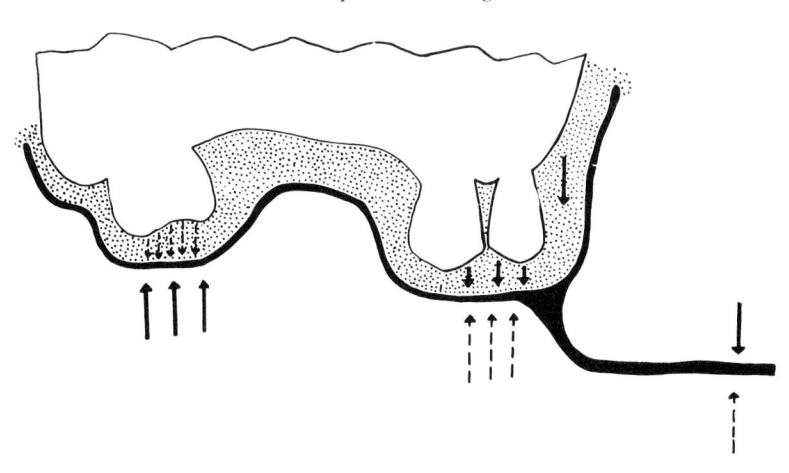

Fig. 15.6. Diagrammatic illustration of alternate compression and tension of alginate if removal from the mouth is attempted by upwards and downwards movement of the tray handle.

Pouring casts

Once the impression has been removed from the mouth it should be rinsed under cold running water in order to move any mucus or blood which may be adhering to the surface. The impression should now be inspected by the operator. In this respect it should demonstrate a well formed periphery with adequate coverage of the denture bearing area, together with accurate reproduction of tooth and soft tissue form. Any air entrapment should be minor and not related to the teeth or major denture bearing area. The tray should not be visible through the impression. If these basic conditions cannot be satisfied the impression should be rejected.

If the impression is satisfactory it should be covered by a damp napkin and a cast poured from it within fifteen minutes of its removal from the mouth. If left longer, dimensional change is liable to occur through syneresis and strain release within the gel. If circumstances are impossible for immediate pouring it should be stored at 100% relative humidity with adequate support and poured as soon as possible. The practice of placing alginate impressions unsupported in a sealed container along with others for pouring at a later stage by a laboratory at some distance from the premises is to be deprecated, as the potential for distortion and dimensional change due to mishandling is considerable.

Distortion of flexible impression materials can be caused during pouring of casts if the consistency of the stone is too thick or if vibration is excessive. For these reasons the recommended water–stone ratio should be adhered to and vibration should not be vigorous. This type of impression must never be inverted and pressed firmly down on to a heap of stone on the bench. This is the *surest way of producing relatively gross distortion* of the impression. Impressions should be filled with stone and the base added later when the stone has set. It is at the pouring stage that unsupported alginate is most liable to distortion. In order to ensure that a cast is produced with the correct peripheral form it is essential to indicate the desired extent of the impression by means of a line drawn on the buccal, labial and lingual surfaces with an indelible pencil (Fig. 15.7). In this way the technician is able to produce a cast recording the correct depth and width of the functional sulcus to which the final denture can be constructed.

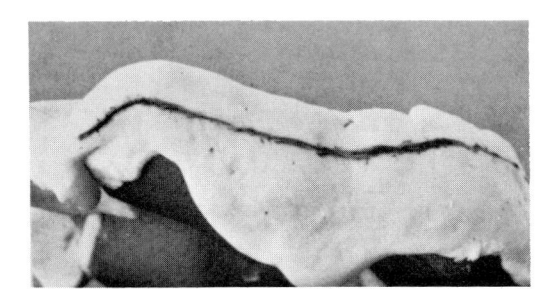

Fig. 15.7. Pencil line marked on alginate impression.

Following pouring of the cast the impression material should be removed approximately one hour later to allow complete setting of the cast material. Prolonged contact between stone and alginate may lead to fracture of teeth on removal of the impression due to contraction of the alginate as it loses some of its water content. Casts should be poured in dental stone in order to ensure satisfactory surface hardness and compressive strength.

Special Impression Techniques

The question of whether it is best to try to obtain displacement of the tissue under a free-end saddle at the impression stage or to take a mucostatic impression (such as is obtained by the alginates) has already been discussed. The usual practice is to employ a rebasing technique.

A dual impression technique for bilateral free-end saddle dentures can be used in an attempt to equalize the loading between mucosa and abutment teeth during function. A close fitting acrylic resin tray is used first to secure a paste impression of the saddle areas and the mucosa between the floor of the mouth and the gingivae of the teeth. After excess material which may have flowed on to the teeth has been cut away, a second impression is taken in alginate with the first impression in position in the mouth. Large holes are made in the saddle areas of the tray used for the alginate so that when this impression is positioned, finger pressure may be applied directly to the saddle area of the first impression. Thus a compressed impression of the mucosa and a mucostatic impression of the teeth are secured at the same time. This technique serves to relate the residual ridge to the teeth as if a functional masticatory load were being applied to the denture base.

This clearly has a disadvantage, in that if the clasps retaining the denture were effective then a constant load would be placed on the underlying denture bearing area of the saddle, which could possibly result in bone resorbtion. Alternatively in a situation where the retentive arms of the clasps were less effective, the recoil of the mucosa which would occur with the removal of the load would tend to raise the denture to a position which was vertically occlusal to its functional position, with the occlual rests out of contact with the teeth. Closure during function would result firstly in contact of the denture teeth, with the occlusal rests becoming effective only following compression of the mucosa of the saddle, a situation which may not be well accepted by the patient.

Similar principles of two part impressions can be applied to the upper jaw when only the anterior teeth are present. A close fitting resin tray is made to cover all the edentulous areas and also the lingual surfaces of the natural teeth. After taking a zinc oxide paste impression any excess that has flowed over the incisal edges is removed. With the paste impression in the mouth, a labial impression of the teeth and sulcus is taken, supported by a labial supporting tray. This part of the impression can be taken in alginate or plaster, according to the dentist's preference.

Elastomeric Impressions

The elastomeric impression materials include the polysulphides, the silicones and the polyethers. Although alginate impression material is generally satisfactory in partial denture construction, in some situations where a particularly high level of accuracy is desired, an elastomeric impression may be preferred. An example might be a cast metal framework with multiple rest seat preparations where accurate adaptation of the metal to unyielding enamel is required. In addition such materials are tougher and more elastic than the alginates and can be used in situations where there are severe undercuts which would result in tearing of the alginate.

The polysulphides are presented as a dual paste system with a base paste and accelerator, which undergoes polymerization after homogeneous mixing. They may be produced in pastes of varying viscosities which are compatible with each other and can be used together, the lower viscosity paste recording fine detail. For partial denture work a single paste of medium viscosity is usually quite suitable. After mixing, the paste undergoes relatively slow polymerization until inserted into the mouth where the process is accelerated by the heat and moisture. To ensure thorough polymerization the material used should not exceed 2–3 mm in thickness, and the impression should not be removed from the mouth until the remainder of the material has set on the mixing pad. An individual tray is therefore necessary and the material is retained by an adhesive produced by the manufacturer. Removal should be rapid to ensure elastic behaviour of the material and 30 minutes should elapse before pouring the cast to allow full elastic recovery.

Silicone materials are also supplied as a base paste and a reactor (which may be either paste or liquid). Setting occurs either by a substitution or addition reaction. In the former, by-products such as alcohol may be produced which may affect the dimensional stability of the impression, whereas in the latter no by-products are formed. Silicone materials have a range of viscosities, from a high viscosity putty to a low viscosity material suitable for a wash impression. In general a medium viscosity material is suitable for partial denture construction and should be used with an individual tray and adhesive as appropriate. The silicone materials are more elastic than the polysulphides and can be used to record deeper undercuts. Although some 30 minutes should be left to allow full elastic recovery before pouring the cast, it should be noted that the silicones are less dimensionally stable in storage than the polysulphides.

Polyether materials are also supplied as a base paste and reactor paste which are mixed together but are not used as commonly as polysulphides and silicones in partial denture work. Some skill is required in their manipulation, and where a large amount of material is being mixed there is a distinct possibility of distortion. When set they are much more rigid than polysulphides or silicones and may be difficult to remove from undercuts without tearing. Similarly, attempted removal from the cast may result in breakage of teeth.

For a more detailed description of the properties of the elastomeric impression materials the reader is referred to an appropriate textbook.

Technique

The patient should be prepared as for an alginate impression. Individual trays are mandatory and should be constructed in acrylic resin which has a rigidity that will limit distortion. Retention of the material to the tray is by means of the manufacturer's adhesive as opposed to perforations.

The tray should have been constructed with its periphery extended to the mucogingival line with any obvious deficiency being restored by low fusing impression compound before taking the impression. In the free-end saddle situation it is useful to include 'stops' of compound or soft red carding wax (Fig. 15.5).

Proportioning and mixing of the base and reactor pastes should be carried out according to the manufacturer's instructions. As reaction between the two pastes is immediate on contact they should be kept separate until mixing is about to commence. A broad bladed flexible spatula should be used and the two pastes mixed thoroughly.

Since the viscosity of the mixed material increases as polymerization proceeds, and this reaction commences as soon as mixing is begun, the tray should be loaded and inserted into the mouth as soon as possible after mixing. Many areas of most impressions will require relatively thin sections of material and if its viscosity becomes too great adequate flow will not be obtained. Owing to the greater viscosity of the elastomeric materials in comparison with alginate, more pressure will be required to seat the impression and a greater degree of tissue displacement may result. The general principles of tray positioning and tissue manipulation should be followed as described for alginate.

Elastomeric materials should not be removed from the mouth until thoroughly set on the mixing pad to avoid possible distortion. For practical purposes they should be kept in position in the mouth for approximately two minutes after they have appeared to set. Although these materials are more elastic and less likely to tear than the alginate, they should nevertheless be removed from the mouth fairly rapidly to maximize their elastic properties. A period of 30 minutes should elapse before pouring the cast to allow full elastic recovery. A completed silicone impression is shown in Fig. 15.8.

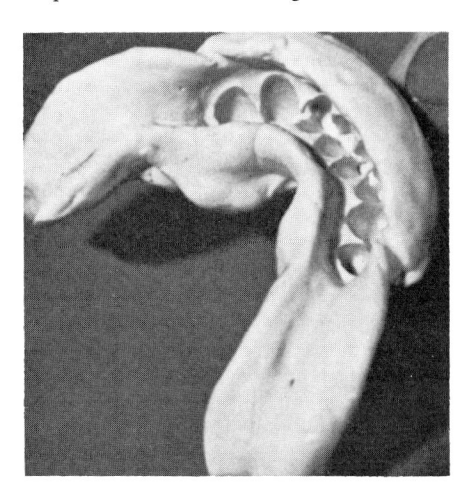

Fig. 15.8. Complete partial lower silicone impression.

The dimensional stability of elastomeric materials after removal from the mouth is greatly superior to that of the alginates. Although it can be assumed that contraction starts after setting it is at least four hours before any dimensional change is measurable, and even then it is hardly of clinical significance. The adhesion of the material to the impression tray is significant in restricting changes in linear dimension and beneficial in reducing possible distortions due to the separation of the material from the tray. When dimensional change can be measured it is found that the material contracts towards the tray and hence the tooth impressions become larger. As a matter of clinical practice it is wise to have the models from all impressions cast not less than four hours after the impressions have been removed from the mouth.

No treatment of the impression surface is necessary before the casts are poured. During pouring there is less danger of distortion of the material than there is with alginate, owing to the greater stiffness. None the less, care should be exercised to ensure that no stress is placed upon the impression material while the model material is setting.

Control of Retching

A few patients are always genuinely embarrassed by having an upper impression taken, because it makes them retch. When such a patient has to have a denture, attention should be paid to the following points. Adjust the posterior border of the tray to be short of the soft palate—in severe cases it must end even further forward. Make sure, by postdamming, that the tray is a close tissue fit at this point. Before inserting the tray the patient may be asked to blow the nose and then be instructed to breathe through it, rather than through the mouth. Rinsing with a mouthwash of sodium bicarbonate will help to remove the viscous mucus often present in these cases and visible as long strands extending back and irritating the soft palate. When inserting the impression seat the posterior portion first and then swing the anterior part up into place, which will bring excess material forwards rather than back onto the soft palate. As a further help in this respect the patient's head should be brought forward and downwards. Preference should be given to impression materials that require the shortest period in the mouth. Although surface anaesthesia is favoured by some operators this is not always effective in controlling the reflex. It does not remove the psychogenic awareness of the patient and in some cases may stimulate retching due to the unusual sensation in the mouth. It may, however, be psychologically prudent to prepare the impression material out of the patient's visual field.

References

BASKER R.M. and SPENCE D. (1976) Some properties and clinical uses of a border trimming material. *Brit. dent. J.* **140,** 138.

HINDELS G.W. (1957) Stress analysis in distal extension partial dentures. *J. pros. Dent.* **7,** 197–205.

KRAMER H.M. (1961) Impression techniques for removable partial dentures. *J. pros. Dent.* **11**, 84.

LAMBRECHT J.R. (1968) Immediate denture construction; the impression phase. *J. pros. Dent.* **19**, 237–45.

MACGREGOR A.R. (1967) Impression trays—a new design. *Dent. Pract.* **18**, 2.

MCLEAN J.W. (1958) Silicone impression materials. *Brit. dent. J.* **104**, 441–51.

MCLEAN J.W. (1961) Physical properties influencing the accuracy of silicone and thiokol impression materials. *Brit. dent. J.* **110**, 85.

OSBORNE J. and LAMMIE G.A. (1954) The manipulation of alginate impression materials. *Brit. dent. J.* **96**, 51–58.

PHANKOSAL P. and TAYLOR T.D. (1984) Repairing torn irreversible hydrocolloid impressions with cyanoacrylate adhesive. *J. pros. Dent.* **51**, 722.

SKINNER E.W. (1946) *The science of dental materials*, 3rd edition. W. B. Saunders Co., Philadelphia.

SKINNER E.W and POMES C.E (1947) Alginate impression materials: technique for manipulation and criteria for selection. *J. Amer. dent, Ass.* **35**, 245–56.

TOMLIN H.R. and OSBORNE J. (1958) Some observations on silicone impression materials. *Brit. dent. J.* **105**, 407–12.

TRYDE G. and BRANTENBERG F. (1965) Den sublinguale barr. *Saertryk af Tand.* **69**, 873–85.

WILSON H.J. and SMITH D.C. (1963) Alginate impression materials. *Brit. dent. J.* **114**, 20.

WILSON H.J. and SMITH D.C. (1963) Bonding of alginate impression materials to impression trays. *Brit. dent. J.* **115**, 291.

16
REGISTRATION OF JAW RELATIONS

For the partially edentuous patient jaw relations must be recorded at an early stage in treatment. This allows preliminary casts to be mounted on an articulator for the clinician to study the relation of the upper and lower teeth in both the intercuspal position and in limited eccentric movements of the mandible. In addition, it affords the facility of viewing the relationship of the teeth from 'inside the mouth' via the rear of the articulator. It is only from the understanding of these relationships, together with information from a preliminary survey, that a satisfactory design can be developed.

Registration of jaw relations for a partially edentulous patient may be relatively straightforward, perhaps only involving location of the upper and lower casts in the intercuspal or tooth position by means of the standing teeth. Alternatively, in a situation where many posterior teeth have been lost, the technique may be similar to that for an edentulous patient. The basic principles remain the same, however, namely the recording of correct vertical and horizontal positions of the mandible relative to the maxilla, together with any necessary face bow recordings, lateral and protrusive jaw relationships, followed by the selection of an appropriate shade, mould and material of tooth.

At this stage it is necessary to establish an occlusion which is in harmony with the occlusion of the remaining natural teeth. If this is not the case, excessive stresses may be transmitted to the natural teeth by components of the partial denture due to cusp locking or excessive load in working occlusions. The stress transmitted to the teeth and residual ridges will be related to the denture design and occlusion developed.

An effective method of developing a satisfactory occlusion without cuspal interference on excursion is by the use of an adjustable or semi-adjustable articulator. In order to be confident of achieving this, however, it is necessary that accurate reproduction of mandibular movement can be obtained, and although some jaw movements may be reproduced accurately, it is not possible to record precisely the whole range of functional movement. So, although the use of an adjustable articulator may be helpful in enabling some assessment of jaw movements, it cannot be accepted that perfect occlusal balance can be achieved, which in any event is only rarely present in the natural dentition. The movements of the articulator are mainly used, therefore, to ensure that there is minimal cuspal interference from the artificial teeth during functional movements, and that they are set in a position in which they are in harmony with the natural occlusion. This harmony must always be improved by additional occlusal adjustment when the dentures are inserted into the mouth. Unlike complete dentures, which may have their occlusion perfected following remounting on an articulator after processing, the final occlusal adjustments to partial dentures are best carried out intra-orally due to the differential compressibility between the supporting oral mucous membrane and the periodontal ligament, and the limitations in articulator theory.

In the majority of cases, therefore, an average movement (fixed condylar guidance angle) articulator is satisfactory. If it is decided to employ a fully adjustable articulator then, in addition to recording the intercuspal or tooth position, the operator must also obtain a face bow recording together with left and right lateral and/or protrusive records to enable the technician to set the individual condylar guidance angles and to position the maxilla correctly in relation to the intercondylar axis.

The Clinical Approach

For the purposes of recording jaw relations, partial dentures may be divided into three main categories:

1 Where one jaw is edentulous and the other is to be restored with a partial denture; the commonest example being an edentulous upper and bilateral free-end saddle lower.
2 Where partial dentures are required in one or both jaws and where there are insufficient teeth present to indicate the intercuspal or tooth position. Examples are situations where there has been extensive loss of posterior teeth.
3 Where there are sufficient teeth present in both jaws to indicate the intercuspal or tooth position.

The record blocks

During registration it is essential that the base of the record block is not only adapted accurately to the underlying tissues, but is also sufficiently strong and rigid at mouth temperature to avoid distortion. It is essential therefore, that all blocks have a strong shellac or acrylic resin base, although this should not extend into undercut areas or the surface of the cast will be damaged during removal and replacement of the block. For free-end saddles the base should be finished short of the distal end of the saddle area in order to facilitate trimming of the rim in situations where there is a limited inter-ridge distance. If necessary, blocks can be stabilized by the use of clasps on the abutment teeth or wrought bars around the standing teeth (Fig. 16.1). The rim of the record block is normally formed in wax, preferably a hard variety of paraffin wax in order to minimize distortion.

Chapter 16

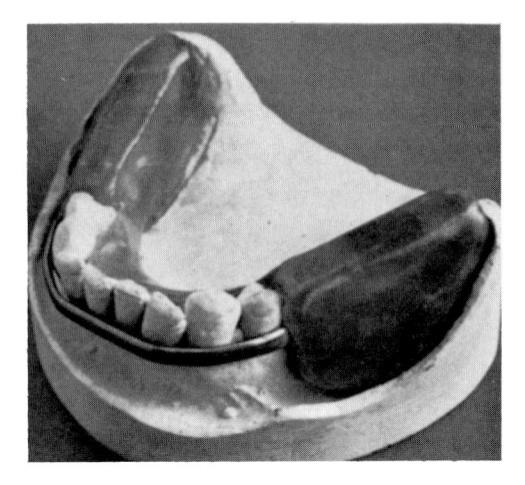

Fig. 16.1. Wrought wire to stabilize a partial lower record block.

In the construction of record blocks it is necessary to consider whether they are required for both jaws or whether the record can be obtained satisfactorily by the use of one block alone. In this respect it should be appreciated that a minimum of three disparate contact areas between the jaws are desirable, bilaterally in the posterior region and singly in the anterior region. If only one block can be used patients are generally more tolerant and co-operative, and so the possibility of an incorrect record is decreased.

Clinical procedures

The basic principles of recording the jaw relationships or occlusion are similar in each category as is the clinical approach.

The edentulous upper and partially edentulous lower. The patient should be seated comfortably in the dental chair with the head upright and in line with the trunk. The upper block is tried in the mouth first and assessed with respect to fit, retention and stability. Particular attention should be given to the periphery of the base and the position of the posterior border, to ensure that it is extended correctly on to the compressible tissues of the hard palate where the posterior seal will be developed.

The wax rim should be carved or moulded to the labial and buccal contour that will be required in the finished denture. In the anterior region this will be determined by the amount of lip support that is desired for the patient. In this respect the appearance desired by the patient and indeed the operator may not be compatible with function and it is often necessary to effect a compromise. For instance the rim often has to be modified to ensure that the pressure exerted on the denture by the lip will not displace it from its basal seat. If the denture is replacing one which has already been satisfactory, due consideration must be given to the tooth position of the previous denture and the relationship to the lower anterior teeth, together with its labial contour in order to avoid any gross alterations in appearance and established neuromuscular patterns. Duplication of the previous denture may be considered in such a situation.

If the patient has been without a denture since the natural teeth were extracted, the position of the anterior teeth may be more difficult to determine. If they are set directly below the residual ridge then lip pressure on the denture will be negligible, however, this will invariably be at the expense of aesthetics and possibly also tongue space. Improved appearance obtained by setting the teeth anterior to the residual ridge may result in instability of the denture. In this respect the use of biometric guidelines for tooth placement is useful, with the labial surface of the central incisors being placed 10 mm anterior to the mid point of the incisive papilla. When correctly contoured, the block should support the lip at an approximate naso-labial angle of 90 ° with the vermilion border of the lip clearly visible. It must be emphasized, however, that these are guidelines only, and that the prominence of the anterior teeth and the amount of lip support will also depend upon factors affecting the likely retention of the upper denture, such as the size and form of the residual alveolar ridge, the consistency of tissues overlying the bone, and the type and amount of saliva present. It must be remembered that the age of the patient, and therefore the elasticity of the tissues, will also influence the manner in which the lip will accommodate to the presence of a denture.

In partial dentures, as opposed to complete dentures, the length and inclination of any natural lower teeth present may have a significant effect on the positioning of the upper teeth. Proclined lower anterior teeth are an embarrassment to both the patient and the operator. If proclination of the lower teeth necessitates excessive proclination of the teeth on the upper denture its stability and retention may be adversely affected. In such cases it may be necessary to compromise between appearance and function, or alternatively to alter the lower teeth by grinding both incisally and interstitially.

Once the anterior part of the block has been moulded it is necessary to establish the level and angulation of the occlusal plane. Wherever natural teeth remain there is some guidance present, and in some cases the occlusal plane is dictated completely by the position of remaining teeth. In the situation where only six lower anterior teeth are present the occlusal plane should be determined initially by the lower rim. In the natural dentition the retromolar pad lies in immediate superior relationship to the last molar tooth, and since resorption in this area is minimal, the anterior part of the retromolar pad may be useful as a guide in indicating the occlusal level in this region. The record block should be trimmed accordingly to a level indicated anteriorly by the abutment teeth and posteriorly by the base of the retromolar pad (Fig. 16.2). At this stage the peripheral extension and buccal and lingual contours of the lower block should be checked and modified where necessary. This can be done lingually by having the patient raise his tongue and execute lateral and protrusive movements, and buccally by movement of the cheeks. These should not be excessive, and the periphery can be adjusted until functional displacement of the block is minimal.

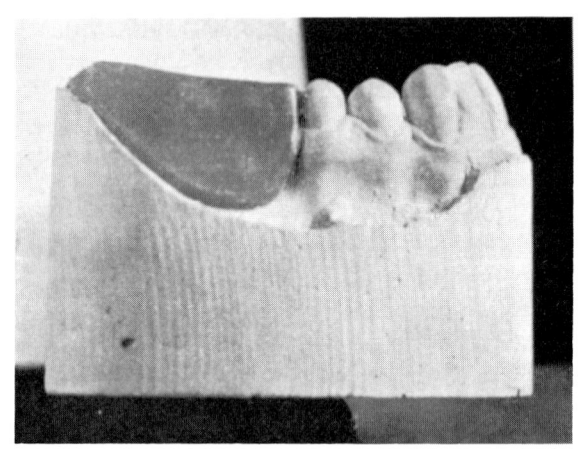

Fig. 16.2. Lower record block curved to the orientation of the occlusal plane indicated by the standing teeth.

Where extensive peripheral adjustment is necessary however, this is indicative of an inaccurate impression, and in such circumstances a new impression should be taken with particular attention given to functional border moulding. The lingual and buccal contours of the lower block in partial denture construction are also of considerable importance to enhance stability, and the contours of the block should be modified in such a way that it resembles the anticipated shape of the finished denture in relation to the tongue and cheeks.

When the lower block has been trimmed satisfactorily, the upper block can be re-inserted and the occlusion modified until even contact is achieved so establishing the position of the upper occlusal plane. Once this has been completed the vertical dimension of occlusion can be recorded.

It has been observed that more dentures fail from incorrect vertical jaw relations than any other cause, and although partial denture construction is dependent upon accuracy and precision at all stages, there is no more important record to be obtained correctly than the vertical dimension of occlusion. An insufficient vertical dimension of occlusion will result in poor aesthetics with inadequate facial and lip support, loss of height in the lower third of the face, impaired masticatory performance and disorders in the temporomandibular joint. Conversely an excessive vertical dimension will result in discomfort in the load bearing tissues, a strained facial appearance, difficulty with speech and mastication, and accelerated ridge resorption due to continuous pressure from the dentures.

The correct recording of vertical dimension is dependent upon the provision of an adequate interocclusal clearance, which is the space existing between the occlusal surfaces of the upper and lower teeth when the mandible is in the rest position. The size of interocclusal clearance varies but on average is between two and four millimetres, and unless provision is made for this clearance the denture will be unsuccessful.

If the patient already has dentures which have been satisfactory this will give an indication of the most suitable vertical dimension of occlusion for the replacement dentures, although some allowance may have to be made for occlusal wear and resorption of the residual ridge which has occurred since the original denture was inserted. In either event the procedure for establishing the vertical dimension of occlusion is similar, and is dependent upon being able to measure the vertical dimension at rest.

With only the lower block in position the patient is asked to relax into the mandibular rest position. Prior to this, however, references are placed in the midline of the face, one on the tip of the nose and one on the chin. The distance between these marks can be determined using a pair of dividers which are then locked to provide a reference measurement, the precise value of which is of no significance. The upper block is then inserted into the mouth and the patient encouraged to close in the muscular or in some cases the retruded contact position and the dividers repositioned against the references on the face. If the distance between the references is the same as before then the vertical dimension of occlusion of the dentures is the same as the rest vertical dimension and there is no interocclusal clearance. If the reference on the chin is more distant from the one on the nose, then the recorded vertical dimension of occlusion is in excess of the rest vertical dimension. If it is closer to the reference on the nose by some 2-3 mm, then the vertical dimension of occlusion is less than the rest vertical dimension, and some interocclusal clearance will be present between the occlusal surfaces of the upper and lower teeth with the mandible in the rest position.

Alternatively a similar result can be achieved by transferring the marks to a card held in front of the patient's face (Fig. 16.3). In this illustration the patient is at the vertical dimension of occlusion with the blocks in contact. The difference between the two lower marks on the card is the difference between the vertical dimension of occlusion and the rest vertical dimension, that is the interocclusal clearance.

Earlier suggestions were made for obtaining a relaxed state when recording the rest position of patients with standing teeth in both jaws. A similar approach should be made in the cases now being considered.

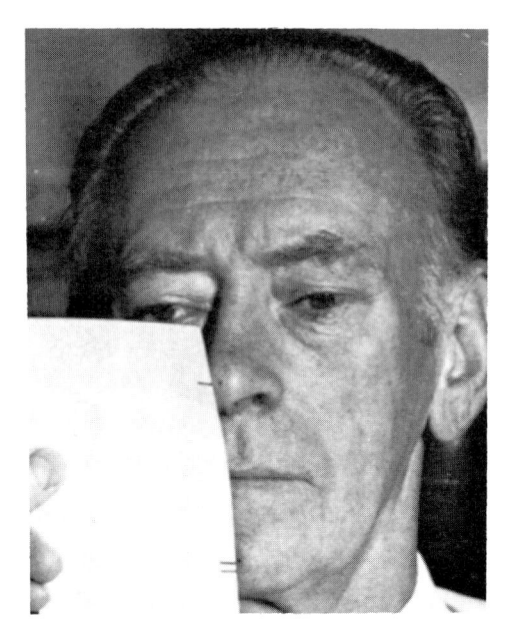

Fig. 16.3. Use of card to record vertical dimension.

Estimation of the interocclusal clearance may be helped by the use of phonetics. Before asking the patient to carry out phonetic tests the lingual and palatal wax of the record blocks should be reduced to allow free tongue movement. It is also important that the blocks remain stable during these tests, and it may be necessary to ensure this by means of gum tragacanth.

If the patient is asked to say 'M' the lips are brought into unstrained contact and no pressure applied. If this sound is made by the patient with the blocks in the mouth, it will possible to observe whether the lips can come into this unstrained relationship. The patient may also be asked if this 'M' sound can be made without the blocks coming into contact.

Another valuable phonetic guide to the interocclusal clearance is to ask the patient to say the words 'thick' or 'thin'. The tip and lateral margins of the tongue may enter the space between the teeth when these words are pronounced, and if the interocclusal clearance is correct, the tongue may be visible between the blocks.

Again it has been found that when the letters 'F' and 'V' are pronounced, the lower lips makes a definite contact with the incisal edges of the upper teeth. If the interocclusal clearance is absent or if the upper anterior teeth are incorrectly placed, the patient will be in difficulties with words such as 'five' or 'valve'. The test is perhaps best applied at the try-in stage since it can then be used as a check on tooth setting as well as vertical dimension.

By use of the phonetic tests, allied to general experience and common sense, it should be possible to check the pressure of the interocclusal clearance and, consequently, the vertical dimension. However, it must be appreciated that a patient who has been partially edentulous for several months will not be able to pronounce words and letters with normal clarity with the record blocks in the mouth, even though the interocclusal clearance is correct. Hence, in common with all other methods of vertical dimension assessment, phonetic tests should not be regarded as always infallible and accurate.

It now remains to unite the blocks together in the muscular or retruded contact position. If the vertical dimension is correct, this should not be a difficult matter. However, it must be appreciated that the success of this procedure depends upon the ability of the operator to induce in the patient a state of complete relaxation. When the patient is relaxed, the upper and lower blocks are inserted and the patient asked to close on the posterior teeth. If this can be repeated to a consistent position, locating notches can be cut in the blocks and the procedure repeated to check the relationship. This can be checked further by feeling some contraction of the fibres of temporalis which occurs with clenching at the muscular position.

Sealing the blocks together is best done by placing a very thin layer of bite registration paste over the occlusal surface of the upper block before final closure is made. Any natural teeth present in occlusion will make an indentation through this material and the surfaces of the two blocks will be united. Prior to placing the paste on the block, apply a thin smear of petroleum jelly to the wax rim so that the upper block may be separated after removal from the mouth and used for subsequent records, such as the face bow.

The centre line must be marked on the upper block. This line should indicate the mesial contact of the two upper centrals and this may not be in alignment with the corresponding teeth in the lower jaw. If the lower centre is not in the midline it is usually better to place the upper centre in the correct position and ignore the fact that it does not coincide with the lower. To the lay eye this is far less noticeable than an upper centre that deviates from the midline.

A registration of jaw relationship recorded in this manner will be suitable for use on an average movement articulator. If a fully adjustable articulator is to be used then several additional records are required.

The first of these should be the face bow recording. The face bow is an instrument which records the relationship of the maxilla to the intercondylar axis of the patient, so that the upper cast may be mounted within the frame of the articulator in a similar relationship to its intercondylar axis. Unless this relationship is established there is little advantage in using this type of articulator.

Initially the face bow is adjusted to the patient. The heads of the condyles are located and their estimated positions marked with a skin pencil. The surface marking of the condyle is approximately twelve millimetres anterior to the tragus of the ear on a line drawn from the point of the tragus to the outer canthus of the eye (Fig. 16.4). Palpation over the condyles or within the external auditory meatus may be used to confirm this position. The condylar rods of the face bow are adjusted so that their ends touch these surface markings with equal pressure. The calibrations should be equal on both sides before the rods are locked in position. The face bow is now removed from the patient.

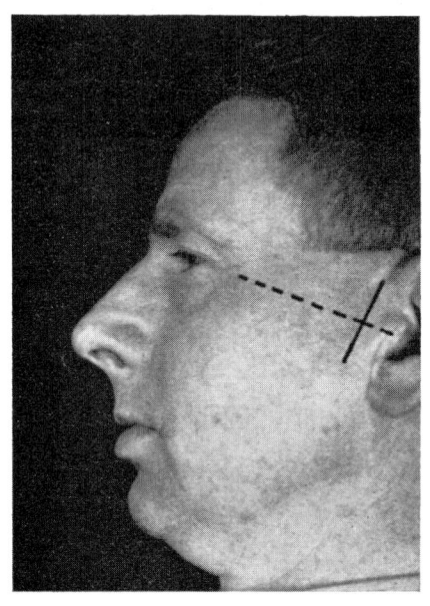

Fig. 16.4. Surface marking of the condyle.

The prongs of the face bow fork should now be covered with wax to a thickness of approximately half a centimetre. Before placing this is in the mouth the record blocks should be inserted after being coated lightly with petroleum jelly.

Whilst the wax is still soft, the face bow fork is inserted between the record blocks, and the patient is instructed to close until it is held securely in position. While the patient is closing, the operator should hold the stem of the fork to ensure that it projects forward in the saggital plane and parallel to the occlusal plane. The forward projection, whilst being horizontal, should be a little off centre to allow for closure of the articulator when mounting the upper cast.

The face bow is now returned to the patient allowing the stem of the fork to be engaged in the clamp as the bow is fitted into position. A check of the position of the condyle rods should be made before tightening the clamp to unite the bow to the fork. The Dentatus articulator provides an additional indicator for aligning the occlusal plane in its correct relation to the Frankfort plane. This consists of a pointer, which is placed in contact with the infra orbital foramen and attached to the face bow by a clamp (Fig. 16.5). When this has been done the whole assembly should be removed carefully and set aside ready for mounting the upper cast on the articulator.

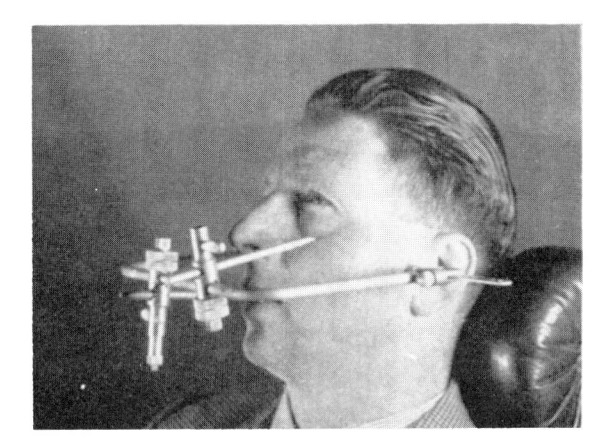

Fig. 16.5. Dentatus face bow in position.

To enable the condylar guidance on both sides to be set on the articulator it is necessary to have records of the mandible in a position where the condyles are moved into a forward position on the articulator eminence. Such a position is that of protrusion, in which both condyles have moved appreciably in the direction desired. These records are obtained by asking the patient to close in the protrusive or lateral positions with a wafer of wax interposed between the record blocks. The wax wafers should be shaped to conform to the arch and should be approximately half a centimetre thick. Three layers of ordinary paraffin wax reinforced with a layer of dental napkin between each of them is very suitable, the napkin providing a strengthening layer. Before placing them in the mouth the occlusal surfaces of the record blocks should be smeared with petroleum jelly to prevent the wax sticking. The surfaces of the blocks should also be notched in such a way that the wafers can be located accurately at a later stage.

With both blocks in the mouth the softened wafer is placed over the lower block and teeth, and the patient instructed to close with the mandible in protruded relation. At least half a centimetre is necessary to provide sufficient condylar movement to make a usable record. Care must be taken to ensure that the movement is protrusive only and that there is no deviation laterally. To this end a check on the alignment of the upper and lower centres when the protrusive closure has taken place is helpful. If this is satisfactory the wax wafer is chilled in the mouth to reduce the risk of distortion during removal.

When a definite protrusive relation of the desired degree cannot be secured it is necessary to obtain left and right lateral records. In any case, it may be considered advisable to take lateral records as a check, when setting the condylar guidance on the articulator, on the accuracy of the protrusive record. Two wafers are required for this purpose, and they are inserted one at a time and the patient asked to close in left and then in right lateral positions.

When face bow and other records are necessary they must be obtained before the recording of the muscular or retruded contact position since the bite registration paste must remain on the lower block to record this relationship. After the casts have been mounted on the articulator the set paste can be removed to allow positioning of the protrusive or lateral wafers.

Before the patient is dismissed, a decision must be made regarding suitable teeth. The principles of tooth selection are discussed fully, later. In general the selected shade of the artificial teeth should blend with that of the natural lower teeth, although a darkening of shade towards the canine region is often desirable. Consideration should also be given to the labial contour of the artificial teeth to ensure that this is of similar form to the lowers.

Tooth selection is assisted by having a representative selection of six upper anterior teeth mounted on handles so that they may be 'tried in' at this stage. A decision will have to be made between porcelain and acrylic resin teeth. The merits and demerits of these tooth materials have been listed in Chapter 9.

Partially dentulous in both jaws. When teeth are standing in both jaws a somewhat different approach to the recording of occlusion is required, particularly when insufficient teeth are standing to indicate this relationship. There is a wide variation in the types of cases that come into this category, some showing marked loss of posterior teeth as in Fig. 16.6, and others where the vertical dimension is maintained by the occlusal contact of several teeth, but the position cannot be determined merely by placing the casts in occlusion.

Before discussing the technique to be followed in these cases mention should be made of two problems which may require consideration prior to recording the

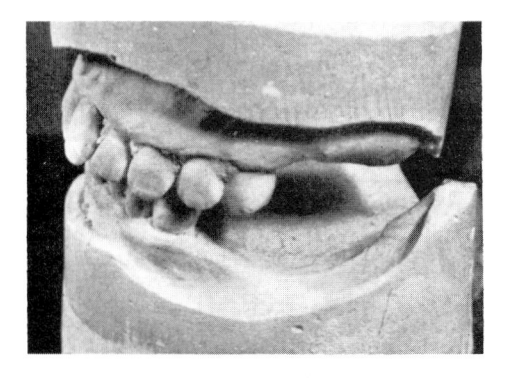

Fig. 16.6. Case with loss of posterior teeth.

occlusion. First, the case may be one in which the muscular position and the tooth position are not coincident. This problem has been discussed fully in Chapter 4, to which reference may be made.

Second, owing to the loss of posterior teeth the vertical dimension of occlusion may be reduced and consideration will have to be given to the manner in which this has occurred and the degree to which it can be restored. It is possible to differentiate three types of case where overclosure of the mandible has occurred. The first is where the loss of posterior teeth has removed the only occlusal stop and the mandible is able to move upwards, on the muscular path, without teeth coming into contact. Such cases have a marked anterior horizontal overlap, as shown diagrammatically in Fig. 16.7a. The second type of case is one where, prior to the loss of posterior teeth the lower incisors did not make contact with the upper incisors in the tooth position. When the posterior teeth are lost the mandible moves upwards, usually to a small extent, and incisal contact is made (Fig. 16.7b). In the third group the upper anterior teeth show evidence of periodontal disease and incisal contact due to the loss of posterior teeth has resulted in labial migration resulting in further upwards movement of the mandible and reduction in vertical dimension (Fig. 16.7c). If untreated by the

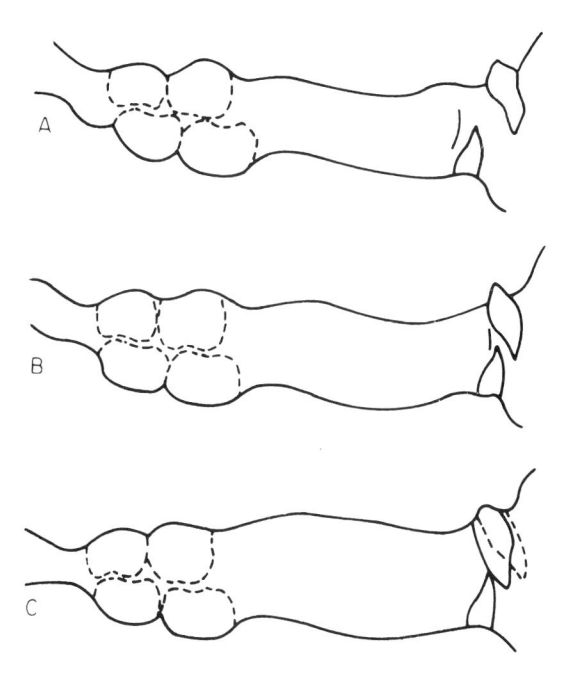

Fig. 16.7. A Mandible moves upwards without incisive contact.
B Mandible makes almost immediate incisive contact.
C Incisive contact causes splaying of the upper incisors and further upward movement of the mandible occurs.

provision of partial dentures such a condition rapidly leads to the loss of the upper anterior teeth. Needless to say, other periodontal treatment is also indicated.

One other category of cases showing reduction in vertical dimension of occlusion should be mentioned. A number of patients exhibit a marked shortening of the lower third of the face and an occlusion which shows attrition of the incisal edges of the anterior teeth but little wear of the occlusal surfaces of the posterior teeth. The interocclusal clearance is often excessive being five to eight millimetres in the incisor region. A reduction in this dimension and the establishment of a new tooth position by means of removable onlay appliances or fixed restorations not only improves the appearance but provides increased comfort to the patient. The condition is one which should have been treated by orthodontic therapy in earlier life (Fig. 16.8).

When the registration of jaw relationship is to be carried out, the interocclusal relationship of the natural teeth should be observed without the blocks in the mouth. If this is accepted as correct it is necessary to record a similar relationship with the record blocks in place.

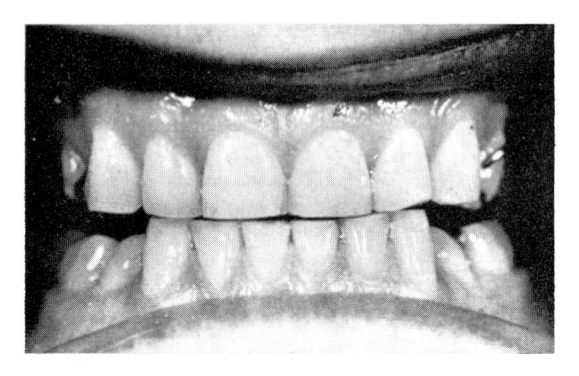

Fig. 16.8. Attrition of incisal edges in a patient aged twenty-three years. The interocclusal clearance is greater than normal.

In all cases when an increase in vertical dimension of occlusion is to be carried out it is essential, in the first instance, to construct some form of temporary appliance which will enable the changed dimension to be assessed. Such temporary appliances should have their occlusal surfaces made of acrylic resin which can be easily reduced by grinding or added to with cold cured resin to alter the new dimension should this prove intolerable to the patient or insufficient for its purpose.

If the vertical dimension is to be increased it is essential to take a measurement of the tooth position, which can then be compared with the proposed new position; this is most readily done with some simple form of gauge as shown in Fig. 16.9. It should be appreciated, however, that measurements taken in this

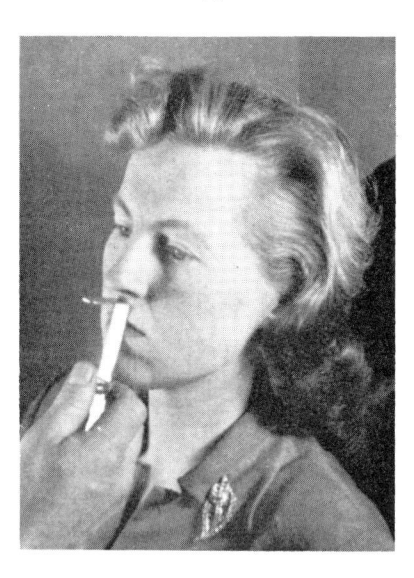

Fig. 16.9. Use of the Willis gauge.

manner are only approximate and that variations can occur even between successive measurements taken by the same operator.

One of the record blocks is now inserted and the occlusal plane trimmed to the correct level. Which block is selected depends upon which jaw will be the greatest help in aligning the occlusal plane. If a posterior molar is standing the plane is adjusted to the level indicated by this tooth. If no posterior teeth are standing, the methods described previously are followed. When the plane is judged correct the patient should be asked to close and any points of contact of the opposing teeth with the record block noted. It is possible that these may necessitate adjustments to the occlusal plane which may have to be trimmed locally to accommodate the cusp of, for example, a lower molar. Alternatively, grinding of the cusps of the opposing teeth may be indicated.

If no increase in vertical dimension of occlusion is required this trimming must be continued until the patient can close together in the position first noted. The other block is then inserted and adjusted until a similar condition can be obtained with it in position. In a number of cases it will be found possible to obtain an accurate recording by the use of only one block and wherever this is possible it should be done.

When two blocks are being used they should be trimmed to allow complete closure without any pressure being applied to them. Final recording of the tooth position can be secured by placing a thin layer of bite registration paste over the occlusal surface on one or both blocks and having the patient close again. This serves to equalize the pressure throughout the occlusion.

It may happen that the vertical dimension of the finished dentures is greater than that recorded at this stage. This may be due to the displaceability of the mucosa of the saddle areas allowing the record blocks to be displaced into these soft tissues. This is particularly liable to occur in the lower jaw when free end saddles are present (Fig. 16.10). This can be minimized by using a cast denture framework embodying appropriate support units as a base for the record block, or by using a 'mucostatic' registration material such as impression plaster to secure the final interocclusal relationship.

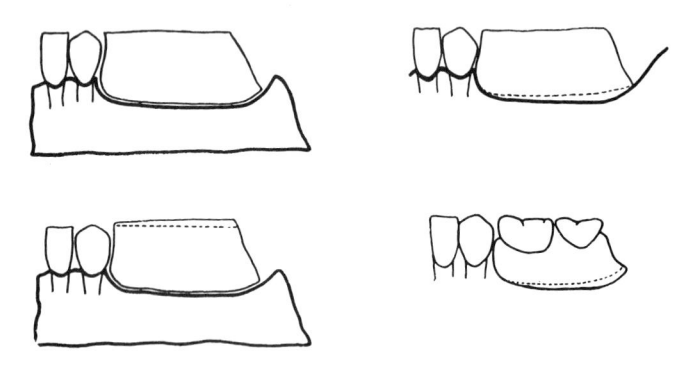

Fig. 16.10. Lower record block compressing the saddle area resulting in a raised occlusion of the finished denture.

This situation is normally restricted to dentures supplied for the lower jaw. In upper dentures it is unlikely to be appreciable owing to the relatively incompressible nature of the normal hard plate. However, excessive pressure applied during recording can result in localized compression and blanching of mucosa at the peripheries of the blocks. If the blocks themselves are freed from direct contact and the final location carried out with bite registration paste under light pressure by the patient, little trouble should be expected in the normal case.

Although this problem has been mentioned in connection with recording the occlusal for cases with teeth standing in both jaws it is, of course, equally applicable to the full upper and partial lower type of case considered previously.

Some of the possible sources of error in recording the occlusion where natural teeth are present is shown in Fig. 16.11. These are discussed below.

(A) If closure in the mouth is made with any force the wax rims themselves may be distorted.

(B) If soft wax is used between the blocks to equalize the pressure there is a danger of its elastic recovery when the pressure is removed. It is also possible that soft wax may be distorted when the models are being engaged into the blocks.

(C) The anterior teeth may fail to make contact due to over-extension of the

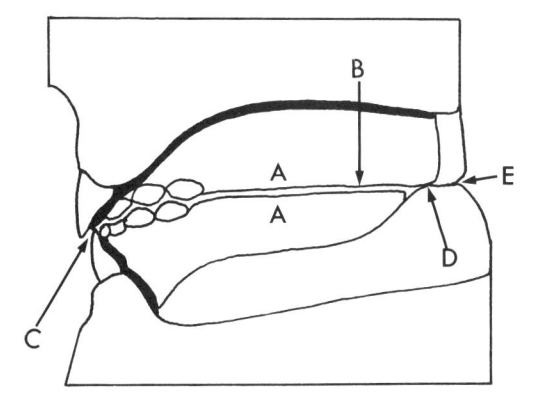

Fig. 16.11. Some possible sources of error when recording the occlusion (from Saunsbury, 1957).

base plate of the upper block on to the cingula of the anterior teeth. In cases of deep anterior vertical overlap this may be difficult to detect. As a routine measure the upper base plate may be kept away from the anterior teeth.

(D) The posterior margin of the upper wax rim may have been in contact with the retromolar pad and displaced the mucosa in this region when closure was made. When the blocks are transferred to the casts no such displacement is possible. Consequently the wax rim must be trimmed in this region before the models can be related correctly. If it is suspected that such a situation exists in the mouth the upper block should be trimmed out of contact with the retromolar pad before the occlusion is recorded.

(E) Excess cast material posterior to the areas recorded by the impressions may prevent the casts engaging the blocks to the full extent.

In many cases of this type it will be necessary to use an adjustable articulator, and particularly so when it is necessary to increase the vertical dimension. Similar records will be required to those discussed in the previous section of this chapter.

The face bow record can be obtained in the same way, the face bow fork being held between the natural teeth and one record block or between a combination of teeth and blocks according to the particular case. Protrusive and lateral records are obtained as before.

Teeth in occlusion in both jaws. In a proportion of cases requiring partial dentures in one or in both jaws, the tooth position can be determined quite definitely by placing the two casts in occlusion. When this relationship is demarcated with certainty there is no necessity to take any recording of tooth position from the patient, but a visual check should be made to see that the cast relationship is, in fact, that exisiting in the patient. The minimum requirements to enable the position to be located from the casts are tooth stops anteriorly and bilaterally posteriorly to determine vertical dimensions, and sufficient intercuspation to determine the antero-posterior and lateral positions.

If an average movement articulator is being used, the casts can be mounted immediately. If however, a fully adjustable articulator is to be used then a face bow recording is required. This is done as described earlier, the fork being held between the natural teeth. Protrusive and lateral records should also be taken in the usual manner.

At the visit of the patient when recording of occlusion is carried out it is often opportune to confirm or adjust the previous decisions regarding the design of the dentures. Normally the general, and in some cases the detailed, plan of the denture design will have been decided earlier in order that the mouth preparation can be carried out and the impression technique decided upon. However, it may sometimes be necessary to defer final decisions until the occlusion has been recorded.

References

APPLEGATE O.C. and NISSLE R.O. (1951) Keeping the partial denture in harmony with biological limitations. *J. Amer. dent. Ass.* **43**, 409.

BECKETT L.S. (1939) Accurate occlusal relations in partial denture construction. *Proceedings of the Xth Australian Dental Congress*, 456–63.

BERRY D.C. (1960) The constancy of the rest position of the mandible. *Dent. Pract.* **10**, 129.

CHAMBERLAIN J.B. and BASKER R.M. (1967) A method of duplicating dentures. *Brit. dent. J.* **122**, 347.

COLLETT H.A. (1951) Balancing the occlusion of the partial dentures. *J. Amer. dent. Ass.* **42**, 162–68.

LAIRD, W.R.E. (1974) Intermaxillary relationships during deglutition. *J. dent. Res.* **53**, 127.

SAUNSBURY P. (1957) Progress in partial denture prosthesis. *Irish dent. Rev.* **3**, 73–82.

WATT D.M. (1978) Tooth positions on complete dentures. *J. Dent.* **6**, 147.

17
THE TRIAL DENTURE

At various stages during the construction of partial dentures it is necessary to assess the work by examination in the patient's mouth. In the majority of cases this is necessary on only one or two occasions, but it should be a general principle that a denture is tried as many times as may be required if there is any doubt on the part of clinician, technician or patient, prior to its being completed.

The dentures should firstly be examined mounted on the articulator to ensure that the instructions to the technician have been carried out correctly. A denture that is unsatisfactory in any way on the articulator and master casts will not be satisfactory in the mouth. Firstly the adaptation of the base to the master cast should be examined, particularly where cast metal is being used, and in this respect it is advisable to try the metal framework separately before teeth or any other additions have been placed.

Once the clinician is satisfied with the appearance, fit, and general construction of the trial denture on the articulator and casts, it can then be examined in the patient's mouth. Particular attention should be paid to the following aspects of design and construction: (1) adaptation of the base and components such as rests and clasps; (2) occlusion; (3) aesthetics; (4) shape of the polished surfaces.

Adaptation

(a) Metal based dentures

If the denture has been designed using a metal base, it is advisable to examine this in the mouth initially without any teeth attached to it. In this way it is easier to obtain a satisfactory view of the actual fitting contact between the metal and the standing teeth than it is if artificial teeth and wax are also present. It is also easier to carry out any minor adjustments to the metal should these be necessary. In this respect attempts at modifications and alteration are neither practicable nor successful; either the base fits or it does not. In the latter case the only sound policy is to start again, unless the discrepancy can be definitely located and is easily remedied. If a discrepancy in fit is suspected it is useful to paint or spray a disclosing agent over the fitting surface in the suspect area. Any areas of excessive pressure will disturb the disclosing agent and a limited amount of grinding can be carried out in these areas in order to correct the error. Where it is decided to construct a new framework it is necessary to be aware of the reason for the misfit before recording a new impression. A metal base or framework which fits the master cast but does not fit the mouth indicates errors in impression taking or pouring of the cast, and if the new framework is to be successful, these errors should not be repeated. Reasons for inaccuracies and distortions from impression have been suggested earlier (Chapter 15).

In the examination of a metal base it should first be inserted gently into the mouth. Tactile sensations will usually indicate whether the general fit is satisfactory, and also the degree of antero-posterior and lateral stability. If this appears to be satisfactory then a detailed examination of the seating and adaptation of the support units (rests) should be made using a mirror and probe. In the upper jaw the tissue fit of palatal connectors should be examined and also the relationship of a posterior bar or the posterior border of a plate, to the junction of the hard and soft palate. If a bar is used it must always be on the hard palate, its antero-posterior position being determined by the design of the particular denture. The patient may be asked to assist in this respect by checking the position with his tongue.

In the case of the lower metal framework there are further specific points which must be considered. The relationship of a lingual bar to the mucosa should be such that whilst food cannot be trapped, there is no trauma to the tissue, particularly at the junction between the bar and the saddle. The relationship of the upper border of the bar to the gingival margins of the standing teeth should permit a cleansing action of these areas by the tongue and the saliva. If the bar is too near the necks of the teeth then food will be packed on to the gingival margin and crevice, and in this respect it is useful to use a bar with a pear-shaped cross section. In addition the bar should not impinge on the floor of the mouth as this would result in tissue ulceration and displacement of the denture during function. The point of entry of the bar into the saddle area should be such that no sharp angles are formed which would be irritating to the patient.

Where labial and buccal bars have been used as connectors these must be checked carefully for freedom of impingment from movable soft tissue structures in the functional sulcus, and for mucosal tissue fit. During their construction they should be relieved from prominent and incompressible areas of the alveolar ridge particularly in the area of the abutment teeth. If this is not done pressure areas will develop leading to pain, inflammation and eventual ulceration.

Where a metal framework incorporating a plate connector has been constructed, particular attention must be given to both the tissue fit and to the contacts of the margins of the plate with the standing natural teeth. In the upper framework, inspection of the margins should reveal no space that would allow entry to food particles which would become packed between the plate and the teeth so increasing the susceptibility to dental caries and periodontal disease. In addition lingual plates should be inspected particularly in their relation to the floor of the mouth and the lingual frenum.

Partial dentures using a metal plate connector will often be mucosa borne designs, and their retention is therefore dependent upon close tissue adaptation. The presence of spaces at the margins of the plate will affect retention adversely. In addition the relationship of the plate connector to the standing teeth of the opposing jaw should be examined with particular attention being given to situations where there is considerable vertical overlap of the incisor teeth, which may result in premature contact and excessive loading of an upper plate connector in the anterior region.

Where metal frameworks have been constructed for both upper and lower arches examination of the occlusion should be undertaken for each separately, prior to checking the occlusion with both in position. Occlusal errors should be rare if the correct principles in relation to design and construction have been followed, but any now present must be corrected. When it has been decided that the framework is satisfactory, it should be returned to the laboratory for the addition of the necessary teeth in wax, prior to re-examination of aesthetics and occlusion.

Retention must also be checked by making certain that the frame remains firmly seated at all times. On insertion it should become progressively firmer as it is seated into position; under no circumstances must it be allowed to go into position with a 'click'. Such an occurrence involves considerable trauma to the natural teeth and is usually caused by the middle third of a clasp or clasps being allowed to pass below the survey line. The patient should be asked to talk and to move the lower jaw in protrusive and lateral excursions and the stability of the frame noted. If there is displacement under these conditions it may be due to incorrect placing of the retentive portions of the clasp arms or to occlusal interference. A check on the latter should first be made by placing blue articulating paper or spray between the jaws and getting the patient to close, first in the intercuspal position and later in protrusive and lateral positions, and observing whether there are any premature contacts at each stage. Grinding may be necessary to reduce these, either on the denture frame or the enamel of opposing teeth. Grinding should normally be done on the metal and the blue marks will be more easily seen on, for example, occlusal rests, if the high polish is first removed from the alloy by light stoning. Enamel should not be ground if this is likely to disturb the balance of the occlusion. If the original diagnosis and technical work have been accurate, there should be only a minimum amount of grinding required.

If there is no occlusal interference but retention is not satisfactory, then the fault will lie in the retentive portion of the clasp arms. These will usually be found not to engage sufficiently far into the undercut area or to have insufficient resilience to engage correctly. Minor adjustments may be made with pliers but care must be taken not to strain the metal. This is particularly so with cobalt chromium although to a lesser extent with cast gold. Wrought metal clasp arms may be adjusted with greater freedom.

When the clasp arms and the denture frame are made of dissimiliar metals—for example, wrought gold clasp arms and chrome cobalt base—it is common practice to attach the clasps by inserting their tags into the acrylic resin of the saddle. In these cases the metal frame should be tried in without the clasps, these being added before the denture is finished.

Clasps must also be checked from the aesthetic viewpoint, but a decision on this should have been made at an earlier visit. If it has been decided that it is desirable to clasp an upper canine or first premolar, then this should be explained to the patient and his or her consent obtained. Some patients will object to a display of metal when they are speaking or laughing, and the design may have to be modified accordingly, and the patient advised of the limitations of the denture.

Where a free-end saddle frame is concerned it should be noted whether the metal work in the region of the saddle has been made to fit on the model, or whether, as is desirable, it has been relieved to allow denture base material to flow around the metal. In any case, if the impression has been taken with a mucostatic material, the frame will rock if pressure is placed on the saddle (due to displacement of the mucosa), but if it has been relieved the movement will be much greater. This point must be remembered when the frame is tried in the mouth.

The retention of frames that incorporate one or two free-end saddles may not be efficient until the finished periphery is added. In such cases occlusion and clasping should be checked as above, but it may be necessary to build up the periphery in wax to check the added retentive effect in the saddle areas.

(b) Plastic base dentures

If these appliances are tried in as wax based dentures there is difficulty in avoiding distortion of the wax during this process. To prevent this it is desirable that the dentures should be set up on shellac or acrylic resin bases. A hard wax should be used for mounting the teeth to mimimize softening in the mouth, but in any case dentures must not be allowed to remain there for any longer than is necessary. Frequent removal, re-adaptation to the master cast and chilling in cold water are desirable.

In these cases a check on the fit is carried out with all the teeth in position, and it is not possible, owing to this fact and the softening of the wax, to asses fit in detail. However, a general impression of saddle fit may be obtained by the overall stability of the denture. Fit of the wax around standing teeth should be observed, and any discrepancies compared with the fit on the model.

Where it is intended that such dentures will incorporate clasps to provide retention or rests to provide support, it is inadvisable to attach them to the trial wax denture. At best they are likely to move within the wax during insertion and removal which makes their functional assessment impossible, and at the worst they may even become detatched from the denture presenting a hazard to the patient.

(c) Clasps

In a correctly designed partial denture each clasp, and indeed part of the clasp, will have been placed for some specific purpose such as retention, bracing, support or reciprocation. In assessing the fit of a clasp the particular function of each part must be borne in mind. A check should first be made for the fit against the tooth when the denture is in position. Note particularly if the retentive portions of the clasp arms are engaging correctly, thus indicating that they possess sufficient resilience to pass over the survey line area and engage in the undercut. This can also be assessed by tactile sensation while the denture is being inserted. If the retentive function of the clasps is correct the denture should be positively retained.

Rigid clasp arms, placed to provide bracing against lateral movement and to reciprocate the retentive pressures of the resilient arms, must be checked for fit and for their position relative to the survey line. Such arms must never pass below the survey line, otherwise, as they are rigid, they will traumatize the tooth and themselves be deformed during insertion and removal.

The relation of the arms to the ridges and gingival tissues must be observed. Occlusally approaching arms should not impinge upon the gingival attachment since this will cause pain. It may also lead to a traumatic inflammatory reaction, either chronic or acute, in the gingival tissue. Gingivally approaching arms must be relieved during laboratory construction from the ridge prominence overlying the roots of the clasped teeth and must not extend into tissue undercuts. If such arms are not relieved, or if the clearance is insufficient, pressure on the tissue may lead to ulceration during function.

The patient should be asked to check the position of clasp arms in relation to his tongue movements. Minute roughness of the edges can be detected better by the patient's tongue than by any other means. This type of check should be applied particularly to ring clasps on lower molars, and to any clasp arms fitted on the lingual aspect of a denture.

Occlusion

The first check on the occlusion should be made as the patient closes gently and slowly into the intercuspal position, or in the case of bilateral upper and lower free-end saddles replacing all the posterior teeth, the muscular or occasionally the retruded contact position. If the latter position is recorded occlusal modifications will be required at insertion to accommodate to the natural muscular position of the patient. If a metal-based denture is involved, a check on the occlusion of the metalwork will have been carried out as described previously. At this stage, therefore, it should only be necessary to check the tooth relationship. In all cases the patient must be warned not to exert heavy pressure, as the teeth are only supported in wax. When occlusal contact is made in the intercuspal position, visual observation will reveal if this is identical with that on the articulator. If it appears to be so, the occlusal contact should be tested by inserting the thin blade of a spatula between the cusps and attempting to rotate it. If contact is not firm it means that the dentures are not seated on their support, and the teeth will be prised apart easily. It must be assured that the patient maintains definite but gentle occlusal pressure during this test.

Should an interocclusal deficiency be revealed in this manner, or if the intercuspal position is incorrect in either antero-posterior or lateral directions then a new recording of occlusion must be made. Such errors usually necessitate the removal of all or most of the teeth, their substitution by wax and the re-recording of this position. Unilateral lack of contact may be corrected occasionally by adding wax or registration paste to the occlusal surface of the teeth on the side where the deficiency exists, together with a thin layer of a similar material on the opposite side to aid location.

If the original recording of occlusion was carried out with record blocks that had no tooth support, and excessive pressure was exerted during the sealing of the blocks together, mucosal displacement may lead to a premature occlusion at the try-in stage. When mucosally supported record blocks have been used, a careful check must be made to ensure that the occlusion is not premature when only light closing pressure is used. If heavy pressure is used by the patient the same error will be repeated and will then not be detected until the finished dentures are fitted.

When checking the occlusion of dentures with no metal base the same general principles and techniques are still applicable. More care must be taken to avoid possible distortion and the use of rigid bases will be helpful in this respect.

Aesthetics

This aspect of the try-in is considered after fit and occlusion, but it should not be regarded as any less important. Indeed for many patients and their families, a pleasing appearance of the dentures is much more important than function or sometimes comfort! However until fit and occlusion are correct, no serious detailed consideration can be given to aesthetics. Therefore, when considering the aesthetic problem, due attention must be paid to the functional purpose of the denture, and in certain cases functional demands may mean some sacrifice of aesthetic perfection.

Consideration of aesthetics at the try-in should be a check on the decisions taken previously, together with any minor modifications in tooth position that may be necessary. If it is decided, for example, that a tooth shade is incorrect or that a tooth should be ridge lapped, then the work must be returned to the laboratory for these alterations before the patient is given an opportunity of examining the dentures.

It must be realized that so far as the patient is concerned the appearance of the dentures is the most important aspect. The patient should be told that at this stage it is possible to make alterations to tooth position, mould, or shade, but that this opportunity will not occur again. It is often advisable to have another person present, such as the wife or husband of the patient, to comment upon the aesthetics.

The patient will view the appearance in a mirror so it is sensible for the dentist also to view the dentures in a mirror so that he sees the same image as the patient. Taking the patient from the chair to stand before a wall mirror in company with the dentist is often helpful.

Before sending the dentures to the technician to be finished a definite expression of satisfaction with their appearance should be obtained from the patient.

The whole subject of the aesthetics of partial dentures is dealt with in the following chapter.

Polished Surfaces

Although retention is assisted by the use of clasps and indirect retainers, it is still necessary that the surrounding musculature should play a role in partial denture retention. Shaping the polished surfaces so that this can be achieved is therefore necessary.

A careful inspection should therefore be made of the peripheral extension of the saddles to ensure that they do not impinge on the mucosal reflection in the depth of the sulcus. This should be carried out with the mouth half open and no gross distortion of buccal or labial musculature. Peripheral overextension will result in either denture displacement or tissue ulceration. The former is more common in free-end saddle situations where retention may be dependent upon border seal, with the latter more likely in the clasp retained bounded saddles. Careful observation is necessary to detect such errors at the trial stage. If tissue displacement is obvious then a new master impression will be required.

The polished surfaces must also be checked for their general angulation. In the mandibular arch the lingual surfaces must face inwards and upwards, so that the tongue may act as a retaining element. If the surfaces face inwards and downwards the tongue will be able to exert an upwards thrust on the saddle and it may be wholly or partly lifted from its basal seat.

The buccal surface of a posterior lower saddle must face upwards and outwards so that the cheek musculature may lie upon it and assist in retention. These buccal surfaces must not be bulky and prominent, but should be hollowed to allow optimum muscular assistance in retention. Anterior lower saddles may have no labial flange, but when they do it must be kept as thin as possible and shaped so that the lip assists retention.

In the upper denture the polished surfaces should not be excessively bulky and the palate should be of uniform thickness. In order to ensure maximum retention of the free-end saddle denture the periphery should be extended around the tuberosity region.

At the trial stage therefore, it is necessary to examine adaptation, occlusion, aesthetics and denture form. If these are considered to be satisfactory from a clinical point of view the opinion of the patient should be sought regarding aesthetics. This is essential to avoid possible disappointment and embarassment at insertion. It is relatively easy to make alterations at the trial stages, and in this respect it is advisable to meet the request of the patient regarding aesthetics, always provided that this would not affect function adversely.

References

SWOOPE C.C. (1970) The try-in—a time for communication. *Dent. Clin. N.A.* **14,** 479.

HOLMES J.B. (1970) The altered cast impression procedure for the distal extension removable partial dentures. *Dent. Clin. N.A.* **14,** 569.

18
AESTHETICS

Although all patients will expect their partial dentures to restore efficiently their powers of mastication (when these have been depleted), they will also expect a high standard of aesthetic restoration. This is a justifiable expectation and one that must be satisfied if partial denture service is to be complete. It has been emphasized throughout this text that partial dentures are not merely appliances for replacing lost teeth in the dental arch, but should contribute towards the maintenance of oral health as a whole. One of the surest methods of stimulating the patient's necessary co-operation in this measure is the provision of the highest standard of aesthetic restoration that is possible. The patient, by virtue of pride in his or her appearance, may be stimulated to keep the appliance clean and the natural tissues in a healthy condition. Hence, whilst a 'beauty service' is in itself a necessary and desirable part of partial denture prosthesis, it may also help to stimulate the patient's co-operation in the maintenance of oral hygiene.

The appearance of a denture depends on the artistic sense and ability of the operator. Unfortunately, unlike the acquisition of biological and technical knowledge, artistic sense cannot be taught easily. However, two factors may be considered in relation to such teaching. The first is the ability to observe detail accurately, a faculty in which there is considerable variation between individuals, but one which may be trained and improved. The second is that more elusive sense of artistry or artistic appreciation which is, to a large extent, inborn, but which can be acquired to a certain degree. In this connection the dentist should try to develop an appreciation of harmony and beauty in the human face.

A satisfactory aesthetic result depends upon a combination of artistic ability and powers of observation, and in these respects the technician, no less than the practitioner, must play a major part. It is desirable to allow the technician to see the patient when the occlusion is being recorded so that he knows at first hand the aesthetic problem on which he is working. The first consideration of aesthetics may arise when the initial decision regarding treatment planning is being made. In most normal cases, however, aesthetics are first considered at the stage of recording the occlusion when decisions must be taken regarding the type of teeth, the mould, size, and shades, and whether they shall be fitted to the ridge or a labial flange employed. Problems of staining or other modifications must also be considered at this stage.

The anterior saddles of partial dentures may be of varying lengths. A long saddle may extend from one premolar region to the other and in such circumstances many of the principles that apply to full dentures may well be relevant. On the other hand short saddles of one or two teeth present very different problems. Accordingly it is appropriate to consider the two types of saddles under separate headings.

The Long Anterior Saddle

The problems of aesthetics in relation to the long partial denture saddle can be discussed under the following headings:
1 General position of the teeth.
2 Character of the teeth.
3 Particular position of the teeth.
4 The labial and buccal flange.

The general position of the teeth

From the aesthetic viewpoint two positions require study, the resting position of the face and the smiling position. These are not the only positions during which assessments are made of appearance, but, from a clinical standpoint, if both these positions are considered it is probable that good aesthetics will result in all the multitude of human facial activities. The two positions are essentially different. In the resting position the facial and masticatory musculature is in a relaxed state, the predominant contribution to good appearance being lip and cheek form and the relationship of their outline to the other characters of the whole face. Skin quality also requires consideration in the resting state. In contra-distinction the smile position is one of active contraction of the facial musculature and the predominant feature is the display of the teeth.

When consideration is being given to the antero-posterior positioning of upper and lower anterior teeth, function and aesthetics must be considered concurrently. It is often maintained that these two demands may be conflicting but on critical analysis generally this is not the case and especially when it is understood that the aesthetic aim is the provision of a natural, congruous, and harmonious appearance. If the patient is young a youthful appearance must be established; if, however, the patient shows facial evidence of ageing no attempt should be made to re-establish what is lost for ever. To attempt to do so is likely to produce a non-retentive, unstable appliance which, far from enhancing appearance, only produces a caricature and tell-tale incongruity. Demands from the patient for a restoration of youthful facial form must be met with the reply that this is not possible and that real happiness can now only be achieved by accepting a philosophy of growing old graciously. When it is realized that the best aesthetic result lies in the creation of a harmonious facial form, then the demands of function and appearance may clash very little.

To appreciate fully the principles of general positioning of the teeth it is necessary to describe the atrophic changes in lip and cheek form which take place in ageing. Ageing here refers to a biological and not a chronological concept; one patient of fifty may maintain youthful characteristics while another of the same age may display marked facial atrophy.

Epithelial tissues, musculature, and bone all display change as a result of ageing. The following examples illustrate this in reference to edentulous persons but the principles are applicable equally to long anterior saddles in partial cases. Reference to Fig. 18.1 shows that little change of facial form has accompanied the change to the edentulous state in a young person. The lips maintain their fullness with a slight eversion and exposure of a normal rounded contour of red mucosa. The pronounced labio-mental angle, too, is preserved. The face has not 'fallen in', a youthful contour being preserved by the maintenance of skin, mucosa and muscle properties as well as by minimal resorption of the alveolar ridge.

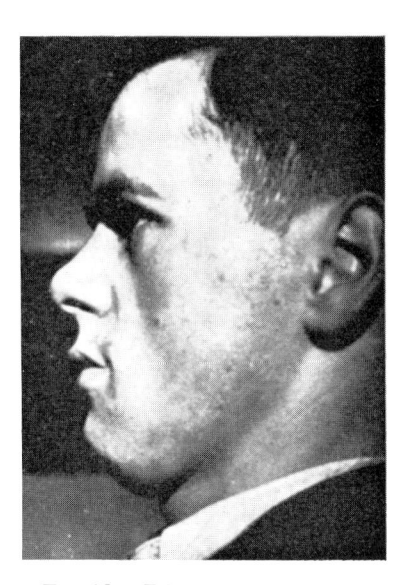

Fig. 18.1. Edentulous young adult.

Fig. 18.2 depicts an edentulous adult who shows some atrophic change but whose biological age (in comparison with his chronological age) is reflected by a loose wrinkled type of skin which has maintained a remarkable degree of elastic quality. The musculature, whereas it may show some hypertonicity giving a tight lip, maintains its ability to adapt, by reduced tonicity, to the accommodation of the teeth and a thick labial flange between the lip and the residual ridge. Although the fullness of the previous contours cannot be restored completely, a fully harmonious profile can be obtained by setting the anterior teeth forward of the ridge with some anterior inclination.

In contra-distinction Fig. 18.3 shows a very atrophic condition. In terms of facial outline, inversion rather than eversion of the lips is seen, only a thin red lip margin being in evidence, the oral aperture has decreased in size, and the labio-mental angle has disappeared. Forward traction on the upper and lower lips reveals tightness, indicating the complete loss of elastic quality. The skin of this patient does not show the wrinkles described in all geriatric texts; it is a thin tight skin, the reduction in surface area of which has caused formidable facial changes. There has in all probability been marked change in the musculature, the elastic tissue of which is replaced by fibrous tissue as part of a change which is irreversible. In such a case there is always a large loss of bone, and the denture must be adapted to the limitations of the tissues. Any attempt to 'build out' is doomed to failure on the grounds of stability and retention as well as appearance. It is not possible to place a thick labial flange between the lip and the ridge and to use a tooth position well in advance of the crest of the ridge, without the development of a reactive force which will cause denture displacement or stress to any remaining teeth that may be clasped. Nor, even, if function were disregarded, could the resultant aesthetic effect be anything but ridiculous. The lip, displaced acutely rather than smoothly, would be unduly emphasized and only

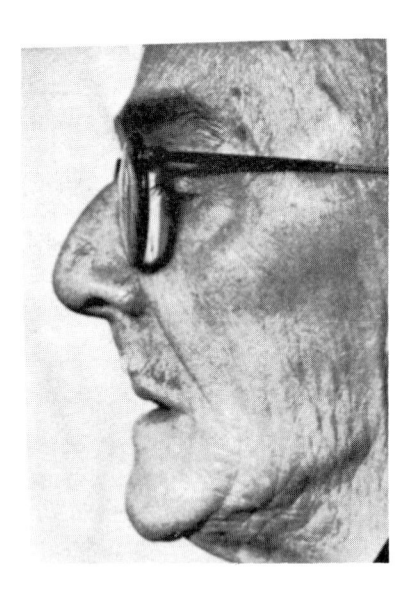

Fig. 18.2. Edentulous adult, biologically young.

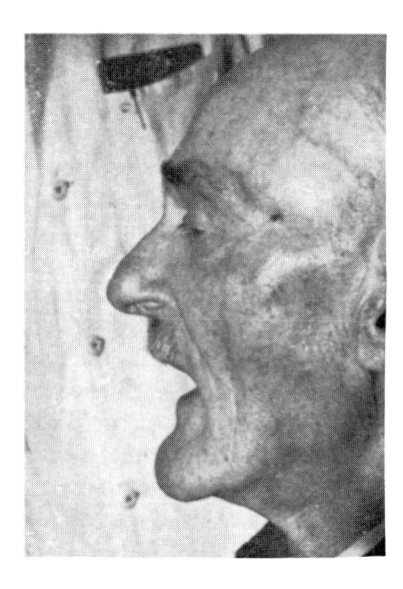

Fig. 18.3. Edentulous adult, biologically old.

call attention more to the taut, pale, parchment-like skin. The only acceptable functional and aesthetic result will be obtained by using a thin labial flange and giving an inward rather than an outward slope, this being more necessary in the lower. If this backward placement of the upper teeth is necessary in the incisal area it becomes even more necessary in the canine area. Here any impingement of the teeth into the line of action of the altered levator anguli oris muscle can only lead to displacement. Thus, in ageing, the upper anterior teeth may have to be set on an arch of reducing radius and a change in arch form from a square to a definite tapering arrangement may be necessary.

The character of the teeth

The individual tooth contributes less to aesthetics than either its general or particular position. However, teeth should be selected with due consideration to their form, size, colour and material of manufacture.

The work of Frush and Fisher offers a convincing basis on which to select and arrange teeth. The basic criteria of selection are the sex, personality and age of the patient.

The male form is built on a cuboidal pattern, the term cuboidal being preferred to square, since it is three dimensional. On the other hand the female form is essentially spheroidal. To obtain aesthetic harmony, a cuboidal tooth form is required for the male and a spheroidal form for the female. Nevertheless it should be remembered that there are varying degrees of masculinity and feminity, requiring all grades of tooth form. Nor is the outline form as viewed from the front the only consideration. Most artificial teeth have a labial surface which is too flat; an increased degree of convexity on this surface always gives a more realistic tooth form. The male tooth should be modified by depth grinding on the mesial and distal edges as depicted in Fig. 18.4, whereas the female tooth should show a smoother convexity. Male and female teeth also differ in the detail of the labial surface, the vigour and hardness of the male requiring vertical crests and ridges, whereas the female tooth should be somewhat smoother. It should not, however, have a uniformly smooth surface as this gives an even reflection of light, rather than a scattering which enhances the colour qualities of the tooth.

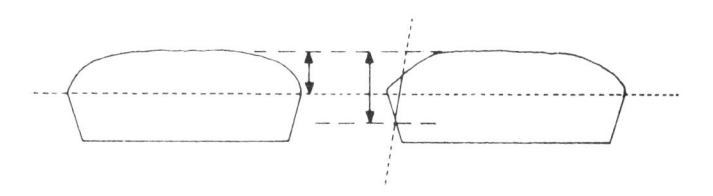

Fig. 18.4. Diagram showing how grinding of the mesial (and distal) aspect of an incisor tooth increases the degree of convexity of the labial surface.

Personality should be regarded as a criterion which modifies the sex factor. Frush and Fisher suggest the application of a personality spectrum, ten per cent of the population being accommodated at its vigorous end, and five per cent at its delicate end. The vigorous personality requires the cuboid tooth form and the delicate the spheroidal form.

Next the age factor must be considered. This is most important in the treatment of the incisal and gingival areas of the teeth. As a result of attrition a straight incisal edge is produced, which later loses its translucent quality as the enamel cap is worn away. A vigorous effect in the ageing male can be produced by grinding local incisal concavities. When natural anterior teeth are present in the opposing jaw the incisal edges of the artificial teeth should be ground to match the attrition that has occurred (Fig. 18.5). The gingival area will be considered together with the labial denture facing.

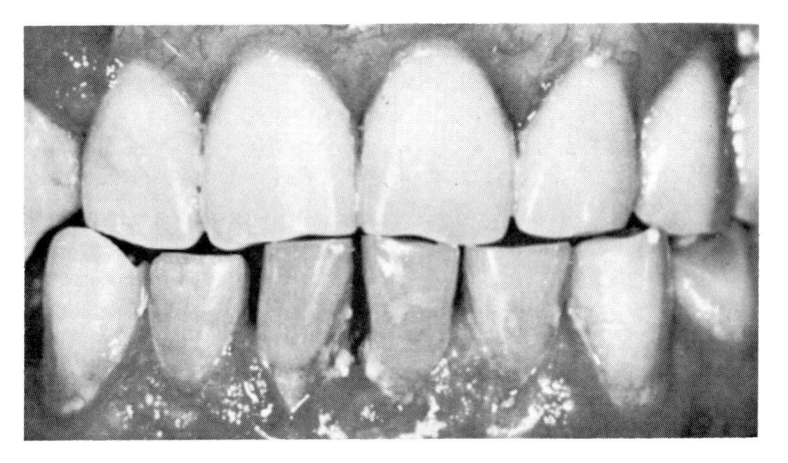

Fig. 18.5. Teeth on a long saddle showing grinding of the incisal edges to match the lowers.

The shade of the selected teeth should be based on the colouring and age of the patient. The colour of the skin and hair are the most reliable indices, dark hair and skin requiring yellow teeth, and blonde hair and fair skin light teeth with a suggestion of blue in them. Age affects the tooth colour, a darker shade with deeper yellow pigmentation and the addition of some grey being indicated with advancing years. The use of *small* gold fillings, *slightly* discoloured composite filling reproductions, and sometimes the inclusion of brown vertical stained lines to simulate enamel cracks, should be used only when the patient desires. In long partial denture saddles the shade of the abutment teeth will dictate the general range of tooth shades to be used. Often a pleasing effect is obtained if the shade progressively lightens from behind forward, centrals thus being lighter than canines. In many cases a long upper anterior saddle will be opposed by natural teeth in the lower jaw, and the upper teeth must be a matching shade.

The size of the teeth is an important factor. Too often teeth that are too narrow are used. It is suggested that the best index for the width of the tooth is the horizontal distance between the two zygomatic arches (De Van). The bi-zygomatic width of the face divided by 16 will generally result in a pleasing width of upper central incisor. If the size of the teeth is related to the size of the face it is more likely that a pleasing effect will result. Even in long saddles the size of the teeth may be influenced by the space available between the abutment teeth. Modifications are best made in the size and position of the lateral incisors when the space does not allow the use of a set of anterior teeth. The laterals can be changed for wider or narrower counterparts or they may be overlapped or spaced in relation to the centrals or canines. Interstitial grinding can also be used when the available space is small but care must be exercised in doing this otherwise the character of the teeth may be altered unfavourably.

The material of which the tooth is made may be either porcelain or acrylic resin. An important point to bear in mind in this connection is the quality of tooth used in both cases. However, the original form of the tooth should only be considered a starting point which may be modified by grinding. Thus it is important that porcelain teeth must be capable of being polished after grinding; a rough surface as well as feeling unpleasant to the tongue, also tends to stain readily. The finest grades of vacuum fired teeth may be polished after grinding to give a satisfactory surface. The disadvantage of acrylic resin is undoubtedly its low abrasion resistance. Not only is minute tooth irregularity lost in this process, but a series of fine scores are made on the surface which become stained and require the use of cleaning abrasives, which again cause loss of tooth detail and leave an unpolished surface. The use of cross-linked polymers may add to the abrasion resistance of acrylic teeth.

The particular position of the teeth

Whereas the general tooth position is more important when the patient is viewed at rest, the particular tooth position is critical when smiling. More pleasing effects are secured by harmonious irregularity rather than by regular and symmetrical arrangements. Moreover, it must be remembered that irregularity is toned down in the mouth and consequently it must be over-emphasized on the articulator. This is comparable to the make-up used by an actor; the caricature effect of the cosmetics is reduced to normality by the stage lighting.

Just as sex, personality and age are important in the selection of the tooth form so do they influence the setting of the upper anterior teeth. In this regard individual artistic flare is important but to give the beginner a starting point a basic setting and some useful modifications will be described. Fig. 18.6 gives a

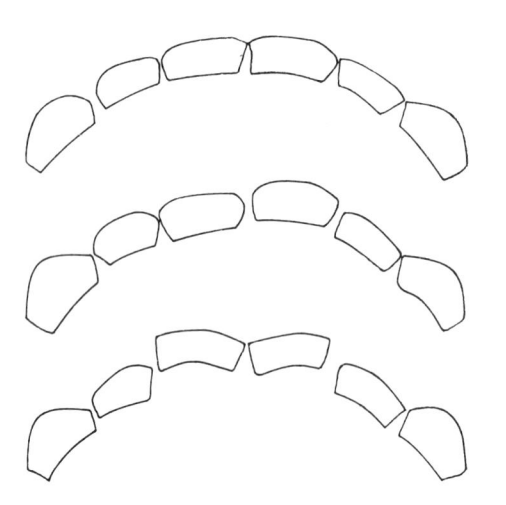

Fig. 18.6. Diagrammatic outline of normal upper anterior tooth position (top); two modifications in the position of the central incisors (middle and bottom).

diagrammatic guide to tooth positions. Aesthetically the central incisors are probably the most important teeth in the arch and the basic arrangement shows them in a symmetrical relationship, placed vertically but with the distal angles somewhat posterior to the mesial. Such a setting must be considered essentially soft and feminine. Graded degrees of hardness and masculinity may be produced by using the two variations depicted in Fig. 18.6. In the first the incisal edges are maintained in symmetrical relationship but the neck of one tooth is displaced outwards. A bolder effect can be achieved by rotating the distal edges of the two central incisors forward.

Although the lateral incisors are less conspicuous than the centrals they are influential in giving a spherical or square form to the arch. A soft feminine arrangement is produced by rotating them distally and a harder masculine effect is secured by rotating them mesially. It is generally desirable to maintain a pleasing asymmetry in these variations.

Although the canines give considerable character to the arch form, neither marked deviations in tooth position or gross asymmetries should normally be used. The neck of the tooth is basically prominent and only for really hard effects should the tip be given prominence. As with the laterals the degree of distal or mesial rotation can be varied to give delicacy or vigour. Distal rotation allows the bulbous shapes of the buccal surfaces of the two premolars to be seen and emphasizes a delicate arrangement. It is important in such an arrangement to make sure that the lengths of the premolars and canines are similar, particularly if the former are abutment teeth. Nothing is so displeasing as an obvious discrepancy in these relationships.

The curvature of the incisal edges, or what De Van calls the 'skyline', is an important contributory factor to aesthetics. An upward slope from the centrals back to the canines emphasizes the spheroidal arrangement, whilst a cuboidal effect is given by lowering the canines.

Two important variations may be used in the ageing patient. First, it is during this period that small diastemas make their appearances. This variation may be used effectively between the lateral and the central, as well as between the two centrals where it is more conventionally employed (Fig. 18.7). Second, the exposure of a larger clinical crown emphasizes the different axial inclinations of the various teeth as the patient becomes older. This illusion may be emphasized by actually tilting the incisor teeth to varying angles from the vertical.

The labial and buccal flange

The natural appearance presented by the labial flange of a long saddle is dependent upon the shaping of the gingival papillae, the shaping of the gingival margins, the overall contouring of the flange as a whole, and its colouring and shading.

In shaping the gingival papillae, the space between the teeth should be filled. The resin representing the papilla may then be lightly polished to give a surface which is readily self-cleansing. Where, on the other hand, a deep recess has been created between the necks of artificial teeth, the resin surface can neither be polished nor cleaned in use; accordingly stains appear readily between the teeth.

As well as the correct shaping of the gingival papillae, attention must be given to the shape of the entire gingival margin. In the natural dentition this gingival 'line' varies in its shape from one tooth to another and when long anterior saddles are being waxed this variation should be reproduced. The line is usually more sharply curved if the neck of the tooth is not prominent, but is higher and straighter if the neck is prominent. A more vigorous expression may be obtained by emphasizing the convexity of the gingival margin. The whole area of the gingival margin should be polished highly to avoid food debris accumulating round the necks of the teeth.

In ageing, both the interdental papilla and the gingival margin require modification. The papilla is positioned higher on the neck of the tooth, and the gingival margin regresses up the root of the tooth and a pointed rather than a curved form should be used, especially at the neck of a prominent tooth such as the canine.

Contouring of the labial flange should be carried out to simulate the development of bony prominences over the roots of teeth and interdental depressions (Fig. 18.7). The degree of prominence given to the canine eminence depends not only on the squareness of the arch setting, but also on the reaction of the levator anguli oris muscle to forward displacement; a canine eminence should never be developed to an extent that it interferes with retention. Stippling of the attached gingivae, as well as giving a pleasing natural appearance, has been found to restrict lip movement in some cases. However, it is not easy for the patient to keep clean.

The lateral margins of labial flanges must be reduced to wafer thinness and be extended over the root eminences of the abutment teeth. The thin edge allows the colour of the flange to blend more naturally with the mucosa (Fig. 18.8).

Whereas harmonious individual contouring effects can only be secured by wax carving, preformed labial plastic patterns emphasizing natural contouring may be used in some cases.

Colouring and shading of labial flanges must be combined with correct contouring and shaping if the optimum effects are to be achieved. It is necessary to have some system of colour matching so that the flange may blend harmoniously with the natural tissues of the patient.

The actual techniques for colouring and shading the acrylic resin are many and varied. Aspin *et al.* have described a method of painting, in which the paint is contained between two thin layers of resin. Many manufacturers supply acrylic materials containing coloured fibres, to which may be added additional stains and shaded polymers. Cold-cure resin polymerized under pressure after being flowed into position over the necks of the teeth can also be used.

Experience on the part of the technician is necessary before consistently good results can be guaranteed, and each person will develop his own preferences for particular methods and materials.

The Short Anterior Saddle

Many points mentioned in the previous section are applicable to the short anterior saddle, but some additional factors will be discussed under the following headings:
1 Tooth position.
2 Tooth characteristics.
3 The labial and buccal flange.

1 *Tooth position.* Tooth position in a short anterior saddle is usually easier to assess since it must conform to the existing arch. The labial surfaces of the artificial teeth must be in line with those of the natural teeth, except where a slight deviation is considered aesthetically desirable. This is indicated if the labial surfaces of the remaining standing teeth present a somewhat uneven appearance. The length of the teeth must be adjusted to correspond with the natural incisal edge level and careful grinding is often necessary in this connection.

18.7

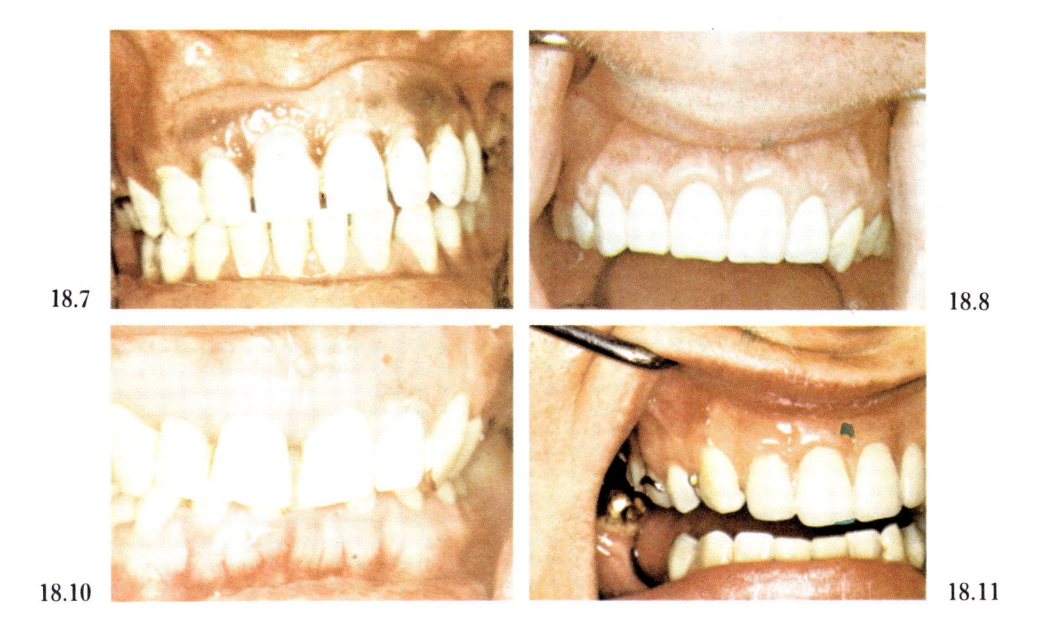

18.8

18.10

18.11

Fig. 18.7. A long saddle made for a coloured lady. Note (a) diastema, (b) the pigmented flange.

Fig. 18.8. A contoured labial flange, colour blended to match the mucosa. Note the thinning of the flange over the necks of the abutment teeth.

Fig. 18.10. The improved result in the case shown in Fig. 18.9, where a small labial flange is used.

Fig. 18.11. Lateral margin of the labial flange thinned over the root eminence of the canine abutment.

The angle that artificial teeth make to the centre line must conform to the general angulation of the natural teeth. A central must be tilted to match its opposite number whilst laterals should follow this angle unless the same tooth on the other side is differently placed. In this case discretion is allowed as to whether it shall match its opposite number or not. The tilt of the canine should differ little from the angulation of the opposite canine since any unbalance in this respect is aesthetically objectionable, giving a one-sided appearance to the dentition.

It is often difficult to decide whether anterior teeth on a partial denture should be gum-fitted or not. A gum-fit is often only possible by using a longer tooth than is really indicated, which is unsightly when the necks of the teeth are revealed by the patient (Fig. 18.9). Usually it is better to use a small flange if possible since this can be very thin and discreet and nearly indetectable at normal conversational distances (Fig. 18.10). The use of a flange also increases the saddle area which is desirable whenever possible. Fitting to the gum is recommended in some cases where the first premolar has to be replaced and the canine is still standing. The ridge just posterior to the canine is often quite prominent and the tooth angulation will be better if no flange is used. In addition, a flange in this area is often noticeable when the patient smiles.

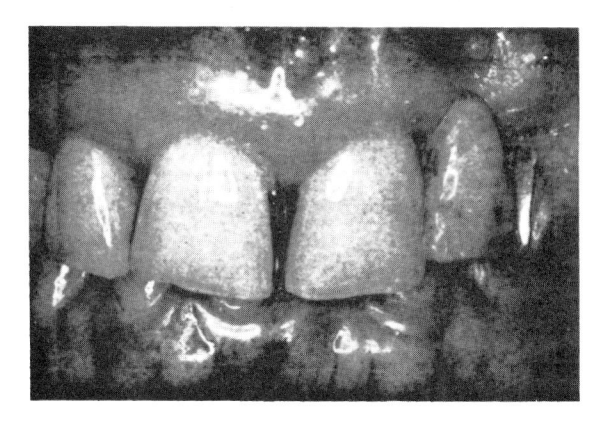

Fig. 18.9. Unsightly result of gum fitting a lateral incisor.

2 *Tooth characteristics.* Again mould and size, shade, and material of manufacture require consideration.

When only one or two anterior teeth are being replaced their size and mould must match the natural teeth adjacent to them. Outline form and labial contour must be followed exactly, and it may be necessary to grind teeth to achieve this.

A possible complication is a mesio-distal reduction in the space available, brought about by movement of the natural teeth subsequent to extraction. Such cases present a difficult aesthetic problem. When the space lost is small it may be overcome by using teeth slightly narrower than the width indicated by the natural teeth. Overlapping of the teeth may be helpful, but this should not be done if the remaining teeth show no evidence of such irregularity. Judicious interproximal grinding of the natural teeth bounding the space may be employed but care must be taken not to destroy their natural contours. This problem usually arises in the younger patient and it may be possible to improve the situation by orthodontic treatment. In extreme cases, when the space is reduced considerably it may be necessary to sacrifice another natural tooth to obtain even a reasonable aesthetic result.

If only one or two teeth are missing from the front of the mouth then the matching of shade is not usually difficult. The decision should be made by using a shade guide of the make of teeth which it has been decided to use. Shades should be matched only after the natural teeth have been polished. The shade guide tooth should be moistened and the patient should be facing a good light. When matching acrylic shades remember that the thickness of the shade guide tooth will affect the result. Only if the tooth to be used is approximately the same thickness as the guide tooth will the shade be identical. If the tooth on the denture has to be reduced in thickness because of close occlusal contacts then its shade will be lightened. Remember also that metal behind teeth, particularly acrylic, affects the shade by making it appear greyer and less translucent. This effect may be minimized by polishing the surface of the metal that comes into direct contact with the acrylic, or by using an opacifier.

It sometimes happens that the natural teeth bounding a space are not the same shade. This may occur particularly when a lateral is to be replaced and it is found that the canine is conspicuously darker than the central. In such cases a compromise in shade between the two may be chosen, or the shade may be matched with the central as this is the more obvious tooth.

If abnormal shade conditions such as enamel striations, hypoplasia, or marked staining are present in the natural teeth and it is decided to match these in the artificial teeth, then acrylic resin teeth will normally be used. Such modifications are not impossible with porcelain teeth, but are more easily carried out with acrylic. In any case, it is helpful to make a sketch of the tooth or teeth at the chairside, indicating the position of the abnormalities, to serve as a reminder to the technician. Preferably he himself should see the patient and make his own notes.

When teeth are to be modified by the technician, an indication must be given of the relative shades required in the body of the teeth, at the neck, and at the incisal edges. Some teeth may also require incisal edge translucency to be removed by grinding to match the natural condition.

When checking at the try-in, view the patient from various angles before deciding whether the shade is correct or not. Do not be satisfied unless the artificial tooth is an exact match or perhaps slightly darker. Any tooth that at first inspection appears lighter will certainly be obviously artificial during use. As with all other aspects of aesthetics the patient's own opinion must be obtained by inspection of the denture, when in the mouth, in a sufficiently large mirror.

3 *The labial and buccal flange.* The general principles discussed in relation to long saddles apply equally to shorter ones.

The junction between artificial and natural gum tissue is more readily seen in the case of the short saddle, and consequently every effort must be made to secure as unobtrusive a blend as possible.

The artificial papilla adjacent to the abutment tooth must be shaped to match the natural contiguous papilla, whilst the shape and contour of the gingival margin must likewise be similar to that of the natural teeth.

One of the most difficult problems is to blend the margins of the flanges into the natural tissues. These margins must be reduced to wafer thinness, and whenever possible, extended over the eminences of the abutment teeth (Figs 18.8 and 18.11). Such thin edges not only blend inconspicuously with the natural tissues, but allow their colour to show through.

In order that such extensions to the facings can be used, it will be necessary to employ a path of insertion that will allow the thin acrylic to pass over the eminence. Patients must be warned of the necessity for care in handling and cleaning when such a denture is supplied.

References

ASPIN M.E., TOMLIN H.R. and OSBORNE J. (1960) Aesthetics of denture gumwork. *Brit. dent. J.* **109**, 271.

BUCHNER R.C. (1963) Cosmetics in denture prosthesis. *J. Amer. Dent. Ass.* **66**, 787.

DE VAN M.M. (1957) The appearance phase of denture construction. *D. Clin. N. A.*, W.B. Saunders Co., Philadelphia and London.

FRUSH J.P. and FISHER R.D. (1955) Introduction to dentogenic restorations. *J. pros. Dent.* **5**, 586–95.

FRUSH J.P. and FISHER R.D. (1956) How dentogenic restorations interpret the sex factor. *J. pros. Dent.* **6**, 160–72.

FRUSH J.P. and FISHER R.D. (1956) How dentogenics interprets the personality factor. *J. pros. Dent.* **6**, 441–49.

FRUSH J.P. and FISHER R.D. (1957) The age factor in dentogenics. *J. pros. Dent.* **7**, 5–13.

POUND E. (1951) Esthetic dentures and their phonetic values. *J. pros. Dent.* **1**, 98.

POWERS J.L. (1953) Brush-on technique in natural colouring of cured cross-linked plastic artificial denture materials. *J. pros. Dent.* **3**, 350.

PROCTOR H.H. (1953) Characterization of dentures. *J. pros. Dent.* **3**, 339.

19
DENTURE INSERTION

When the technician has finished the dentures they should be left in water until they are fitted in the mouth. Acrylic resin contracts if it becomes dry, and therefore this precaution is important particularly when there is no metal frame. If the dentures have been processed on duplicate casts they must be fitted to the master casts and the occlusal relationship perfected when completed.

Before placing in the mouth the denture should be dried and inspected for any surface roughness and sharp margins which may be potentially traumatic. The inner aspect of clasps, bars, plates and saddles should also be inspected, together with surface polish. A high level of polish is desirable since this will result in improved tolerance of the appliance and will minimize the deposition of dental plaque or food debris. It will also avoid soreness to the tongue, cheeks, or mucosa which might result from a rough surface or sharp margin.

When the patient is in the chair the denture should be taken from its water bath and inserted carefully into the mouth. If the surveying, the decision regarding path of insertion, the elimination of under-cuts, and all the further details of the technical process have been carried out correctly, the denture should go into position without further adjustment. This will normally occur if the base or frame of the denture has been made in metal, since the fit of this will have been determined at an earlier visit. However, when an all-acrylic denture, or one that has a considerable surface of acrylic making contact with standing teeth, is being inserted it may be found that some slight adjustment is required before the denture can be seated. Processing on duplicate casts will reduce the chairside time required for these adjustments to a minimum, since the dentures can be fitted to the master cast in the laboratory.

If the denture cannot be fitted because of some obstruction no attempt should be made to force it into place. It should be inserted as far as possible and careful observation made, with a mirror, to locate the point, or points, of premature contact. A check should be made that the denture is being fitted in its correct path of insertion.

If it is doubtful, by visual examination, exactly which part of the denture is causing the trouble, it should be removed and disclosing wax flowed over the general contacting area in question. Re-seat the denture as far as possible, remove it, and note the points where the wax has been removed.

When the area causing the obstruction has been detected the acrylic should be removed from the fitting surface towards the polished surface until the denture can be inserted correctly. It is important that the contact point between denture and tooth is not destroyed, otherwise food packing will occur with consequent gingivitis or caries.

General stability must be checked by applying pressure anteriorly and posteriorly alternately. The denture should exhibit no movement under this test, or when the pressure is applied first on one side and then on the other. Free-end saddles are an exception to this since it may be possible to displace them against the underlying mucosa if mucostatic impressions have been taken and rebasing has not been carried out. If stability is correct an examination should be made of the fit of the various component parts, such as bars, clasps, and occlusal rests, and of the peripheral margins. It is quite possible for a denture to be stable and yet one of the clasp arms, for example, to be positioned incorrectly. The patient's opinion regarding the comfort of the denture should be sought at this stage.

A check must now be made of the occlusion in the tooth position and in lateral and antero-posterior positions. Blue articulating paper, occlusal indicator wax, or occlusal spray should be placed between the upper and lower teeth and the patient asked to close in the tooth position three or four times. Points of occlusal contact may be seen with a mouth mirror. In normal cases the occlusal contact must be evenly distributed between the natural teeth and the denture. Any concentration of load at the distal of free-end saddles must be reduced so that the load is transferred as far forward on the saddle as possible. It is also important to reduce any excess pressure on occlusal rests or clasp shoulders as this may result, quite apart from pain, in fracture of these components.

When occlusion in the tooth position has been corrected the patient is asked to make lateral, protrusive and retrusive movements, the range of which should be that normally used by the patient in mastication. Any cuspal contacts that interfere with free gliding excursion from lateral or protrusive contact to the tooth position must be removed by grinding.

When all positions of occlusion have been checked the aesthetics must be considered. It may be necessary to grind incisal edges or to modify contours slightly, but decisions on aesthetics should have been taken at the previous visit. The patient's opinion of the aesthetics should be ascertained before they leave.

When the clinician is satisfied that the dentures are satisfactory he should demonstrate to the patient how to insert and remove them. This is essential, otherwise the patient may not be able to remove the dentures at all, or if successful in this, be unable to re-insert them. Patients should be discouraged from using clasp arms as a means of removing dentures. Most patients, if not told otherwise, will do this, and in time the metal may become distorted and the clasps non-functional. Dentures can usually be removed by pressure at the buccal saddle peripheries instead of by the clasps.

A large proportion of free-end saddle dentures should normally be rebased immediately on fitting. The procedure for this is described in the next chapter.

It is essential that every patient should be informed regarding the possible difficulties that may be encountered during the early period of denture wearing. Advice must be given regarding eating, talking, cleaning, and wearing at night, and provision for review at an early date. The following points must be explained to the patient in suitable lay terminology.

Review

The period that elapses before the patient is reviewed will vary according to circumstances, but it should not normally be longer than one week. The dentures should be examined in the light of the patient's comments and any necessary adjustments carried out. Inspection should also include all other aspects of the dentures, about which the patient may have no comment. Clasp arms, rests, occlusion, and aesthetics should all be examined, irrespective of whether the patient has any comments concerning them.

At this point it is convenient to consider some of the more common complaints with which a patient may present after a short period of wearing his partial denture.

Complaints

Normally it should be expected that the dentures will be satisfactory and that any complaints will be of a minor nature. Sometimes, however, even with the greatest care, skill, and technical ability, a patient will have a serious complaint. This will be, to the patient, real and genuine regarding the denture, but in fact it may be due to a lack of understanding on his part, indicating the importance of adequate instructions and appreciation of the difficulties of denture wearing.

The first step in dealing with a complaint is to ascertain its possible cause. For example soreness at the periphery of a saddle may be due to faulty occlusion, and not to over-extension or roughness of the peripery itself; before adjusting the saddle, the occlusion must be checked.

In making a diagnosis the operator may not be helped by the terminology used by the patient to describe the complaints. The lay person may express this in terms that may be misleading. For example, a locked occlusion may be described as 'The dentures are no good for eating', 'They get mixed up with food', 'The plates hurt at the edges' or 'The dentures don't fit'. If the occlusion is unbalanced it may be said that 'The teeth do not meet on one side at all', 'They are noisy', 'They hurt me on one side', or 'They move about in the mouth'.

On first hearing these descriptions it may not be easy to associate them with the actual problem. Many different symptoms may all be due to one error such as one high cusp, but this, as such, is never named by the patient. To arrive at the truth it is necessary to examine the denture in the mouth and to question the patient on his denture-wearing experiences.

The various complaints that may be made will be considered under their appropriate headings.

1 Pain

There are many causes of pain produced by partial dentures.

(a) *Soreness at saddle peripheries.* This usually produces an inflammatory or ulcerative area at the site of the tenderness. If the dentures have been fitted recently it may be due to over-extension of the periphery, which has not been detected at the trial stage. Basically this is often due to insufficient care being taken when defining the periphery of the impression. Roughness or sharpness of the saddle margin may also be the cause.

Before any reduction of the periphery is undertaken it is essential to check the occlusion in all tooth contact positions. Any interference in occlusion during lateral or protrusive excursions may result in a lateral or posterior thrust on a lower partial denture, or a lateral or anterior thrust upon an upper. Reference to Chapter 11 will indicate the areas and structures that resist these thrusts. Consequently, the site of the soreness may indicate the area of the occlusion that requires attention.

If the occlusion is adjusted it may also be necessary to relieve the denture periphery. Whenever any adjustment is made to the base material, the surface must be polished before the denture is fitted again.

The most common sites for discomfort related to the denture periphery are in the lower lingual region in the area of the mylo-hyoid ridge, the buccal region at the anterior part of free-end saddles, and buccally in partial upper dentures where the palatal connector is not rigid. In fact, any non-rigid connection between saddles is likely to lead to peripheral pain brought about by flexing of the connector and consequent rotational movement of the saddle. Discomfort related to the periphery may also arise from faulty laboratory technique. Lack of care when pouring a cast from an alginate impression, for instance, may result in distortion and an inaccurate peripheral form in the finished denture.

Mucosa borne partial dentures may produce painful peripheries after either a long or short period. As these dentures transmit all the load directly to the ridges it is not uncommon for them to be reduced in size by resorption, as described in earlier chapters. When this happens the denture saddle moves from the narrower higher area of the ridge to the broader lower region. This results in excessive compression of the mucosa and consequent pain. Adjustment of the saddles should be only a temporary measure since a denture that has reached this condition should have the saddles rebased as soon as possible.

(b) *Soreness under saddle.* This complaint may be associated with soreness at the periphery and in some cases the causes are the same.

Damage to the master cast through mishandling may be responsible and the saddle must be inspected for any obvious prominences resulting from such damage. Small pimples of acrylic resin may sometimes be left on the fitting surface and will cause considerable pain if not removed.

The occlusion must be checked as before to ensure that there are no cuspal interferences. When the pain is under the saddle rather than at the periphery, the cause may be uneven contact in the tooth position and this must be checked also.

This complaint is more common with free-end saddles than with bounded saddles that are tooth supported, since the ridge is taking a higher proportion of the load. In these circumstances any abnormal condition of the mucosa or underlying bone will be likely to cause pain during function. It has been pointed out that when the ridge is covered by a thin atropic mucosa and submucosa, pain may be experienced posteriorly and lingually where the mylohyoid ridge is inadequately covered to resist the pressure of the saddle. Treatment of such a condition may be the surgical reduction of the bony prominence or the use of a resilient lining to the saddle.

The general condition of bone under free-end saddles should be assessed by radiographs and any evidence of a progressing osteolysis will indicate an unfavourable prognosis for denture comfort. Sharp, irregular ridges, will receive an excess of pressure and will be painful. A narrow, high ridge may not resist without discomfort the vertical or lateral stresses placed upon it during mastication. This will especially be so when natural teeth are providing the occlusal contacts.

All these contacts strengthen the case for reducing the area of the occlusal table in order to minimize the load falling on the ridge under the free-end saddle. The patient will often be much more comfortable after this has been done.

It is sometimes helpful in these cases, when the patient complains of pain under a saddle, to provide a resilient lining. Of the materials available, the silicone rubbers are probably the most effective although they may give rise to other problems such as infection due to the ready growth of *Candida albicans* on their surface, or frictional irritation due to reduced wettability.

Excessive displacement of the mucosa during impression taking may lead to pain under the saddle. This may arise if the impression tray is pressed through alginate to impinge directly on the ridge tissue. Pain arising from this cause will be continuous if the clasping is rigid enough to prevent the saddle 'easing off' the mucosa when not under load, or intermittent if the clasping allows such movement to occur.

If the vertical dimension is too great, pain under the saddles may be expected. Such an error is not common when one partial denture is made, but may occur when a complete denture is made for the upper jaw and a partial denture for the lower. In such cases, excess vertical dimension will cause pain under the lower saddles since the lower ridge will be called upon to bear a greater proportion of load per unit of surface area than the upper. Treatment will usually mean remaking one or both dentures so that the vertical dimension is corrected.

(c) *Pain in or around standing teeth.* A complaint of this nature is serious since it usually indicates that a continuous load in excess of the physiological limit is being placed upon the tooth or teeth concerned. If allowed to persist it may mean their loss. Although the seriousness of this complaint may be realized, a diagnosis of the cause may not be easy.

The patient must be questioned regarding the incidence, nature, and duration of the pain. The possibility of undetected caries or a leaking restoration must not be forgotten. If these are eliminated it is usually found, if the denture is the causative factor, that the pain is periodontal in nature.

If a denture is rocking on an occlusal rest this may cause pain in the tooth; this error is easily detected (the complaint of pain is associated with one regarding movement of the denture) and the rest must be removed and replaced in correct position or the adjacent saddles rebased. Adjustment of the fitting surface of the rest is not advisable, and rarely improves the condition. Pain should not normally be caused in this manner since such instability should be detected when the denture is fitted.

It may be found that a clasp arm, usually one used for retention, is exerting too much pressure which is not being adequately reciprocated by the opposing arm and excess stress is applied to the tooth. The most likely conditions under which this may arise are, that the denture has had a clasp arm displaced accidentally during construction, or that a flexible arm has been displaced by careless handling on the part of the patient. Treatment may be to adjust the clasp arm, but often it will be necessary to make a new clasp.

Flexible connections between saddles may allow the denture to exert a lateral thrust on a tooth or teeth when the full occlusal pressure is applied. The use of rigid saddle connections must be regarded as essential, except when stress broken designs are used.

The occlusion must always be checked in the region of a tooth that is painful. A denture in the opposing jaw may impose a lateral or antero-posterior thrust upon the tooth. Adjustment of the occlusion must be carried out if interference of this sort is found.

Excessive movement of a free-end saddle that has rigid connections to the clasp may cause pain to the clasped tooth by stress transmitted via the clasp. Rebasing of the saddle may be indicated or possibly a change to a stress-broken design. Complaints of this nature will arise after a period of wear when some bone resorption may have occurred under the saddle.

Electrolytic action between the metal components of a denture and metallic restorations may be a cause of tooth pain. In such cases the pain is located in a restored tooth when a dissimilar denture alloy is present. In the electromotive series both cobalt chromium and gold alloys are sufficiently apart from amalgam to provide an electric stimulus. Cobalt chromium is further removed than gold, but the number of cases that occur are few. When it occurs with cobalt chromium it is very transient and this may be due to the non-conducting film that is developed on the surface of an amalgam restoration after a very short period in the mouth. In severe cases of electrolytic action either the denture material or the restoration must be changed.

If the denture design is faulty in that it allows food debris to be packed against the gingival margin then pain may be caused at these points. An example of this may be found if a lingual bar is placed with its upper margin too near the gingival margins of the natural teeth.

(d) *Tongue or cheek biting.* Biting of the cheek is the commoner of the two conditions. It is more likely to occur in older patients when loss of tone of the cheek musculature is more advanced. It often occurs when the buccal cusps of the upper and lower posterior teeth meet in an edge-to-edge occlusion. Such a lack of posterior horizontal overlap causes the buccal mucosa to be caught up easily between the teeth. The cure is to reset the teeth into normal relationship if this is practicable. If the upper teeth cannot be moved buccally nor the lowers lingually, the buccal cusps of the lowers should be reduced about 2 mm in a lingual direction and repolished.

Correct shaping of the buccal flanges of the dentures will be helpful in preventing this complaint, since they can be designed to keep the cheek mucosa away from the teeth.

When natural posterior teeth meet in occlusion, cheek biting may be caused if one of the lower teeth is clasped, to provide retention for a free-end saddle on the opposing side of the arch. The thickness of the clasp arm may obliterate the effect of the natural horizontal overlap and the cheek becomes trapped between the palatal slope of the upper buccal cusps and the superior surface of the clasp arm. In some cases the clasp arm will have to be removed or transferred to another tooth. In other cases grinding of the upper tooth may eliminate the discomfort.

Tongue biting may be due to the teeth being set too far lingually, allowing insufficient tongue space. Moving the teeth or judicious grinding is the method of treatment. In the case of upper and lower free-end saddle dentures in opposition or a complete denture in one jaw opposing a partial denture in the other, the level of the occlusal plane may be too low.

2 Movement

A complaint that a denture moves may often be associated with complaint of pain and, therefore, the two conditions may have to be considered together. In this section, however, the possible causes of movement alone will be considered.

The most common complaint is that the denture moves during mastication. The retention of most partial dentures is sufficiently good to resist displacement in any other circumstances, but the patient may find it inadequate during eating.

The patient should be questioned as to whether displacement occurs on both sides alternately or only unilaterally and whether it is anterior or posterior. This may help to locate the cause which is commonly a defect in the occlusion. This should be checked and any cuspal interference or premature contacts reduced. Usually the fault will be found on the opposite side of the mouth to that where the displacement occurs. It may be helpful in locating the displacing force to place the fingers on some buccal area of the dentures while the patient occludes and carries out masticating movements.

If no error can be detected in the occlusion, the clasp arms should be examined for their position in relation to the undercut areas in which they are supposed to engage. Arms used for retention may be found not to engage far enough into the undercut in relation to their resilience. For example, a wrought wire which does not engage a sufficient depth of undercut may be so resilient that it allows itself to pass over the survey line. To prevent this it may have to engage the undercut area to a greater degree.

It is undesirable to try to prevent partial denture movement by 'tightening' clasp arms so that the denture 'clicks' into position. This may prevent movement, but only at the expense of over-stressing the teeth and possibly fracturing the clasp. Adjustment of clasp position *can* be carried out at the chairside, to make an arm engage deeper into the undercut, for example, but indiscriminate 'tightening' is not desirable. Any minor adjustments of this sort should be made out of view of the patient. It suggests that the original workmanship may have been inaccurate (it has, but the patient need not know!) and also the patient may be inclined to repeat the treatment himself if he sees what is done.

If no fault is found with either occlusion or clasp positions the cause of the movement may be over-extension of the saddle peripheries. Such over-extension will result in movement or soreness, but the former is only likely to occur with long free-end saddles. If retention is good then pain results, but if retention is not so efficient then the saddle is displaced. Such an occurrence can take place in the region of free-end saddle in the upper or lower jaws. Detection of the offending area is not easy, but the patient should be asked to carry out lateral and protrusive movements with the mouth about half open. Movement of the denture may be seen. If not, then asking the patient to open and close the mouth widely may reveal the area. Over-extension on the lingual aspect of a lower should be located if the tip of the tongue is moved to the corners of the mouth. When the area of over-extension has been found it should be reduced and repolished.

Denture movement during mastication may also be due to posterior teeth being set in such a position that either the tongue or the cheek muscles exert lateral pressure on the denture. In partial dentures this is not likely to happen with bounded saddles, but may occur with the free-end type particularly if the teeth are set too far lingually.

When retention of the denture is partially dependent upon the establishment of a border seal, such as in a bilateral free-end saddle in the upper jaw, the denture should be inspected to ensure that the saddles are extended to the optimum depth round the tuberosities. This examination may have to be made digitally. Any deficiency at the periphery in this region will have a marked effect on the retention, particularly during mastication.

The occasional complaint of displacement when yawning is only likely with claspless saddles and is due to over-extension of the periphery or over-thickening of peripheral margins.

Spoon design dentures depend largely upon adhesion for their retention and consequently there are limitations to their use for incision. These should be explained to the patient and if they later complain of lack of retention it should be ascertained that they are not making an incisive bite with the teeth on the denture. Such dentures must be examined for their peripheral adaptation to the palate. If this is satisfactory, and for aesthetic reasons an anterior flange cannot be added, and retention is not satisfactory, some lateral extension of the spoon may have to be considered.

3 Difficulties during mastication

These will often be due to movement of the denture as discussed above and will be treated accordingly. Other complaints associated with mastication may be that the patient cannot chew food adequately, that food becomes trapped under the denture, or that it becomes lodged on the denture or between it and the natural teeth.

Inability to chew may be caused by the patient taking too much food into the mouth at once. It should be explained that mastication must be slower and that this is a desirable state of affairs since less stress will be placed upon the remaining natural teeth. The advantage to the patient's digestion may also be mentioned!

If the patient has previously worn dentures with porcelain teeth and now has acrylic resin teeth, he may complain of a relative lack of 'sharpness'. In some cases it may be necessary to change the teeth, but usually the patient will tolerate the change after a short period of wear.

There are very few dentures being worn under which a small proportion of food does not find its way. However, if the amount is sufficient to make wearing of the denture intolerable, it will often be due to slight movement of a saddle away from the mucosa during mastication. This in turn may be caused by unbalanced occlusion or inefficient clasping. A saddle connector that is resilient will allow food to pass under it and this may occur with lingual plates or broad palatal bars. Such connectors must be rigid. Slight saddle movement may indicate the necessity for rebasing, particularly if the denture has been worn for a period.

Food impaction around the denture is annoying to the patient. Its prevention depends to a large extent upon good denture design, and it is a factor which must always be considered. It is obvious that the more complex the design, the greater is the possibility of this complication. The design that is best in this respect is the 'plate' type, either palatal or lingual, since food is easily swept off with the tongue.

Lingual bars may entrap food, but, if they are shaped and positioned correctly and not used in conjunction with continuous clasps, the danger is not great. If a continuous clasp is present the liability of food to lodge between it and the lingual bar is considerable. In the same way, stress-broken designs are an even greater hazard. Some patients will cope with these problems better than others and the temperament of the individual should be considered when deciding upon the design. Complete alteration of the design after the denture has been completed is an unfortunate step to have to take, but it may be unavoidable if the patient is to be satisfied and the denture worn.

The denture should always be inspected to make certain that the polish is good since any rough areas or unpolished crevices will cause food to adhere readily.

4 Difficulties with speech

It should be explained when fitting the dentures that some initial disturbance of speech is to be expected. Should this continue for longer than a few days, and speech remains blurred, the most likely cause is incorrect postioning of the posterior teeth. Such a condition is only likely to occur with larger partial dentures. The bucco-lingual width of the posterior teeth may be too great, even if the teeth themselves are set correctly. They should be ground away on the lingual or palatal side and repolished. Alternatively, they may be set incorrectly and may require removal and replacing. Excessive thickness of the lingual side of a lower saddle may embarrass the tongue, but it is unlikely that a palate would be made sufficiently thick to do so. Continuous clasps may be a source of embarrassment in speaking, particularly when used in the upper jaw. Palatal bars have their minimum effect upon speech if they cross the palate in the region of the first molars but other considerations may make this location unsuitable.

When a number of upper anterior teeth have been replaced with a denture the patient may complain of whistling or lisping. This indicates some interference with the pronunciation of the 's' sound. A correct 's' sound is formed by an escape of air through a slit-like channel on the inner aspect of the palate. This channel is formed by the anterior lateral borders of the tongue curling upwards and making contact with the anterior portion of the palate. If this channel is not the correct shape, if it is round or oval or too large, the air will escape with a whistling sound. If it becomes obliterated the result is the 'th' sound and lisping.

Whistling may occur if the anterior overjet is considerable, and it may be necessary to move the upper teeth backwards. Alternatively, the denture base may be thickened behind these teeth to reduce the size of the channel. Wax may be added at the chairside to decide the amount of thickening required. Lisping may be treated by reducing the denture base thickness in this region, or possibly by moving the teeth slightly forwards.

Speech in general may be influenced by the shaping of the denture base that covers the rugae areas and this should be contoured to reproduce the natural anatomy, as far as possible. The shaping of the palatal aspect of an anterior saddle should also conform to tooth contour whenever this can be done without any danger of a reduction in strength.

Further causes of speech impairment may be unsatisfactory retention or excessive vertical dimension. However, in both these instances the patient will usually complain additionally of other factors, as discussed previously.

5   Noise

A complaint of noise due to interocclusal tooth contact may be due to an excessive vertical dimension of occlusion or to inadequate retention, with a denture continually being displaced from its basal seat and contacting its antagonist. Another cause may be uneven occlusion; the teeth meeting on one side and tilting a saddle on the opposite side so that it meets its opponents with a sharp tap. A complaint of noise is less common with partial than with full dentures. Acrylic resin teeth are less noisy in function than those made of porcelain. Occasionally patients wearing disjunct dentures complain of the denture 'rattling' due to the movement of the saddle component against the tooth supported part.

6   Metallic taste

Although it might be thought that this complaint would only arise when a partial denture carried some metal components, it can sometimes be made when only non-metallic bases have been employed. In such instances it is often a local manifestation of a general condition, usually the menopause, but worry and a state of nervous tension may induce such a complaint. In such cases there is no dental treatment to be prescribed. The possibility that it might be due to some ingredient of the acrylic resin is highly unlikely.

Complaints of a metallic taste with a metal base may be made in respect of either cobalt chromium or stainless steel. In the case of the former any metallic taste that may be noticeable on first insertion usually disappears within a few days. This is thought to be due to rapid accommodation in the susceptible nerve endings. Some patients find the taste of stainless steel so objectionable that the alloy has to be changed. In cases of this sort a check should be made on any welded or soldered attachments that are exposed to the mouth. Inefficient welding or the use of low silver-content solders may cause a metallic taste.

7 Nausea

This is commonly a complaint directed against upper dentures, although it may also be related to the disto-lingual extension of the lower. It is usually associated with hypersensitivity of the patient and awareness of the bulk of the denture in the mouth, and in this respect is more common with complete as opposed to partial dentures.

The areas of the mouth that may appear unduly sensitive are the soft palate, the fauces and the posterior part of the dorsum of the tongue. The patient's symptoms may range from nausea, through retching to frank vomiting, although the latter is rare. The symptomatic cause is multifactorial, although it can be divided into a somatogenic reaction due to physical stimulation of the tissue by the denture, or a psychogenic reaction. That it is not simply tactile is clear from the fact that the patient is able to tolerate food in the mouth, and whatever the precise cause it appears to be dependent upon the patient's awareness of the provoking stimulus. One of the major causes related to denture design appears to be postioning of the posterior palatal border. Palatal bar designs should be free from this complaint provided that they are well fitting, since they will normally be placed far enough anteriorly to avoid resting on the hard and soft palate junction. A palatal plate extending on the soft palate will clearly cause nausea but this should have been detected and corrected at an early stage.

If the post dam of a palatal plate is incorrectly developed and a space exists between the plate and the tissues, then nausea may result due to unreliable retention and movement during function. The cure is to develop an efficient post dam. Nausea may also be caused by excessive thickness of the posterior palatal border, which occasionally occurs with an acrylic resin plate.

Other causes of nausea include the polished surface of the palatal plate which is sometimes described as 'slimy', and the construction of the dentures to an excessive vertical dimension of occlusion. In the former, the surface may be made matt or artificial rugae incorporated, and in the latter the dentures should be remade to a lesser vertical dimension of occlusion.

In protracted cases the use of hypnotherapy can be extremely helpful, and serves to direct the patient's attention away from the provoking stimulus. The use of topical anaesthesia is not recommended as it may only serve to increase patient awareness, so increasing the likelihood of nausea.

8   Excessive salivation

This is usually due to stimulation of the salivary glands by the presence in the mouth of the dentures themselves. It only persists for a short period and the secretion returns to normal as soon as the patient has become accustomed to the dentures.

9   Burning sensation

This is most commonly encountered amongst menopausal and post-menopausal females where a decrease in oestrogen secretion results in both metabolic and vasomotor disturbances, which lead to an increase in the level of neurosis. As such, the complaint is a local manifestation of a general condition although the dentures are often an irritating factor. The situation is commonest in relation to the maxillary denture bearing area, the tongue, and the lips, and its appearance often coincides with the provision of new dentures. It has been observed however that there are often associated faults present in the denture, but once these are eliminated little can be done for the patient from a dental point of view if the situation does not resolve.

Occasionally it is suggested that patients may be allergic to the denture base material. This may be apparent with gold alloys and in nickel containing cobalt chromium alloys, and if an allergy to nickel has been demonstrated the alloy should be replaced. Allergy to acrylic resin is, however, rare and any hypersensitivity reactions are usually ascribed to leachable residual monomer due to an incorrect processing cycle. The symptoms usually disappear on removal of the denture and recur on its re-insertion. Short curing cycles can produce a denture with many times the residual monomer content compared with a long cycle, and this is not removed simply by prolonged immersion in water. It is advisable therefore, always to use a long processing cycle for dentures for such patients. If this does not improve the situation, it may be necessary to consider using an injection moulded pre-polymerized resin.

10   Appearance

A complaint regarding the appearance of the dentures is generally due to insufficient care being taken at the try-in stage, and the operator has only himself to blame. The patient's opinion must be sought at this time, and the dentures should not be passed for finish until the patient has expressed satisfaction regarding the aesthetics.

When a large number of anterior teeth have been replaced, after the patient has been without teeth for some time, the bulk of the denture may cause the patient to imagine that the lips are extended unduly. In these cases no alteration should be made until sufficient time has elapsed to enable the musculature to accommodate to the changed conditions. It may then be found that the patient is satisfied with the appearance.

Arrangements must always be made for periodic re-examination of partial dentures at intervals of approximately six months. A close watch must be kept for the necessity of saddle rebasing and for the continued efficiency of clasps and stress breakers, if present.

References

ANDERSON J.N. and BATES J.F. (1959) The cobalt-chromium partial denture. *Brit. dent. J.* **107**, 57.

AUSTIN A.T. and BASKER R.M. (1982) Residual monomer levels in denture bases. The effects of varying short cure cycles. *Brit. dent. J.* **153**, 424.

FAIGENBLUM M.J. (1968) Retching, its causes and management in prosthetic practice. *Brit. dent. J.* **125**, 485.

FERGUSON M.M., CARTER J., BOYLE P., HART D.M. and LINDSAY R. (1981) Oral complaints related to clinacteric symptoms in oophorectomized women. *J. Roy. Soc. Med.* **74**, 492.

GIUNTA J. and ZABLOTSKY N. (1976) Allergic stomatitis caused by self polymerising resin. *Oral Surg.* **41**, 631.

KROL A.J. (1963) A new approach to the gagging problem. *J. pros. Dent.* **13**, 611.

LAWSON W.A. (1965) Information and advice for patients wearing dentures. *D. Pract.* **15**, 402.

LAWSON W.A. and BOND E.K. (1969) Speech and its relation to dentistry. *D. Pract.* **19**, 150.

MAIN D.M.G. and BASKER R.M. (1983) Patients complaining of a burning mouth. *Brit. dent. J.* **154**, 206.

SINGER F. (1966) Occlusion, functions and para-functions. *Int. dent. J.* **16**, 385.

TROEST T. (1964) Diagnosing minute deflective occlusal contacts. *J. pros. Dent.* **14**, 71.

WOOD J.F.L. (1974) Mucosal reaction to cobalt-chromium alloy. *Brit. dent. J.* **136**, 423.

WRIGHT S.M. (1981) Oral awareness and oral motor proficiency in retchers. *J. Oral Rehab.* **8**, 421.

YLIPPO A. (1955) The effect of dentures on speech. *Int. dent. J.* **5**, 225–40.

20
REBASING

In previous chapters reference has been made to the necessity for rebasing the saddles of partial dentures. Such a procedure may be required at any time from the first insertion of the denture to any subsequent period of its use. It is however more likely to be necessary with free-end rather than bounded saddles owing to the displaceability of their mucosal support.

As has been explained previously, free-end saddles during function will produce a damaging torque on the abutment tooth if this is clasped, and will initiate an inflammatory reaction in the gingival margin adjacent to the saddle. If this condition continues it may lead eventually to loss of the abutment tooth.

In addition to the use of specific principles of design which have been discussed already, the functional stability of the free-end saddle denture can also be improved by clinical techniques. This may be achieved by using the altered cast technique in which correction of the cast is made before the denture base is finally processed, by rebasing the denture at the time of insertion, or by rebasing the denture at varying periods throughout its life.

Altered Cast Techniques

The edentulous saddle area may be recorded in two forms, either an anatomical form where the contour of the tissues is recorded under minimum load, or a functional form where load is applied to the tissues during impression taking. If the master impression is taken in a conventional manner using a relatively mucostatic impression material such as alginate in an individual tray, then the mucosa of the edentulous saddles will be recorded in its anatomical form. The major support of the denture, if a free-end saddle design, will be provided by the saddle area with some additional contribution from the teeth where support units have been used. As the compressibility of the periodontal ligament and the oral mucosa is dissimilar, functional loading of the saddle will result in movement of the denture.

The load applied to the tissues underlying the denture saddle will not be distributed evenly, however, with certain areas receiving more load than others. Movement of a distal extension base into the mucosa of the saddle is unavoidable and even where stress breaking devices have been employed some rotational movement is to be expected. It is important, however, that this load is distributed as uniformly as possible both to protect the underlying tissues and to improve the stability of the denture during function. In order to achieve this it has been suggested that the anatomy of the teeth and the saddle areas should be recorded independently, as in the altered or corrected cast technique.

In this technique the cast framework of the partial denture is first constructed on a master cast poured from an alginate impression. The framework is then tried in the mouth and examined to ensure that it is satisfactory. When this has been completed the framework extending over the saddle area (with which it is not in contact) should be covered with autopolymerizing resin to form a custom built 'tray'. This tray will be used to hold the material for a further impression of the edentulous saddle area (Fig. 20.1).

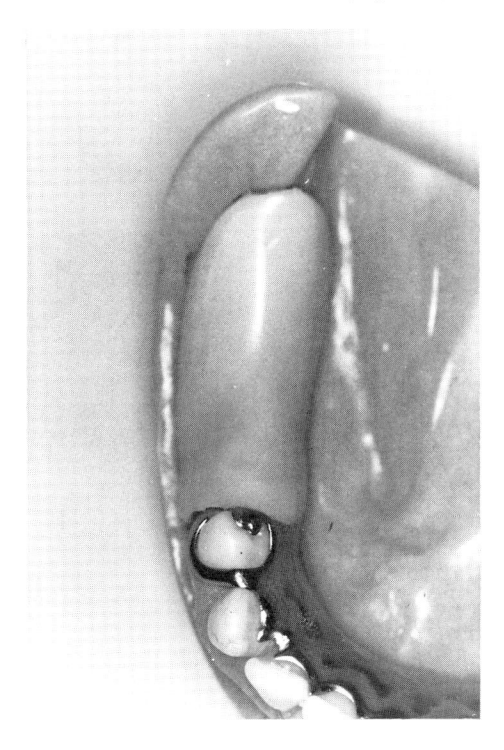

Fig. 20.1. Free-end saddle of framework covered to form a tray.

The choice of impression material for this purpose is between zinc oxide paste, light bodied polysulphide or silicone material, and impression wax. It has been shown, however, that impression wax gives the best results in terms of stability of the denture during function. The wax selected should be capable of a high degree of flow at mouth temperature, in order to avoid overdisplacement of the tissues and ensure that only those tissues that are readily displaced will be recorded in a different form. The wax should also be capable of accurately recording the peripheral form of the base. A suggested formula for such a wax is given by McCrorie, 1982 as:

Yellow beeswax 25 per cent

Paraffin wax 75 per cent

The wax is prepared in a tray over a thermostatically controlled water bath and is painted on to the fitting surface of the metal framework tray. When sufficient wax has been added, it is tempered in water at 45°C before insertion into the mouth. When inserted, the framework should be held firmly in position, by pressure applied to its tooth-supported components. No direct load is applied to the edentulous saddle area.

The framework should be held in position for at least four minutes, so that the wax may flow under the indirect load applied. After removal, the surface of the wax should be inspected and any areas that do not show a glossy surface should be built up by painting more wax over them. The denture must then be reinserted for a further two or three minutes (Fig. 20.2).

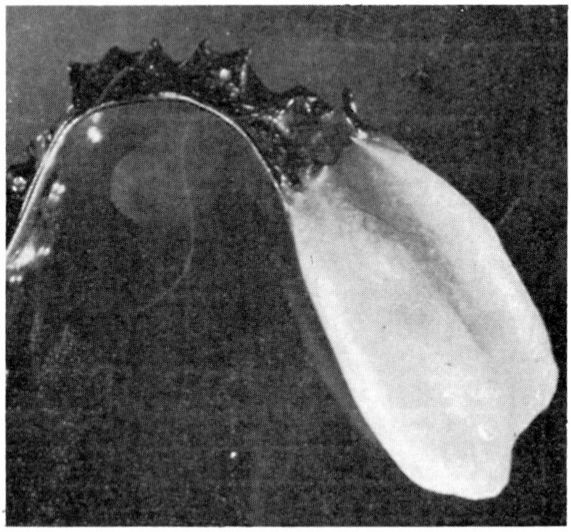

Fig. 20.2. Even glossy wax surface indicating that uniform pressure has been applied.

When the entire wax surface is glossy it may be assumed that the pressure applied to the mucosa has been reasonably uniform and that in function the denture will have minimal movement.

The framework is now returned to the master cast but before it can be fitted it will be necessary to cut away the area previously underlying the free-end saddle (Fig. 20.3). When this is done, the denture can be seated on the cast, secured firmly in position and a new free-end saddle area cast in position (Fig. 20.4). On

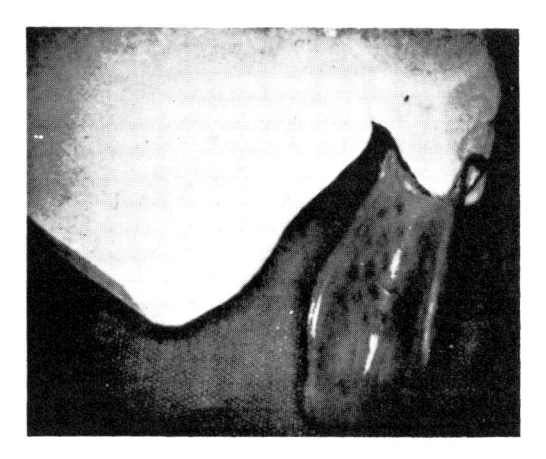

Fig. 20.3. Master cast cut to allow seating of framework and wax impression.

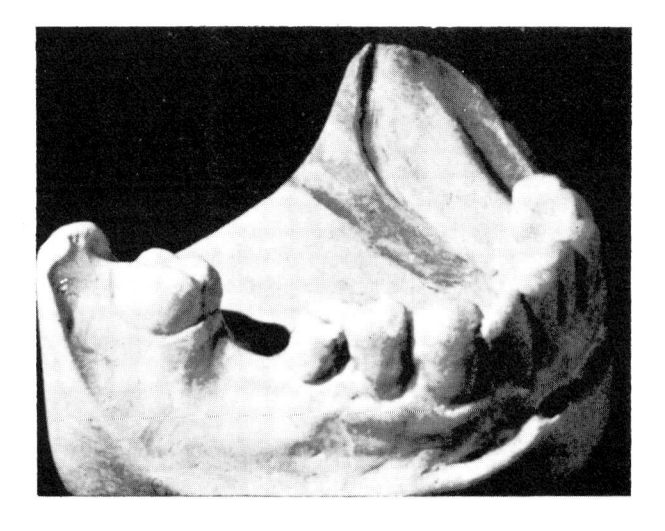

Fig. 20.4. The modified model ('altered cast').

the modified or altered cast the denture base material is processed and hence corresponds to the wax impression surface.

Rebasing New Dentures

In this situation the denture has been processed on the master cast with the knowledge that the fitting surface of the free-end saddles will still require modification. The most suitable impression material is usually a zinc oxide and eugenol paste, although a functional impression material or tissue conditioner could be used.

The denture should be fitted as described previously. When the fit is satisfactory the denture should then be examined to ensure that the saddles are not depressed at any of the positions of occlusion. This is accomplished most effectively by using an occlusal indicator spray the thickness of which is negligible. The teeth on the saddles should then be adjusted as appropriate until the majority of occlusal pressure is being taken by the natural teeth which are in occlusion. The occlusal contact of the saddle should be such that the teeth meet lightly without any heavy pressure. If there are no natural teeth making contact, then a 'stop' in compound must be provided so that the occlusal pressure on the free-end saddles can be adjusted as described.

It is necessary that there is sufficient space beneath the saddle to accommodate the impression paste. Obviously, the ultimate thickness of the paste under the saddle will vary according to the displacement of the mucosa and the degree of pressure applied to the saddle. As a routine procedure it is helpful if a space is created deliberately so that the thickness of the paste is approximately 1 to 2 mm. This allows an equal thickness of denture base material to be packed and minimizes the possibility of the saddle being thickened and the occlusion disturbed during processing, which often occurs if only a very thin layer of acrylic resin has to be packed.

There are three possible methods of providing this space. Firstly, the impression paste may be placed directly on to the saddle, which is exactly as processed on the duplicate of the master cast. This method may be satisfactory if the degree of tissue displacement is marked and a considerable thickness of paste is required to achieve stability. If, however, the ridge is firm and the mucosa is only very slightly displaceable there is a danger of disturbing the occlusion, and also of producing too great a degree of compression in localized areas of the ridge.

Secondly, the space beneath the saddle may be predetermined by placing a strip of metal foil 1 mm thick over the edentulous ridge on the master cast prior to its duplication. This will give a uniform space into which an adequate thickness of paste can be placed.

The third method is to remove from the finished saddle a thickness of denture base material adequate for the purpose. This can be done with large burs or stones, but is a time-wasting and haphazard method compared to the foil method.

If the foil method is used the acrylic surface may require slight roughening before the paste is applied to it, although union is normally satisfactory if the base material is thoroughly dried with the air syringe before the paste is placed in position. Any saddle that is to be rebased must have a 'lattice work' type of metal frame to allow proper union between old and new denture-base material.

Three possible combinations of conditions may present at the rebasing stage: (*a*) one lower denture, (*b*) one upper denture, or (*c*) two dentures. All these dentures may have one or more saddles to be rebased.

(a) Lower denture

Mix the paste to the required consistency and apply it to the saddle or saddles that are to be rebased. If more than one saddle is to be treated they must be rebased at the same time. An attempt should be made to place the bulk of the paste on the buccal and lingual walls of the saddles to avoid a concentration of pressure on the crest of the ridge. In practice, this is not easy to accomplish, particularly with small saddles.

The denture is placed in position, care being taken to make certain that all tooth-supported components fit accurately into place. No pressure should be applied to the saddle area, but the denture should be held firmly in position by pressure on the occlusal rests or any other tooth-bearing components until the paste hardens. The patient is then asked to close, before the denture is removed, and the occlusal pressure on the saddles is re-checked to ensure equal distribution of load during function.

(b) Upper denture

The basic procedure is exactly the same as described for the lower, but the position of the denture and the saddle can be determined by making sure that the bar, or other palatal portion, is in its correct relationship to the tissues. Owing to the reduced displaceability of the mucosa in the upper jaw, compared with the average lower, it is advisable to mix the paste to a thinner consistency to ensure correct seating of the denture.

(c) Two dentures

When both upper and lower dentures are to be rebased the former should be done first. This then acts as a check on the occlusion when the lower denture is rebased as described previously.

When the displacement of the saddles is slight, it may be preferable to use a functional impression material or tissue conditioner. This should be applied to the fitting surface and the denture and held in position as described previously. When the material has hardened, excess should be removed from the polished surfaces of the denture and a check of the occlusion carried out.

The patient is now instructed to wear the denture for two days. If, at the end of this period, any area of the saddle has been denuded of material, this part should be relieved and the whole procedure repeated. When satisfactory, the saddle is reprocessed to the new fitting surface developed by the functional material.

Rebasing Old Dentures

When examination of a patient who has worn partial dentures for some period reveals the necessity for rebasing, the technique to be adopted will vary according to several factors.

The first factor is the type of saddle that requires rebasing. Normally little bone resorption will have occurred under the saddles of tooth-supported dentures but in dentures requiring any form of mucosal support the discrepancy of adaptation may be considerable after a period of wear. A different approach may be required, therefore, according to the type of saddle and degree of resorption. Secondly, the peripheral adaptation is another factor which has to be considered. Saddles which are underextended will require additions to the periphery to restore maximum mucosal coverage, whereas in situations where sinking of the saddle has occurred due to loss or ridge height, the peripheral form will require to be reduced and re-formed. Thirdly, the occlusion of the artificial teeth will affect the problem; although it is not likely to be disturbed seriously in the case of tooth supported bounded saddles, in free-end saddles it may be affected severely. If rigid clasping is used and a considerable degree of resorption occurs under the saddle, then maintenance of satisfactory occlusion will be achieved only at the expense of the supporting structures of the abutment teeth. Finally, when free-end saddles sink posteriorly not only is the occlusion deranged but the metal framework of a lower denture is rotated. This has the effect of raising the lingual bar and continuous clasp so that they lose contact with the mucosa and the teeth respectively. When the denture is rebased they must be brought into their original positions.

The following techniques in saddle rebasing are based on the degree of resorption that has occurred. It is difficult to quantify what is meant by slight resorption and marked resorption and a clinical assessment of this can only be made with experience.

(a) Bounded saddle with slight resorption

In these cases the periphery should be be examined for its extension. Modifications to this will rarely be necessary, but if so they should be made by adding low fusing impression compound or an acrylic border moulding material and executing border moulding. If there are any undercuts on the fitting surface they should be eliminated by grinding away the acrylic resin. Unless such undercuts are eliminated in the resin, fracture of the investing plaster will occur on separation of the halves of the flask preparatory to packing.

Impression paste of thin consistency should be used for the final rebasing impression but care must be taken to keep it away from the occlusal rests otherwise correct seating of the denture will not be possible.

(b) Bounded saddle with marked resorption

The acrylic resin fitting surface should be ground away so that the whole area may be lined with a thin layer of impression compound in which a preliminary impression is taken. At the same time the periphery of the saddle can be reshaped if this is necessary. Only the minimum thickness of impression material should be used otherwise there will be a danger of over displacement of the mucosa. When the denture is seated care must be taken to see that the occlusal rests are seated correctly and a check should be made of the occlusion; in tooth suported dentures it should not require adjustment. The final impression is taken in impression paste which should be of thin consistency as the space available for it will be minimal.

(c) Free-end saddle with slight resorption

The procedure in these cases is similar to that described for rebasing a new denture. The occlusion should be checked but normally should be found satisfactory. If any additions are required to the periphery these should be made using a suitable border moulding material and any fitting surface undercuts must be removed as in (a) above. A paste impression is taken and the denture is seated by pressure on the abutments; the patient is not asked to close on the denture since this may produce unequal pressure on the ridges as well as possibly rotating the framework out of position. If stability is not achieved with this impression a further layer of paste should be added and the denture reinserted. After the new resin has been processed it will usually be necessary to readjust the occlusion on fitting the denture.

(d) Free-end saddle with moderate resorption

The acrylic fitting surface should be ground away to produce approximately 2 mm space. A thin wafer of compound should be used to take a preliminary impression and when doing so the denture should be seated by pressure on the abutments. After removal and chilling, the occlusion and stability must be checked. If the occlusal discrepancy is gross the case should be treated as one of marked resorption; if the adjustments required are not excessive then they can be carried out by grinding after the denture has been processed. In such cases, if stability is satisfactory, a final impression is taken in impression paste. Should stability not be satisfactory a further addition of compound should be made to the distal area of the saddle before taking the paste impression.

(e) Free-end saddle with marked resorption

These cases will show marked discrepancy of the occlusion and some degree of rotation of the denture framework. The acrylic fitting surface should be ground as above and a preliminary impression taken in compound. Care must be taken to seat the framework into position accurately. On reseating the denture after chilling it will be found that, although the framework may fit correctly, stability will not be satisfactory, and a further addition of compound should be made. When stability is correct it will often be noted that the occlusion is grossly deranged. Should this be so it is better to remove all the teeth on the saddle, obtain a new record of the occlusal relationship and set up the teeth anew. If the occlusion can be corrected by grinding then a final paste impression is taken as before. After processing the occlusion is adjusted in the mouth.

References

APPLEGATE O.C. (1955) The partial denture base. *J. pros. Dent.* **5**, 636.
APPLEGATE O.C. (1959) *Essentials of removable partial denture prosthesis*, 2nd edition. W.B. Saunders Co.
BECKETT L.S. (1938) Bite taking and rebasing for partial denture construction. *Dent. J. Aust.* **10**, 205.
BECKETT L.S. (1971) The rebasing of tissue borne saddles, theory and practice. *Aus. Dent. J.* **16**, 340.
BLATTERFEIN L. (1958) Rebasing procedures for removable partial dentures. *J. pros. Dent.* **8**, 441–67.
HOLMES J.B. (1965) Influence of impression procedures and occlusal loading on partial denture movement. *J. pros. Dent.* **15**, 474.
HOLMES J.B. (1970) Altered cast impression procedure for the distal extension removable partial denture. *Dent. Clinic N.A.* **14**, 569.
KENNEDY E. *Partial denture construction.* Kimpton, London.
LEUFOLD R.J. and KRATOCHVIL F.J. (1965) An altered cast procedure to improve tissue support for removable partial dentures. *J. pros. Dent.* **15**, 672.
LEUFOLD R.J. (1966) A comparative study of impression procedures for distal extension removable partial dentures. *J. pros. Dent.* **16**, 708.
LYTLE R.B. (1962) Soft tissue displacement beneath removable partial and complete dentures. *J. pros. Dent.* **12**, 34.
MCCRORIE J.W. (1982) Corrective impression waxes. *Brit. dent. J.* **152**, 95.
SKINNER E.W., COOPER E.N. and ZIEHM H.W. (1950) Some physical properties of the zinc oxide-eugenol impression pastes. *J. Amer. dent. Soc.* **41**, 449.
STORER R. (1962) Partial denture saddle correction. *Brit. dent. J.* **112**, 454.
WILSON J.H. (1953) Partial dentures—relining the saddle supported by the mucosa and alveolar bone. *J. pros. Dent.* **3**, 807.

21
PERIODONTAL PROSTHESES AND MOUTH PROTECTORS

As a result of current improvements in dental health together with educational programmes aimed at increased motivation towards maintaining a healthy dentition, practitioners may be called upon to construct appliances for which there has been little demand in the past such as periodontal prostheses (veneers) and mouth protectors. Although these are not partial dentures in a definitive sense, their construction is often based upon similar principles.

Periodontal Prostheses

These appliances, which are essentially aesthetic in nature, are often required following surgical treatment of periodontal disease, particularly in the anterior region of the mouth. Such surgery is invariably undertaken in order to eliminate pockets that have become established, the elimination of which will permit the patient to develop a more effective technique of plaque control than would otherwise be possible. The inevitable exposure of the root of the tooth from this procedure results in lengthening the clinical crown and the development of interdental spaces. Whilst this may be relatively unimportant in the posterior region of the mouth, in the anterior region it is often aesthetically unacceptable to patient and clinician alike. This is more apparent in the upper rather than the lower arch due to the position and protective nature of the lower lip which reduces visibility of the lower teeth.

In such a situation the lost gingival tissue may be restored prosthetically by the construction of a thin acrylic veneer, which can be placed over the necks of the standing teeth and the labial aspect of the alveolar ridge. Careful attention to detail will not only restore the pre-operative level of the gingival margin if this is desired, but also the shape, contour, and colour of the tissues together with a certain amount of gingival function in relation to food deflection and protection against thermal insult.

In the construction of such an appliance an opposing cast is not required. A preliminary impression of the relevant dentition, extending to include the first premolar region is obtained using alginate impression material in a stock tray. In cases where there is a considerable amount of interdental spacing in the cervical areas of the teeth, it may be necessary to obliterate these areas with soft carding wax prior to taking the impression in order to avoid tearing of the material on removal. A stone cast is poured from this impression, upon which is constructed an individual tray in acrylic resin (Fig. 21.1). This tray extends vertically from the incisal edge of the standing teeth to the reflection of the functional sulcus, and laterally a short distance distally to the canine teeth. It is designed to be inserted and removed from the mouth in a labio-palatal direction only, and to enable the recording of the labial and buccal surfaces of the teeth and alveolar ridge.

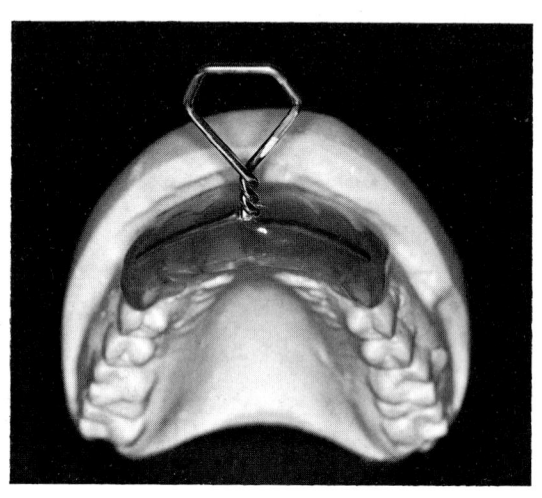

Fig. 21.1. An individual tray in acrylic resin suitable for recording an impression prior to the construction of a periodontal prosthesis.

The master impression may be obtained in either an alginate or silicone based impression material with interdental spaces being obliterated by wax as appropriate. A master cast is poured in stone on which can be indicated both the desired outline of the new gingival margins and interdental papillae, and the peripheral extension of the veneer. Any obvious interdental spaces or undercuts should be masked out in plaster so that projections of hard acrylic do not extend interdentally as this may result in discomfort to the patient. Shading of the veneer in order that it will blend with the tissues of the mouth is achieved by the use of preformed acrylic disc shade guides, which have been prepared using known ratios of pink, tinted, veined and clear acrylics. Further personalization of the appliance can be done by hand tinting if required. The veneer is waxed upon the master cast and processed directly on to that cast in the normal way. It should be kept as light as possible for comfort and aesthetics, and should be thinned at its distal and superior borders so that it blends with the natural tissues.

These appliances are easily removed and inserted by the patient, and their retention and appearance is good (Fig. 21.2a and b). The patient should be instructed to remove the appliances and to clean both the labial and the fitting surface after meals. They should not be worn when sleeping, being stored in water overnight with an appropriate denture cleanser added. Patients who require such treatment have often had a history of inability to maintain an adequate level of oral hygiene. It is essential therefore, that where a periodontal prosthesis is prescribed the patient should be aware of the increased importance of oral hygiene procedures in respect of the natural teeth. The regular use of woodsticks, floss and an interdental toothbrush or water irrigation device is mandatory.

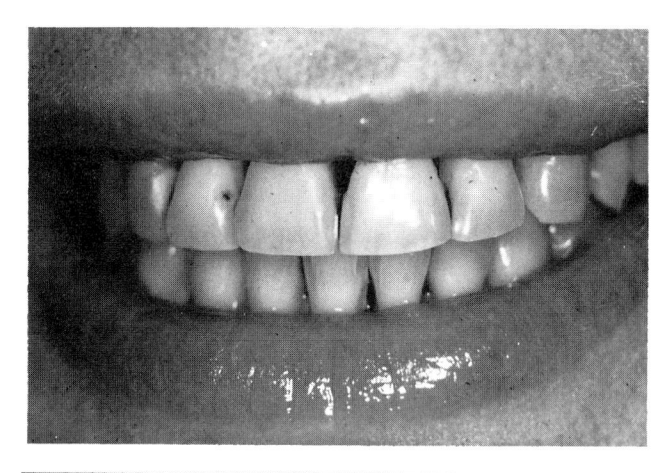

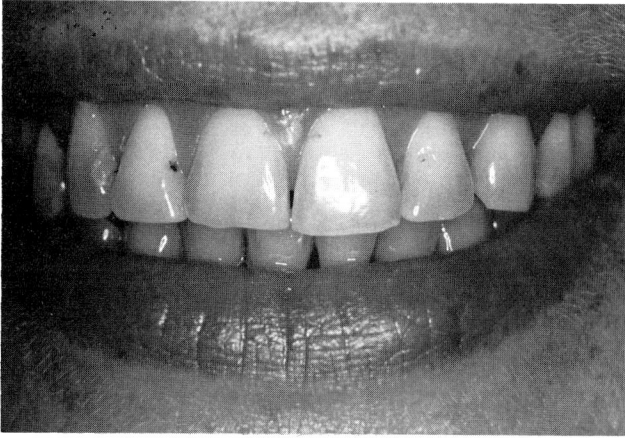

Fig. 21.2. a The appearance of the upper incisors of a patient following periodontal surgery.
b The same patient with an anterior periodontal prosthesis.

Mouth Protectors

Mouth protectors are worn commonly during contact sports such as boxing, hockey and rugby football in order to prevent or minimize injuries to the oral and dental tissues. They may also be used in post-traumatic therapy such as in the stabilizing of avulsed teeth, or in preventive dentistry for the delivery of topical fluoride gels.

Dental injuries are common in contact sports and it has been shown that the incidence and severity of such injuries can be reduced if well-fitting individually constructed mouth protectors are worn by the participants. In order to be acceptable and readily worn, however, a mouth protector should be comfortable, easily retained and not interfere with breathing or speech. In this respect it is desirable that it should be custom made for the individual rather than using preformed or mouth-formed appliances often available from sports shops and mail order companies. A properly designed and constructed mouth protector should not only protect the teeth but also the soft tissues of the lips, cheeks and tongue. Laceration of tissues can be prevented by the presence of a resilient flange and impact shattering of teeth by the presence of an interocclusal 'pad'. The latter will act as a shock absorber and also serve to reduce impact transmitted to the temporomandibular joint and the cranium.

For reasons of stability and retention, mouth protectors are always worn in the upper arch, and common materials used in their construction are soft vinyl or acrylic polymers, or pre-vulcanized latex rubber. In the construction of such an appliance it is necessary to take an impression of the upper arch using alginate material in a stock tray. A cast should then be poured in dental stone. It should be noted that if a partial denture is worn this should be removed prior to taking the impression, as its wear would be contra-indicated during sporting activity.

The details of construction of the appliance vary according to the preferred material. One simple and convenient method involves the use of discs of plasticized poly-vinyl chloride which are thermoplastically adapted to the master cast by means of a vacuum. The resultant appliance (Fig. 21.3) should then be trimmed some 2–3 mm short of the functional sulcus, and also in the palatal region to provide horseshoe coverage. The periphery can be trimmed and rounded with conventional abrasives and finally smoothed by wiping with monomer.

Such an appliance is both tough and pliable and will resist tooth penetration whilst also cushioning impact. In spite of its undoubted protective nature however, many sportsmen discard their mouth protectors, mainly due to discomfort and interference with breathing. In this respect efforts should be made to motivate such patients towards the benefits of long-term preservation of their dentition.

After use, the mouth protector should be cleansed with soap and water, dried,

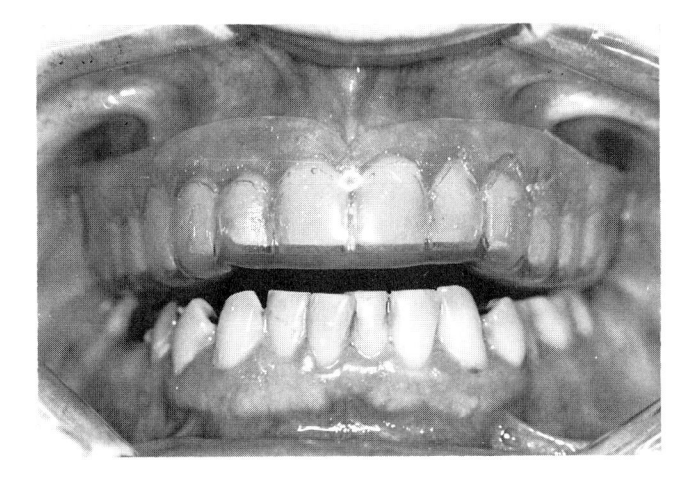

Fig. 21.3. A plasticized poly-vinyl chloride mouth protector worn on the upper arch.

and returned to the master cast which should be supplied to the patient with the appliance. The protector should be stored in the dry state in order to minimize possible dimensional changes.

References

DAVIES R.M., BRADLEY D., HALE R.W., LAIRD W.R.E. and THOMAS P.D. (1977) The prevalence of dental injuries in rugby players and their attitude to mouthguards. *Brit. J. Sports Med.* **11**, 42.

GOING R.E., LOEHMAN R.E. and CHAN M.S. (1974) Mouthguard materials: their physical and mechanical properties. *J. Amer. dent. Ass.* **89**, 132.

L'ESTRANGE P.R. (1966) Prosthetic restoration of the postoperative periodontal contour. *Dent. Pract.* **16**, 176.

SEALS R.R. and DORROUGH B.C. (1984) Custom mouth protectors; a review of their applications. *J. pros. Dent.* **51**, 238.

THOMSON J.C. (1962) Mouth protectors for amateur boxers. *Brit. dent. J.* **112**, 253.

22
INSTRUCTIONS TO PATIENTS

Once the partial denture has been inserted and is to the satisfaction of both the patient and clinician, specific advice and instructions should be given to the patient in respect of functional limitations of their new denture, care of the appliance, continuing care and maintenance of the natural dentition, and the need for regular review. Time spent on this will be well rewarded and it should be regarded as an essential aspect of patient treatment and management. Although the information can be given verbally, it is useful to support this with a prepared sheet of instructions which the patient can study at leisure.

In general the patient will have reasonably high expectations from his denture and will certainly expect it to improve both his appearance and his masticatory performance, although he may in some instances express some doubt in respect of his ability in managing the new appliance. Unless the various aspects of partial denture wearing are explained, difficulties may arise by the patient's failure to appreciate the problems of denture wearing, and to understand their own responsibilities following its insertion. Many patients expect much more from dentures than it is possible to achieve, and indeed some expect their appliances to last a lifetime with few, if any, return visits to the dentists. If the appropriate advice and instruction is not presented to them they may be disappointed later with what they may regard as an unsatisfactory standard of treatment.

Functional Limitations

Artificial teeth are not the same as natural teeth and it is perhaps not unrealistic to regard any prosthesis as a substitute for no teeth rather than a substitute for teeth. Initially the partial dentures may seem large and cumbersome, but gradually will become more comfortable and easily tolerated, as the patient learns new skills and adapts to them. This will naturally entail a period of learning, the length of which will vary according to the age of the patient and his ability to adapt to altered circumstances. In this respect a younger person will become accustomed to denture wearing more rapidly than an older one.

Earlier in the text the significance of inherent patterns of the masticatory musculature was stressed, and it was considered that no matter how many teeth were lost, these paterns remained. Consequently, as long as the muscular and intercuspal or tooth positions are co-incident then the acquired masticatory patterns and the occlusal relationship will not be in conflict. In such circumstances the period of patient re-education on denture insertion is relatively short. In the majority of partially edentulous patients, there will have been little disturbance of the relationship between the muscular and tooth positions, such as may occur in the edentulous person. Most, therefore, will accomodate rapidly to partial dentures. Nevertheless it should be emphasized, that initially food should be taken in small portions and chewed slowly, and incision into food with the anterior teeth should be avoided until the patient has learned to control the denture and has gained in confidence.

The larger partial denture will often cause some embarrassment due to interference with speech, but this is a temporary inconvenience which is usually overcome in a few days. Any persistent trouble of this nature usually indicates too great a denture thickness or an incorrect anterior tooth position.

In general most difficulties related to adaptation will resolve themselves with practice, patience and perseverance. The patient should also be advised, however, that in the first few days of wearing the denture they may experience some low grade discomfort related to their natural teeth. This is relatively uncommon where a replacement denture has been constructed, but with a first denture it is probably due to the reaction of the natural teeth to an alteration in the pattern of loading during mastication. If this persists, however, there is usually some fault in design, or disturbances in blood supply which may necessitate tissue conditioning.

In addition to the problems mentioned, it should be made clear that the new denture may require minor adjustments and modifications in the early stages to perfect the fit, retention, and occlusion, and this can be done at a review appointment. If severe pain and discomfort occur, however, this is a different situation altogether and the patient should be urged to seek further treatment immediately.

Finally it might be an advantage in the early stages to advise the patient to concentrate on one functional activity at a time, and, for instance, not to attempt to combine both eating and speaking.

Care of the Denture

In general, partial dentures can be considered as relatively delicate structures, particularly in relation to their clasp units, and in the case of some, their skeleton type designs. They are therefore easily damaged by mishandling. Patients should be instructed in the removal and insertion of the denture and this should be demonstrated and practised in the surgery with the use of a mirror before their being dismissed. In particular, the patient should learn the correct path of insertion and removal of the denture and should understand that the clasp arms will offer resistance to both procedures. The denture should be inserted and removed by holding the saddle area and not the clasp arms which may become distorted. When the denture is not being worn it should be placed in a suitable container and immersed in water.

Besides avoiding damage to the denture, its care also includes keeping it clean. This is necessary to remove plaque deposits which may occur on the denture surface, which will adsorb food and tobacco stains as well as acting as a substrate for calculus deposition. (Fig. 22.1). Dentures may be cleaned by both mechanical and chemical methods. It has been suggested that simple cleaning with a toothbrush and toothpaste or liquid soap is effective in removing attached deposits and stains. The denture appears relatively wear resistant to such a regime provided there is little abrasive content in the toothpaste. Some toothpastes are now produced specifically for denture cleaning which decrease the risk of abrasion to the acrylic components. These should be used with a properly designed denture brush and not an ordinary toothbrush, and the brush should be replaced as appropriate. It has been noted that less wear is apparent if a brush with long narrow bristles is used.

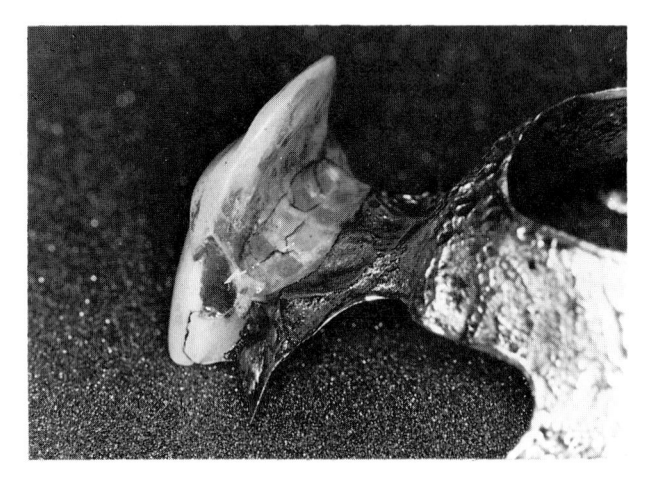

Fig. 22.1. Disclosed plaque on the surface of a partial denture.

Chemical denture cleansers should be able to remove deposits on the surface of the dentures without affecting either their aesthetic or functional properties. The commonest are the immersion cleansers either as oxygenating or hypochlorite solutions. Dilute mineral acids may also be used, often by direct application. The oxygenating cleansers have no serious disadvantages although they may cause some deterioration of resilient lining materials. They are most effective when used in an overnight soaking regime, being less effective over a short period. Hypochlorite solutions are effective in the removal of both stains and dental (denture) plaque. They are also both bacteriocidal and fungicidal and by dissolving the organic matrix of plaque they may also inhibit calculus formation. The major disadvantage of such solutions is the fact that they may have a corrosive effect on components of the denture that are constructed in cobalt chromium alloy or stainless steel. In the mildest form this will result in surface discoloration or tarnishing, but it may also affect the physical properties of the material, resulting in increased flexibility of clasp arms and consequent looseness of the denture. If used in high concentration they may also cause bleaching of the matrix acrylic.

The use of dilute acids, whilst enabling chemical removal of stains and calculus deposits, will also cause corrosion of metal components. Dentures must be washed thoroughly after using such cleaners.

Partial dentures, of course, are relatively difficult to clean, particularly due to difficult access to fitting areas of clasps and rests, and anatomical contours of the appliance. Efficient cleaning also requires a degree of manual dexterity.

It would appear, therefore, that the simplest and most effective method may well be brushing with a denture brush and a toothpaste formulated for use with dentures. In this respect the patient should be encouraged to use disclosing tablets or solutions to stain plaque and debris so facilitating its removal. If possible, dentures should be brushed after every meal and rinsed vigorously before re-insertion. If brushing is impractical, then rinsing alone is better than nothing. In addition, dentures that are removed overnight can be soaked in an appropriate chemical denture cleaner, with the denture being thoroughly rinsed afterwards to avoid any possible tissue damage due to the chemicals. It should be noted, however, that soaking in chemical cleansers alone is not normally sufficient to remove all plaque and debris, and any soaking regime should be supplemented by brushing, in order to clean the denture completely.

The Dental and Oral Tissues

In many instances the wearing of a removable partial denture has been implicated in damage caused to the remaining oral tissues. This is commonly associated with accumulation of dental plaque around the teeth and on the denture, resulting in caries, enamel decalcification and gingivitis. This is particularly likely to occur where there is a poor standard of oral hygiene, poor patient co-operation and defective appliance design.

The very nature of the design of a partial denture is bound to encourage some degree of food accumulation at points where it comes into contact with the natural tooth surface, as it will interfere with any cleansing effect brought about by the soft tissues such as the tongue and cheeks during masticatory performance. It is also important to appreciate, however, that the mere presence of a prosthesis in the mouth will increase the total plaque accumulation in that mouth, and in general, cause a deterioration in oral hygiene. Whilst increased plaque accumulation will be most evident on tooth surfaces immediately adjacent to the prosthesis, it is not restricted to these areas. In this respect the therapeutic value of the partial denture has been questioned, and it has been suggested that the indications for such treatment should be restricted, on the basis that the denture may have an adverse effect on structures that it is designed to maintain.

More recently, it has been demonstrated that the adverse effects of the partial denture can be avoided, if in addition to careful design, emphasis is placed on the development and maintenance of a high standard of oral hygiene. With very few exceptions however, patients who are wearing partial dentures have often lost their teeth as a result of inadequate motivation and oral hygiene. It is doubtful, therefore, whether the provision of a partial denture *per se* will change either attitudes or customs, and in this respect the patient must be regarded as a major contributory factor to the damage which may be caused to his own mouth by the denture.

Strict attention to all aspects to oral hygiene is essential, therefore, for denture wearers and even the best designed denture will fail in its purpose of restoring and maintaining oral health in the absence of patient co-operation.

In this respect the patient should be motivated and instructed in oral hygiene procedures at an early stage and certainly before denture construction is commenced. This should ideally be carried out by the dental hygienist and should be combined with scaling of the teeth to remove deposits of plaque and calculus. The use of disclosing agents on both the teeth, and the denture, will identify positively to the patient, areas in which plaque has accumulated, and will so aid in efforts at removal. The clinician should be satisfied that the patient is able to maintain a satisfactory level of oral hygiene *before* constructing the dentures.

Following insertion of the denture, the patient should be re-motivated and re-instructed in oral hygiene techniques, and should be particularly receptive at this stage. Advice should be given relating to the increased importance of maintaining a satisfactory level of oral hygiene now that a denture has been provided, with instruction on the use of woodsticks, dental floss or tape, and the various toothbrushes which may be used (Fig. 22.2). An early appointment with the hygienist should be given to ensure that these requirements are being met. In addition to the basic oral hygiene procedures the patients should be encouraged to make use of a toothbrush-applied chlorhexidine gel, if not daily at least on a weekly basis. This will complement the effect of toothbrushing particularly in the areas of the mouth where there is difficulty in access, and will aid both in preventing plaque formation and controlling the incidence of marginal gingivitis.

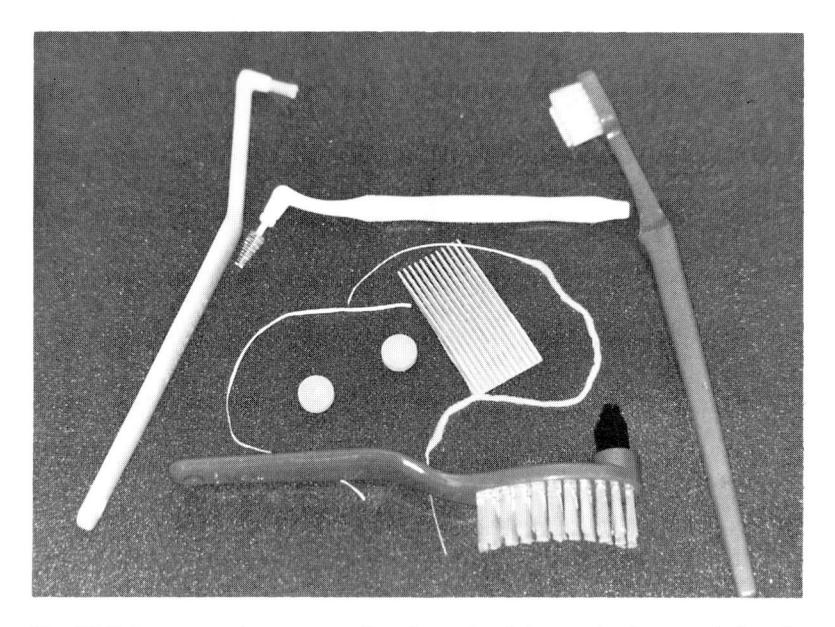

Fig. 22.2. A suggested armamentarium for oral and denture hygiene consisting of disclosing tablets, dental floss, woodsticks, standard toothbrush, interspace brushes, and denture brush.

The patient should also be instructed to use a fluoride containing toothpaste, and in some cases it may be prudent also to apply topical fluoride solution to areas where rests seats have been prepared.

Unless the partial dentures have been provided for the purpose of treating some form of tempero-mandibular joint or muscular disorder, they should not be worn at night, with the exception of the first few days to aid in habituation. With constant wear, abnormal stresses and overloading may be applied to the natural teeth during sleeping, particularly as a result of nocturnal bruxism. With the exception of poor oral hygiene, the wearing of a partial denture at night contributes more than anything else to deterioration of gingival and mucosal tissues. Upon retiring, therefore, the following routine is suggested. The dentures should be removed and areas of plaque accumulation identified using a disclosing tablet or solutions. Dental floss and woodsticks or irrigating devices should be used on the natural teeth as appropriate with particular attention paid to the abutments. The natural teeth should then be cleaned with a toothbrush and toothpaste as instructed. The denture should now also be cleaned using an appropriate brush and paste, care being taken to avoid damage to its component parts, and this should be done over a basin of water to minimize the risk of breakage if the denture should be dropped. It can then be placed in water in a container to which an appropriate chemical cleanser, if desired, is added for overnight soaking. The patient must be warned of the dangers of using hot water or household cleaners on the denture as these may cause irreversible damage.

Apart from the adverse effects on the teeth and their supporting tissues, inflammation may occur in the mucosa covering the edentulous ridges or the palate. When it occurs on the ridges it does so more frequently in free-ended rather than bounded saddles and is usually a result of excessive load caused either by an occlusal error or an ill-fitting base. It is rare in this area for inflammation to progress to chronically inflamed fibrous tissue which is most commonly seen in anterior maxillary saddles in association with the presence of opposing natural lower teeth.

Inflammation of the palate, producing the condition of denture stomatitis, is on the other hand, the more common manifestation of the inflammatory process of the mucosa occurring beneath partial dentures. In particular, this is likely to occur beneath a mucosa borne denture with an acrylic palatal plate, although localized areas of inflammation may be seen under connecting bars of tooth supported dentures.

Denture stomatitis is evident as a bright erythematous area involving all or part of the mucosa underlying the denture. In addition there may be some swelling and oedema present giving a spongy appearance of the tissues. The condition is often asymptomatic, although sometimes the patient may complain of soreness or discomfort. The severity of symptoms is not necessarily related to the degree of inflammation.

Although various suggestions have been put forward for the aetiology of denture stomatitis, including trauma and blockage of palatal mucous ducts, it is generally agreed that infection by the fungus *Candida albicans* is the main causal factor. The environment created by a denture with full palatal coverage is particularly favourable for the proliferation of *Candida albicans*, which may spread to the angles of the mouth resulting in angular cheilitis. The upper denture may exacerbate the problem by mechanical irritation of the surface of the mucosa, and by virtue of its close adaptation preventing free movement of the mucus film at the denture–tissue interface.

Although it has been suggested that there may be some destruction of the protective keratotic layer of the palatal epithelium there is no clear evidence of mucosal invasion by the fungus. The majority of organisms do in fact occur on the surface of the denture rather than on the mucous membrane, their proliferation occuring within plaque which collects on the fitting surface of the denture particularly where there is poor oral and denture hygiene.

Treatment of the *Candida* should, therefore, be directed to the elimination of organisms from the denture surface rather than the mucous membranes. Treatment of the latter by anti-fungal agents alone is seldom successful with early eradication being followed by recurrence with cessation of therapy. Also, the clinician should be aware that other factors such as systemic disorders, debilitating disease and denture trauma may be contributory, and if so, appropriate remedial therapy should also be undertaken together with treatment of the denture surface. This is related to establishing an effective regime of denture hygiene with the use of disclosing solutions as previously described, together with overnight soaking in a hypochlorite solution if appropriate.

Once infection has been controlled and any associated inflammation and oedema resolved, it may be necessary to rebase or remake the denture. In the long term the soft tissues can be kept clean and healthy by regular brushing of the denture bearing mucosa using a soft toothbrush.

Review

A partial denture is not a permanent appliance. Apart from the initial post-insertion review the patient should be seen regularly every six months as a routine. At these visits the dentist will be able to check for any adverse changes that may have occurred in the tissues such as caries, gingivitis, tooth mobility or bone resorption and take any necessary action. Any alterations to the denture such as clasp adjustments or rebasing can be carried out if desired.

At each review appointment the patient should have their natural teeth professionally cleaned, and be re-motivated and re-instructed in respect of oral and denture hygiene. The application of a fluoride gel to the teeth on these occasions will give added protection. It is important that the patient realizes that health of the remaining natural teeth is essential for success of the denture. If any are lost or subject to deterioration the denture will be unable to function effectively.

Attention to the points raised in this chapter will help to maintain the patient's oral health, and ensure that the construction of his partial denture is a contribution to his oral rehabilitation and not simply a transitional stage on the way to a complete denture.

References

ADDY M. and BATES J.F. (1977) The effect of partial dentures and chlorhexidine gluconate gel on plaque accumulation in the absence of oral hygiene. *J. clin. Periodontol.* **4,** 41.

ANTHONY D.H. and GIBBONS P. (1958) The nature and behaviour of denture cleansers. *J. pros. Dent.* **8,** 796.

BASSIOUNY M.A. and GRANT A.A. (1975) The toothbrush application of chlorhexidine. A clinical trial. *Brit. dent. J.* **139,** 323.

BERGMAN B. (1984) Caries, periodontal and prosthetic conditions in patients fitted with removable dentures. A 10 year longitudinal study. *In:* Bates J.F., Neill D.J., and Preiskel H.W. *Restoration of the partially dentate mouth.* Quintessence Publishing Co. Inc., Chicago.

BUDTZ-JORGENSEN E. (1979) Materials and methods for cleaning dentures. *J. pros. Dent.* **42**, 619.
CARLSSON G.D., HEDEGÅRD B. and KOIVUMAA K.K. (1965) Studies in partial denture prostheses IV. Final results of a 4 year longitudinal study. *Acta Odont. Scand.* **28**, 581.
DAVENPORT J.C. (1970) The oral distribution of *Candida* in denture stomatitis. *Brit. dent. J.* **129**, 151.
DAVENPORT J.C. and HAMADA T. (1979) Denture stomatitis—a literature review with case reports. *Hiroshima J. Med. Sci.* **28**, 209.
DERRY A. and BERTRAM U. (1970) A clinical survey of removable partial dentures after two years usage. *Acta Odont. Scand.* **28**, 581.
KASTNER C., SCANDRETT F.R. and TAYLOR T. (1983) Effects of chemical denture cleaners on the flexibility of clasp arms. *J. pros. Dent.* **50**, 473.
LAIRD W.R.E. and GRANT A.A. (1983) Dental bacterial plaque. *Int. J. Biochem.* **15**, 1095.
MILLIN D.J. and SMITH M.H. (1961) Nature and composition of dental plaque. *Nature*, **189**, 664.
NEILL D.J. (1968) A study of materials and methods employed in cleaning dentures. *Brit. dent. J.* **124**, 107.
STIPHO H.D.K, MURPHY W.M. and ADAMS D. (1978) Effect of oral prostheses on plaque accumulation. *Brit. dent. J.* **145**, 47.
WAGNER A.G. (1973) Maintenance of the partially edentulous mouth and care of the denture. *D. Clin. N.A.* **17**, 755.
WICTORIN L. (1972) Effect of toothbrushing on acrylic resin veneering material. II Abrasive effect of selected dentifrices and toothbrushes. *Acta Odont. Scand.* **30**, 383.

23
CLINICAL AND LABORATORY SEQUENCES IN PARTIAL DENTURE CONSTRUCTION

This chapter summarizes the clinical and laboratory sequences in the construction of partial dentures. These have been discussed in detail in previous chapters although not necessarily in the sequence in which they take place. It may be helpful therefore, to list in logical succession, the stages to be followed in the design and construction of a partial denture. It is not suggested that every stage is necessary in every case, and the importance of any one procedure may vary from patient to patient according to the particular clinical circumstances.

1 Examination and treatment planning

- Intra-oral radiographs of both natural teeth and edentulous areas should be available.
- Decisions must be taken regarding extraction of unsavable, unfavourable or unerupted teeth, or retained roots.
- Arrangement must be made for any necessary conservative or periodontal treatment.
- Assessment should be made of the condition of the tooth supporting structures, the alveolar bone in saddle areas, thickness of mucosa and personal factors relating to the patient.
- If occlusal analysis is appropriate, preliminary impressions are required together with interocclusal records and face bow recordings prior to mounting casts on an adjustable articulator. This may also be necessary in deciding on extractions and conservative treatment.

2 Preliminary impressions

- Taken in stock trays in alginate impression material, the trays being modified as appropriate.

3 Preliminary casts

- Casts poured in dental stone.

- Used by dentist, with his knowledge of the clinical condition, supplemented by a preliminary survey, to obtain first ideas regarding design.
- Used to locate areas of teeth which will require occlusal rest seat preparation, or modification of incisal edge, cusp height, or contour.
- Used for purpose of occlusal analysis if this is required.

4 Individual trays

- Constructed in autopolymerizing acrylic resin for necessary strength and rigidity. Perforated as appropriate.

5 Mouth preparation

A certain amount of surgical, conservative, and periodontal treatment will have been completed following the initial examination and before preliminary impressions are taken.

Further mouth preparation may include:

- Occlusal adjustment to establish coincidence of muscular and intercuspal (tooth) positions, and to improve working and balancing occlusion.
- Rest seat preparation to allow the construction of support units of adequate size and strength without interfering with the occlusion.
- Modification of incisal edges where appropriate.
- Reduction of cuspal height to produce an occlusal plane of regular curvature and to reduce lateral loading.
- Modification of tooth contour for purposes of retention, or the establishment of guiding planes.

6 Master impressions

- Always taken in individual trays.
- Either mucostatic in alginate material or polysulphides, or slightly mucocompressive using silicone based or polyether materials.
- Precautions are required against distortion of alginate.

7 Master casts

- Always poured in dental stone.

8 Cast surveying and design

- Decide on the tilt to be given to the cast prior to surveying. Normally this will be such that the occlusal plane is at right angles to the analysing rod.

Clinical and Laboratory Sequences in Partial Denture Construction 457

- Mark survey lines on teeth.
- Make final decision regarding design.

The following points should be remembered when deciding upon the details of design:

Bilateral free-end saddle (Class I)

The forces acting upon the edentulous ridges and upon the abutment teeth may be controlled in the following ways.

1 By reducing the vertical load
This is done by reducing the area of the occlusal table.

2 By distributing the load between teeth and ridges
(*a*) By denture design.
- Use *rigid clasping* when saddles are short, ridges well developed and covered by firm submucosa, abutment teeth periodontally healthy with a large root surface. This puts maximal load on the tooth.
- *Flexible clasping*, such as a wrought wire, places less torque on the abutment. Applicable to premolars in good periodontal condition.
- *Bar clasps* place less torque on the abutment and allow the ridge to be more heavily loaded owing to their resilience, which permits a minor degree of stress-breaking.
- *Stress breakers* place least load on the abutments and maximum load on the ridge. Hence they may be used when the saddle is long and the periodontal condition of the teeth is poor.

(*b*) By anterior placement of the occlusal rest.
This will reduce the load on the abutment tooth and increase the load on the residual ridge.

(*c*) By mucocompression.
It is suggested that the mucosa covering the edentulous ridge can be kept under constant light pressure without suffering a trophic disturbance. If heavy pressure is applied to the mucosa, either in the impression or rebasing technique, it must be combined with light clasping or stress breaking so that the tissues can recoil. Constant heavy pressure causes pain on nerve endings and trophic disturbance.

(*d*) By specific design techniques such as disjunct dentures, RPI system, the balance of force system, or the swinglock denture.

3 By wide distribution load
(*a*) The vertical load falling on a free-end saddle may be distributed over more than one tooth by:
- Splinting.
- Compound clasping methods.

- Multiple embrasure clasping.

(*b*) The maximum area of ridge should be covered by the saddle to reduce the pressure falling on any unit area.

Unilateral free-end saddle (Class II)

1 *Short saddle.* The ridge is usually prominent and the covering mucosa firm. Rigid clasping of the abutment tooth and the teeth on the opposite side of the arch is necessary. Rigid connections between the saddle and the retainer unit is satisfactory.

2 *Long saddle.* The ridge will be called upon to accept a greater load and, in cases where the covering mucosa is more compressible, flexible connection between saddle and retainer unit may be desirable. This may be achieved by anterior placement of the occlusal rest which enables the lingual bar to be a semi-flexible structure, or by use of a split casting.

Bounded saddle (Class III)

Unmodified case

1 *Short saddle.* May be treated by a unilateral denture, sectional denture, bilateral denture or fixed bridge as follows:
(*a*) *Unilateral denture.* Normally is only advisable in the upper jaw and only if the anterior abutment is a sound premolar and the posterior abutment either a first or second molar. Instability can be minimized by (i) adequate lingual and buccal cusp contacts, (ii) the use of wide occlusal rests, (iii) adequate bracing, and (iv) adequate retention.
(*b*) *Sectional denture.* Used where suitable undercuts exist in the proximal surfaces of abutment teeth at each end of the saddle and a denture can be designed to utilize these undercuts.
(*c*) *Bilateral denture.* Has the advantage of increased stability and wider load distribution. Preferable in most cases, but particularly when crown shape, root size, or periodontal condition contra-indicates a unilateral denture.
(*d*) *Fixed bridge.* This is often the best form of treatment.

2 *Long saddle.* Load can normally be placed upon the teeth and consequently a skeleton design employed. Sometimes, because of saddle length or condition of the teeth, broad palatal coverage may be necessary to give wider distribution of load.

Modifications of Class III. Designs for these cases will depend upon the periodontal condition of the teeth, the length and number of the saddles, and the condition of the mucosa.

Anterior bounded saddle (Class IV)

1 *Short saddle.* Treatment may be by a denture or a bridge.
Dentures may be of four designs; a simple spoon denture, a skeleton denture, a palatal plate or a sectional or hinge denture.
(*a*) *Spoon denture.* Has the advantage of freedom from gingivae and disadvantage of poor retention. Success can be expected, especially in children, if the mucosa is of average compressibility, the hard palate form is normal, and an anterior flange can be used. Cobalt chromium may be used for cases where there is a deep vertical overlap of the anterior teeth.
(*b*) *Skeleton denture.* Retention should be placed as far posteriorly as possible.
(*c*) *Sectional or hinge denture.* Allows utilization of anterior undercut and lateral extension of acrylic matrix.

2 *Long saddle.* Not a common type of case. Broad palatal coverage and multiple clasping are normally required.

9 Elimination of undercuts

- Wax out all unwanted undercuts on teeth and mucosa and parallel wax in line with the angle of surveying, using wax trimmer on surveyor.

10 Cast duplication

- The waxed out master cast is duplicated in dental stone, or refractory investment material if a casting is required. The final processing is done on the duplicate stone cast.

11 Record blocks

- Make record blocks on duplicate stone casts, using shellac base plates, or the cast metal frame, and wax rims.

12 Recording occlusion

The intercuspal position or muscular position or retruded contact position is recorded as appropriate using wax record blocks. If an adjustable articulator is to be used, a face bow record and lateral and/or protrusive positions must be recorded.

To prevent mucosal displacement and possible alteration in tooth-cast relationship, take final recording under light pressure with free-end saddles, or use rests on blocks for bounded saddles.

13 Articulation

- Mount casts on articulator. Use duplicates if these are in stone.

14 Metal work

- Construct any metal work. This may vary from complete castings for the entire denture frame to a number of separately cast or wrought pieces such as occlusal rests or clasps. Completed framework should be tried in the mouth without teeth attached.

They may be used to record occlusion if wax rims are added.

15 Setting up

- If metal frames are used, add the necessary teeth.
- In other cases assemble any constituent metal pieces and complete the setting up of the teeth.

16 Trial dentures

- Try the dentures in the mouth. Check particularly on aesthetics, stability, retention, and occlusion.
- Observe the position of clasp arms, bars, etc., in relation to mucosa, teeth, and gingivae.
- Obtain patient's opinion on aesthetics. Do not pass for finishing unless completely satisfied on all points.
- Have further trials if necessary.

17 Finishing

- Process in acrylic resin, using duplicate stone casts.
- Fit the finished dentures to the master casts and check the occlusion. Adjust any gross errors due to tooth movement during processing. Ensure that all parts are polished particularly the inner aspect of clasp arms and occlusal rests and over the relieved gingival margins.

18 Assessment

Insert the dentures into the patient's mouth. If duplicate casts have been used and surveying has been accurate, the dentures should require minimal adjustment to accomplish this.
- Check occlusion in all positions by use of articulating paper or occlusal indicator wax and adjust any errors.
- Check retention, stability, and accuracy of fit round standing teeth.

19 Rebasing

- Rebase all free-end saddles, if master impressions have been mucostatic. Zinc-oxide pastes or functional impression materials may be used.
- Check occlusion before removing rebased saddles.

20 Processing rebase

- Process the rebased saddles taking care not to alter the occlusion.

21 Insertion

Insert the rebased denture and re-check the occlusion.
- Give the patient explicit instructions regarding usage and maintenance.
- Instruct patient to return in a few days for examination.

22 Review

Check dentures on all points.
- Deal with any complaints made by the patient.
- Make arrangements for recall of patient at regular intervals.

INDEX

Abrasion, compensatory 121
Abrasive discs 142
Abrasive strips 140
Abutment teeth 162, 292, 293
Acrylic resin 6, 194, 196, 206
Adaptation (fit) of dentures 397
   clasps 401
   metal based 397
   plastic based 400
Aesthetics 405
   trial dentures 402
Age changes 28, 60
Air crews, war-time dental services 2
Alginate impressions 363
   clinical techniques 371
   dimensional accuracy 364
   powder mixing 369
   special techniques 374
   techniques 366
Alloys 160
   choice of 193
Altered cast technique 433
Alveolar bone, crestal 101
Alveolar ridge, preparation 171
Analysing rod 179
Anterio-posterior component of force, free-end saddle 294
Anterior bounded saddles (class IV dentures) 347, 460
Appearance
   complaints 432
   restoration 22
   trial dentures 402
Arch decompression 139
Armed services, dental care 2
Articulators 8, 151, 380, 461
Ascorbic acid deficiency 115
Atrophy, dental apparatus 78
Attrition 109, 392

Back action clasps 245
Balanced occlusion 64, 380

Beckett classification 18
Beryllium, toxicity 189
Beveridge Report 3
Bilateral dentures 339
Bone
   pressure effects of 60, 73, 89
   radiographic assessment of 90
Bounded saddles (class III dentures) 330, 347, 459
   resorption of 439
Bracing of saddles 200, 235, 251
Bridges 21, 131
   composite bonded 357
Buccal bars 285
Buccal flanges 413, 418
Burning sensation 431

Camper plane 155
Candida albicans infections 453
Carbon marker 180
Care of dentures 448
Caries 28, 35
Casts
   altering 433
   master 457
   pouring 373
   preliminary 456
   surveying 5, 173, 457
   surveyor 179
Cheek biting 425
Chemical cleaners 449
Children, treatment 347
Cingulum preparations 167
Claspless denture 345
Clasps 224
   adaptation (fit) 401
   as retainers 225
   back action 245
   bracing effect of 235
   cobalt chromium 252
   combination 248, 255
   compound 254, 255

continuous 266, 285
De Van 249
extended arm 247
gingivally approaching 239, 250
gold 252
historical aspects 4, 7
mesio-distal 248, 249
occlusally approaching 240, 250
passive placement of 232
reciprocation 233
reverse back action 244, 245
ring 244, 245
wrought wire 244
Classification of dentures 13
Cobalt chromium alloys 5, 189, 252
Combination clasps 248, 255
Complaints 421
Compound impression material 4
Connectors 204, 272
Conservative aspects of treatment 132
Continuous clasps 266, 285
Corrosion resistance 192
Crestal alveolar bone 101
Cusps, inclination degree, loading 79

De Van clasps 249
Density 190
Denture base materials
  historical aspects 3
  metallic 5, 189
  non-metallic 6, 194
  properties of 190
Denture stomatitis 453
Design 198
  for children 347
  class I dentures (bilateral free-end saddle) 295
  class II dentures (unilateral free-end saddle) 324
  class III dentures (bounded-saddle) 330
  class IV dentures (anterior bounded-saddle) 352
  problems 204
  system 198
Diagnosis 129
Diastemata 24
Direct retainers 224
Disjunct denture 301
Drug therapy, periodontal disease 147

Economic factors 2
  treatment 40
Edentulousness 2
Elastomeric impressions 375
  techniques 376
Elongation 192
Embrasure hooks 221
Empty movements 57
Endogenous postural position 42
Every denture 343
Extended arm clasps 247
Extraction, changes following 75

Face bow 387
Fitting dentures 419
Flanges 413, 418
Force balance principle 305
Free-end saddles
  bilateral (class I dentures) 289, 458
  problems of 295
  resorption of 440
  treatment of 295
  unilateral (class II dentures) 324, 459
Functional limitations 447
Fungal infections 453

Gingivectomy 149
Gingivitis, chronic marginal 98
Gold alloys 189, 252
Grinding of teeth 104
  interstitial 140
  occlusal 144

Hardness 190
Heat treatment 193
History 1
Hyperplasia, dental 78

Ill health 39
Impressions
  alginate 4, 363
  elastomeric 375
  historical aspects 4
  master 362, 457
  preliminary 361, 456
  rebasing 434
  wax 434

Index

Incentives, denture wearing 38
Incisal edge
 modifications 170
 preparations 169
Indirect retainers 264
Inflammatory process 103
Insertion of dentures 419, 462
Interstitial grinding 140
Ischaemia 105
 causes of 113

Joint symptoms 150

Kennedy classification 14
 class I 14, 289
 class II 15, 324
 class III 16, 330
 class IV 17, 347

Labial bars 285
Labial flanges 413, 418
Lateral loading, free-end saddle 292
Ligmentous position 44
Lingual bars 278
Lingual plates 283
Load distribution 17, 95, 211, 297
 wide 310

Malocclusion 25
Mandibular movements 7, 53
Mandibular positions 41
 coinciding 158
 non-coinciding 66
 overclosure and protrusion 27, 30, 31
 rest 42, 156
Marginal cuff 124
Marginal ligament 101
 breakdown 122
Mastication 53
 difficulties 427
 restoration 20
Masticatory movements 9, 53
Menopause 39
Mesio-distal clasps 248, 249
Metallic taste 429
Modulus of elasticity 192
Mouth preparation 129, 457

Mouth protectors 445
Movement
 pain in 426
 patterns of 51
Mucocompression 307
Mucosa borne 17
Mucosa conditioning 89, 171
Mucostasis 307
Muscular position 46
Muscular symptoms 150

National Health Service 3
Natural teeth, loading 82
Nausea 430
Neuroanatomy and neurophysiology 47
Nickel alloys 189
Noisy dentures 429

Occlusal formation 62
Occlusal grinding 144
Occlusal loading 59, 78
Occlusal plane 383
Occlusal rest seat preparation 164, 218
 anterior teeth 167
 posterior teeth 165
Occlusal rests 200, 210
 anterior placement 303
 dimensions 217
 functions of 210
 effects on teeth 214
Occlusal stop, posterior, loss of 68
Occlusal surface modifications 170
Occlusal table 296
Occlusion 41
 analysis 145, 158
 balanced 64, 380
 checking 401
 close 351
 registration of 380, 460
Onlays 218
Oral health, maintenance 31, 137
Oral hygiene 35, 37, 137, 451
Oral tissue damage 450
Organization, denture service 1
Osteolysis 74

Pain 310, 422
Palatal bars 272

Index

Palatal plates 278
Path of insertion 182
Pathological considerations 62
Patients, instructions 420, 447
Periodontal disease 27, 98
   treatment of 136
Periodontal membrane, histological structure 74
Periodontal prostheses 442
Personal factors 37
Phonetics 386, 428
Physiological considerations 41, 73
Plaque 35, 449
Plaster of Paris 4
Polished surface, shape 403
Polyether impressions 376
Polysulphide impressions 375
Porcelain 196
   jacket crowns 29
Precision attachments 254
Pressure effects
   on bone 60, 73, 89
   on edentulous ridge 84
   on periodontal membrane 74
Prognosis 37
Proportional limit 191

Rebasing 433, 462
Record blocks 381, 460
Rest position, mandibular 42
   radiographic determination 156
Rest seat preparation 164, 218
Restoration 160
Retching control 378
Retention 202, 224, 254
Retruded position 45
Reverse back action clasps 244, 245
Reviewing 454, 462
   timing 421
Ring clasps 244, 245
RPI system 303

Saddles 13, 206
   anterior bounded 347, 460
   anterior designs 347
   area 199, 207
   bounded 330, 440, 459
   bracing 200, 235, 241
   effect on abutments 292, 293
   effect on bone 84, 85
   forces acting on 84, 85, 291
   free-end 14, 289, 440, 458
   long posterior 340
   pain under 93, 423
   retainer unit connection 204
   sectional dentures 336
   support of 200, 210
Salivation, excessive 431
Scaling 138
Sectional dentures 336
Selection of teeth 409, 415
Silicone impressions 376
Skeleton dentures 353
Specialization 11
Speech 386, 428
Splinting of teeth 149, 162, 254
Spoon dentures 349
Stainless steel 189
Stepping of teeth 108
Stereosthoscopy 11
Stillman's cleft 107
Stomatitis 453
Stress breaking 297
Stress, occlusal 58
Sublingual bar 281
Surgical aspects of treatment 133
Survey lines 218
Surveying 173
   principles of 173
   techniques of 180
Swallowing movements 57

Techniques, historical overview 3
Teeth, loading reactions 73
Temporomandibular joint 9
   syndrome 10, 150
Tensile strength 191
Thiokol 5
Tongue biting 425
Tooth borne 17
Tooth contours, modifications 161
Tooth grinding 140, 144, 410
Tooth materials 195
Tooth position 46, 406, 411, 414
Trauma 22
Traumatism, ischaemic 115
Trays 366, 434, 457
Treatment planning 129, 456
   economic factors 40
   periodontal aspects 136
   restorations 160
   surgical aspects 133
Trial dentures 461

Index

Ultrasonic therapy 142
Undercut areas 174
Undercut gauges 180
Unilateral dentures 331

Vertical dimension, recording 155, 384
Vertical loading, free-end saddle 289

Wax impressions 434
Wax trimmer 180, 185, 186
Willis bite gauge 393
Wolff's law 88
Wrought wire clasps 243, 244

ZA anchor 345

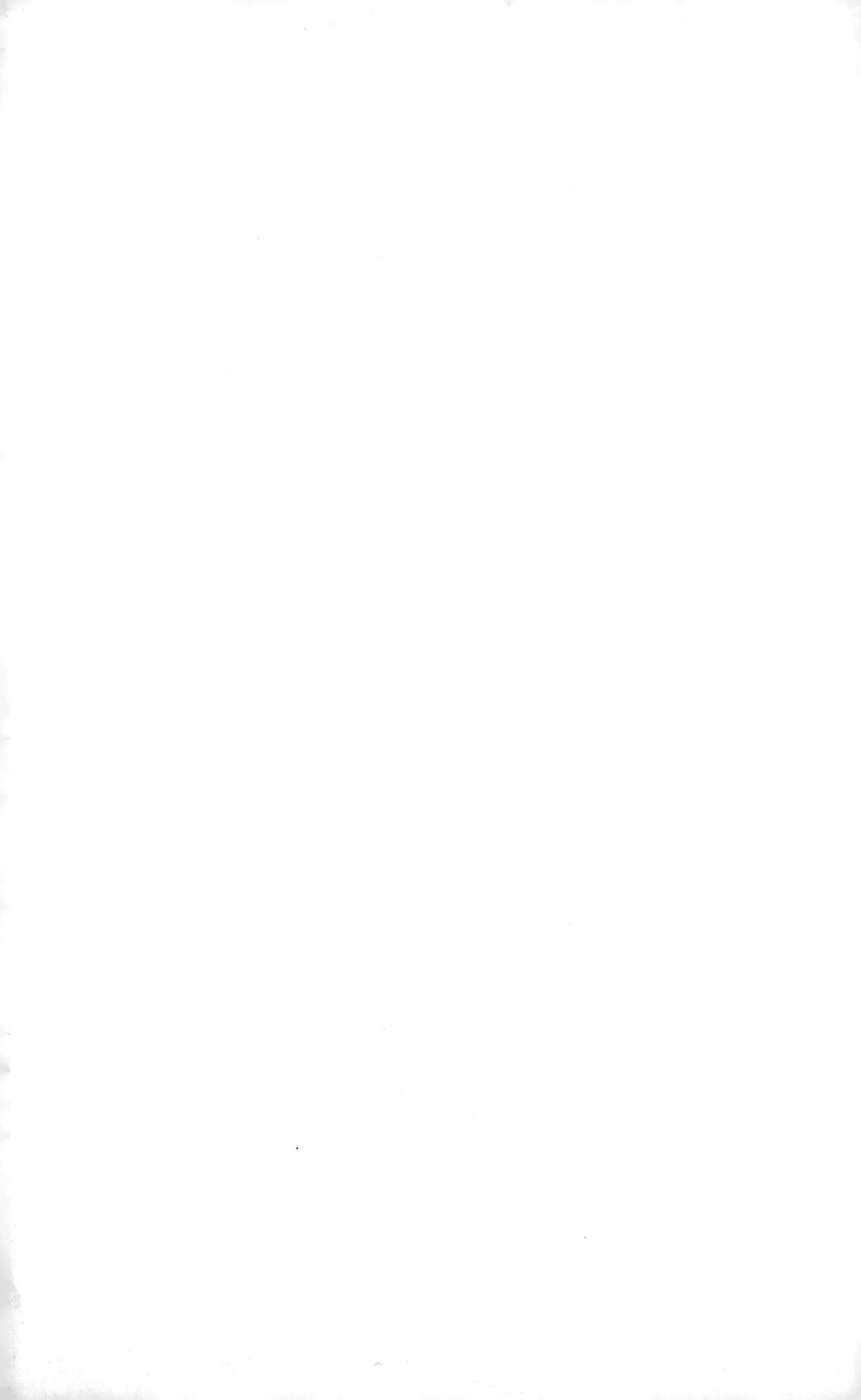